The Women's Health Companion to Maternal-Child Nursing Care

Optimizing Outcomes for Mothers, Children, & Families

The Women's Health Companion to Maternal-Child Nursing Care

Optimizing Outcomes for Mothers, Children, & Families

SECOND EDITION

Shelton M. Hisley, PhD, RNC, WHNP-BC
Assistant Professor of Nursing (Retired)
University of North Carolina at Wilmington
Wilmington, North Carolina

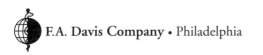
F.A. Davis Company • Philadelphia

F. A. Davis Company
1915 Arch Street
Philadelphia, PA 19103
www.fadavis.com

Printed in the United States of America

Last digit indicates print number: 10 9 8 7 6 5 4 3

Publisher, Nursing: Lisa Houck
Developmental Editor: Beth LoGiudice
Content Development Manager: Darlene Pedersen
Content Project Manager: Christina L. Snyder
Design and Illustration Manager: Carolyn O'Brien

As new scientific information becomes available through basic and clinical research, recommended treatments and drug therapies undergo changes. The author(s) and publisher have done everything possible to make this book accurate, up to date, and in accord with accepted standards at the time of publication. The author(s), editors, and publisher are not responsible for errors or omissions or for consequences from application of the book, and make no warranty, expressed or implied, in regard to the contents of the book. Any practice described in this book should be applied by the reader in accordance with professional standards of care used in regard to the unique circumstances that may apply in each situation. The reader is advised always to check product information (package inserts) for changes and new information regarding dose and contraindications before administering any drug. Caution is especially urged when using new or infrequently ordered drugs.

Library of Congress Control Number: 2015940175

The Women's Health Companion serves as a guide to caring for women across the life span. The broad directives set forth in the Healthy People 2020 national initiative are central in the development and delivery of contemporary medical and nursing education. Today's emphasis on health care has shifted from an illness-focused model to a preventive model grounded in the shared goals of health promotion, health protection, and preventive services for all individuals. Consistent with this model, nursing education today embraces a wellness-centered approach that emphasizes health promotion and maintenance. The women's health information offered in the *Women's Health Companion to Maternal-Child Nursing Care: Optimizing Outcomes for Mothers, Children, & Families* 2nd edition is framed in a health promotion context designed to appeal to nursing educators and students alike. Constructed to complement and enhance the parent text *Maternal-Child Nursing Care: Optimizing Outcomes for Mothers, Children, & Families* 2nd edition, the *Women's Health Companion* is presented in a similar style with special features that parallel those found in the basic book and emphasize the nurse's role in health promotion and community-based care. This information is designed to allow students to increase their understanding about strategies for promoting women's health and enhance their expertise in caring for women of all ages in a variety of settings.

Table of Contents

chapter 5

Promoting Reproductive Health Through an Understanding of Sexually Transmitted Diseases   93

chapter 6

Promoting Reproductive Health Through an Understanding of Cervical Cytology Screening, Human Papillomavirus, and Cervical Cancer   116

chapter 7

Promoting Menopausal Health   144

Promoting Mental Health and Physical Safety Through an Understanding of Intimate Partner Violence

 I Got Flowers Today

I got flowers today.
It wasn't my birthday or any other special day.
We had our first argument last night, and he said a lot of cruel things that really hurt me.
I know he is sorry and didn't mean the things he said.
Because he sent me flowers today.
I got flowers today.
It wasn't our anniversary or any other special day.
Last night he threw me into a wall and started to choke me.
It seemed like a nightmare.
I couldn't believe it was real.
I woke up this morning sore and bruised all over.
I know he must be sorry.
Because he sent me flowers today.
I got flowers today,

And it wasn't Mother's Day or any other special day.
Last night he beat me up again.
And it was much worse than all the other times.
If I leave him, what will I do?
What about money?
I'm afraid of him and scared to leave.
But I know he must be sorry.
Because he sent me flowers today.
I got flowers today.
Today was a very special day.
It was the day of my funeral.
Last night he finally killed me.
He beat me to death.
If only I had gathered enough courage and strength to leave him,
I would not have gotten flowers . . . today.

—Paulette Kelly

LEARNING TARGETS *At the completion of this chapter, the student will be able to:*

◆ Define the term *intimate partner violence* and discuss the significance and scope of the problem.

◆ Describe the different types of intimate partner violence.

◆ Identify a national health goal related to intimate partner violence and discuss how nurses may be instrumental in helping the nation to achieve this goal.

◆ Discuss characteristics of the three phases typically included in a cycle of violence and describe how partners generally react during each phase.

◆ Explain how to conduct intimate partner violence screening and assessments.

◆ Describe the nurse's role in planning and providing care for victims of intimate partner violence.

PICO(T) Questions

The intent of Evidence-Based Practice (EBP) is to provide nursing care that integrates the best available evidence. An initial step in EBP is to write a PICO(T) question that effectively guides the research. A PICO(T) question is an acronym that stands for population (P), intervention or issue (I), comparison of interest (C), outcome (O), and time frame (T). Depending on the question, all or some of the question components are used in the research process. Use these PICO(T) questions to spark your thinking as you read the chapter.

1. What (I) types of abuse do (P) victims of intimate partner violence (IPV) say are the (O) most difficult to endure?

2. What do (P) victims of IPV say are the (O) top two reasons that cause them (I) to attempt to leave the abusive situation?

Evidence-Based Practice

Gerber, M.R., Fried, L.E., Pineles, S.L., Shipherd, J.C., & Bernstein, C.A. (2012). Posttraumatic stress disorder and intimate partner violence in a women's headache center. *Women & Health, 52*(5), 454–471.

The purpose of this study was to examine the relationship between headache and post-traumatic stress disorder (PTSD) in women and to assess for the prevalence of undetected or suspected PTSD and intimate partner violence (IPV) in a women's headache clinic. Previous research has linked the incidence of chronic pain to past traumatic experiences. Headache is considered one of the most common forms of chronic pain, which can account for disability and increased use of services. Research suggests that PTSD can be a factor in the incidence of physical health-related sequelae, and has suggested a prevalence that ranges from 12% to 33% among patients seen in primary care. One large general population study (Peterlin, Rosso, & Merikangas, 2011) found that "the 12-month odds of PTSD in women with migraine were increased three-fold, as compared with women not reporting headache" (p. 456). This study indicated that the prevalence of PTSD among women reporting headaches ranges from 12.5% to 42.9%. The National Intimate Partner and Sexual Abuse Study documented a twofold increase in headache among patients reporting PTSD. PTSD was also reported as a risk factor in the incidence of chronic headache.

IPV is considered a form of interpersonal trauma, resulting in PTSD. IPV is defined by the National Intimate Partner and Sexual Abuse study as "a pattern of coercive behavior in which one person attempts to control another through threats or actual use of physical violence, sexual assaults, and verbal or psychological abuse" (p. 456). This same study indicated that the rate of lifetime IPV is 24.3%, with recent IPV at a rate of 2.7%. When additional, less severe forms of IPV were included, the rates rose to 30.3% (lifetime) and 3.6% (recent) IPV. Because physical abuse often involves the head and neck, abused women have a one and a half to two times higher risk of chronic pain, including headaches. Also, women who have experienced IPV are 60% more likely to suffer headaches than are women who have not experienced IPV. One study found that in the United States, 35% of women receiving tertiary care for headaches had a reported history of lifetime abuse.

The study conducted by Gerber and colleagues included a convenience sample of 92 women referred to a headache center for tension and migraine headaches. The mean age of the participants was 39 years (range 18–66 years); 73% ($n = 67$) were living with an intimate partner and of these, approximately 50% ($n = 46$) were married. The initial assessment included completion of the five-item self-report Migraine Disability Assessment (MIDAS) questionnaire, which assessed headache-related disability during the preceding 90 days as it related to missed paid work/education days, diminished household/family matters productivity, and interference with social/leisure activities. The modified Breslau seven-item screening tool was used to assess PTSD on 17 core symptoms. The three-item STaT (Slapped, Threatened, and Thrown) tool and the Partner Violence Screen were used to assess lifetime IPV. All tools used in this study were previously found to be reliable and valid.

Data were analyzed using various cross-tabulation methods and multivariable regression analysis. Of the 92 participants, approximately 28% ($n = 26$) were positive for PTSD; 9.8% ($n = 9$) had experienced recent IPV; 36.9% ($n = 34$) had experienced lifetime IPV, and a strong association between IPV and headache severity was noted. The participants with a lifetime history of IPV reported nine more days of headache-related disability than did the non-IPV participants.

The researchers concluded that PTSD was significantly associated with the severity of reported headaches. However, neither lifetime nor recent IPV was significantly associated with headache severity, a finding that reaffirmed results from previous studies, and the incidence of PTSD was positively associated with a lifetime exposure to IPV.

---

1. How is this information useful to clinical nursing practice?

2. Based on these findings, what are implications for further research?

See Suggested Responses for Evidence-Based Practice on Davis*Plus.*

Introduction

This chapter focuses on violence against women and the nurse's role in promoting mental health and physical safety for victims of intimate partner violence. Formerly termed *domestic violence* (DV), *intimate partner violence* (IPV) is considered a more modern term that recognizes that in contemporary society, intimate partners do not always share the same household. IPV is a significant public health problem that causes physical and emotional trauma for women, men, and children and leads to a myriad of health problems for the victims. Individuals who have been abused may be subjected to unnecessary diagnostic testing for various chronic problems that may be related to physical and emotional abuse. Although the physical manifestations of abuse

may be treated by the health-care professional, it is incumbent upon the nurse to also address the underlying causes of the injuries and empower the victim with safety information and other appropriate resources (Davila, Mendias, & Juneau, 2013; Wadsworth & Van Order, 2012).

Nurses have long been at the forefront of research in the area of violence against women. Early investigations by Campbell (1986), Parker and McFarlane (1991), and McFarlane and colleagues (1991) helped to raise awareness about this significant public health problem. Nurses who care for women and are advocates for the prevention of abuse are perfectly situated to screen patients and educate others on the importance of screening.

An important *Healthy People 2020* national goal clearly underscores the magnitude of intimate partner violence: *Reduce violence by current or former intimate partners*

(U.S. Department of Health and Human Services [USDHHS], 2011). This includes physical and sexual violence, psychological abuse, and stalking. Nurses can be instrumental in helping the nation to achieve this goal by routinely assessing women and their families to identify those at risk, assisting with counseling or initiating referrals for professional care, and maintaining contact to ensure that appropriate follow-up mechanisms are in place (USDHHS, 2011).

Definition, Incidence, and Impact on Individuals and Society

Intimate partner violence (IPV) is defined as physical, sexual, or psychological harm or social isolation perpetrated by a current or former partner (adult or adolescent), in an intimate or dating relationship. The violence can occur between members of heterosexual or homosexual couples and does not require sexual intimacy. The abuser's actions are intended to instill fear and to intimidate and control the victim (Futures Without Violence, 2013; Ward & Wood, 2009).

Viewed as a potentially preventable public health problem, IPV affected more than 12 million individuals in the United States during 2010. On average, 24 people per minute are victims of rape, physical violence, or stalking by an intimate partner, according to a 2010 survey conducted by the Centers for Disease Control and Prevention (CDC) (Black, Basile, Breiding, Smith, Walters, Merrick, et al., 2011). Around the world, at least one in every three women has been beaten, coerced into sex, or otherwise abused during her lifetime. Intimate partner violence is the most common form of violence directed against women, and according to the World Health Organization (WHO), one of every six women has been a victim of IPV. In many situations, women are victimized more than once by the same partner. In this country, it is estimated that women have a one in four chance of becoming a victim of IPV at some point during their lifetime. During 2007, there were 248,300 rapes/sexual assaults in the United States, more than 500 per day, up from 190,600 in 2005. Also during 2007, IPV resulted in 2,340 deaths; of these deaths, 30% were males and 70% were females (Black et al., 2011; CDC, 2012).

> ❀ *Nursing Insight*— *IPV: appreciating the scope of the problem*
>
> In 2010, the CDC initiated the National Intimate Partner and Sexual Violence Survey (NISVS) to collect detailed information on sexual violence, stalking, and intimate partner violence victimization of adult women and men in the United States. Findings from the survey reveal that these acts are widespread and disproportionately affect women, as underscored by the following highlights (Black et al., 2011):
> - 1.3 million women were raped during the year preceding this survey.
> - Nearly one in five women have been raped during their lifetime, whereas one in 71 men have been raped during their lifetime.
> - One in six women have been stalked during their lifetime, whereas one in 19 men have experienced stalking during their lifetime.

- One in four women have been the victim of severe physical violence by an intimate partner whereas one in seven men experienced severe physical violence by an intimate partner.
- 81% of women who experience rape, stalking, or physical violence by an intimate partner reported significant short- or long-term effects related to the violent experience in the relationship, such as PTSD symptoms and injury, whereas 35% of men report such effects stemming from their experiences.
- Women who had experienced rape or stalking by any perpetrator or physical violence by an intimate partner in their lifetime were more likely than women who did not experience these forms of violence to report having asthma, diabetes, and irritable bowel syndrome.
- Women and men who experienced these forms of violence were more likely to report frequent headaches, chronic pain, difficulty with sleeping, activity limitations, poor physical health, and poor mental health than were men and women who did not experience these forms of violence.

According to the WHO (2013), violence constitutes one of 10 health and social risk factors associated with women's health worldwide. The WHO has suggested that dense urban environments are associated with increased violence perpetrated against women, and women who reside in crowded, low socioeconomic urban neighborhoods are faced with day-to-day threats. A prevailing fear of violence diminishes women's likelihood to engage freely in urban activities and ultimately affects overall quality of life, generating feelings of insecurity, helplessness, and anxiety. Such feelings may lead to social isolation and reduced mobility. The document *Hidden Cities: Unmasking and Overcoming Health Inequities in Urban Settings*, jointly published by the WHO and the United Nations Human Settlement Programme (2010), addresses challenges, opportunities, and health inequities associated with urbanization (Stringer, 2011; WHO & United Nations Human Settlement Programme, 2010).

> ❀ *Nursing Insight*— *Revised rape definition to track statistics*
>
> In 2013, the Federal Bureau of Investigation (FBI) published a revised definition of rape to track statistics for the annual Uniform Crime Report. Previously, rape was defined only as forceful vaginal penetration of a woman by a man's penis. The new definition of rape recognizes that victims and perpetrators may be female or male, and the assault may include oral or anal penetration or penetration with an object. Also, physical force is no longer a requirement of rape. Hence, the definition includes vulnerable victims, those who are intoxicated or otherwise mentally or physically incapable of demonstrating a lack of consent. It should be noted, however, that the FBI's change does not affect definitions under federal or state criminal laws; rather, it applies for statistical purposes only (American College of Obstetricians and Gynecologists {ACOG], 2014; FBI, 2013).

A man with a history of violence often brings violence into the family. The abuser's expressions of violent behavior usually erupt early in the courtship and grow progressively worse. Violence is used to handle conflicts, and the abuser exerts power to elicit a pervasive feeling of powerlessness in those around him. Male abusers frequently have a history of early and prolonged exposure to family violence as children, and alcohol is often associated with the violent behavior (Bull, 2009; CDC, Injury Center: Violence Prevention, 2013).

For victims of IPV, the health consequences of the trauma are far reaching and substantial. Immediate effects include injuries and death; long-term effects include an increased incidence of sexually transmitted diseases including HIV, pelvic inflammatory disease, and unintended pregnancy. Chronic mental health conditions related to IPV include PTSD, anxiety disorders, substance abuse, and suicide. PTSD is characterized by a cluster of symptoms involving reexperiencing the previous trauma, avoidance, and sustaining a state of hyperarousal. Interestingly, the symptoms may not appear for months or even years after the traumatic experience. A multitude of physical conditions such as chronic pain, neurological disorders resulting from injuries, gastrointestinal disorders (e.g., irritable bowel syndrome), sleeping difficulties, and migraine headaches often follow in the aftermath of IPV. Exposure to IPV during adolescence and young adulthood increases the likelihood of tobacco, alcohol, and drug abuse; eating disorders; obesity; poor self-esteem; risky sexual behaviors; and teen depression, anxiety, and suicidality (ACOG, 2014; Gerber et al., 2012; USDHHS, 2012).

Statistically, female victims are substantially more likely than male victims to be killed by an intimate partner. In 2007, females were killed by intimate partners at twice the rate of males: The rate of intimate partner homicide for females was 1.07 per 100,000 female residents, as compared with 0.46 per 100,000 male residents. Females made up 70% of victims killed by an intimate partner in 2007, a proportion that has changed very little since 1993. Overall, females are murdered by people they know. In 64% of female homicide cases in 2007, females were killed by a family member or intimate partner. In 2007, 24% of female homicide victims were killed by a spouse or ex-spouse; 21% were killed by a boyfriend or girlfriend and 19% by another family member (Catalano, Smith, Snyder, & Rand, 2009).

Intimate partner violence reaches across all strata of society and affects persons regardless of economic status, ethnic background, educational level, or religious status. The economic toll of the violence is substantial. It is estimated that the costs of IPV, physical assault, and stalking exceed $8.3 billion per year. Of this amount, more than $4.1 billion is directly related to physical and mental health services. Individuals affected by IPV experience a productivity loss of 8 million days of paid work (the equivalent of 32,000 full-time jobs) and approximately 5.6 million days of unpaid household work each year (CDC, 2012).

Cultural Diversity: Intimate Partner Violence

According to Tjaden and Thoennes (2000), in the United States, the groups found to have the highest prevalence of IPV are American Indian and Alaska Native women and men, black women, and Hispanic women. From 2001 to 2005, the annual rate of nonfatal IPV was generally higher for American Indian and Alaska Native females, and similar for black females and white females. In 2007, black female victims of intimate partner homicide were twice as likely as white female homicide victims to be

killed by a spouse (0.96 and 0.50 per 100,000, respectively), and black females were four times more likely than white females to be murdered by a boyfriend or girlfriend (1.44 and 0.34 per 100,000, respectively). The rate of IPV for Hispanic women peaked at ages 20 to 24 (Catalano et al., 2009). Latinas are known to underuse traditional intervention services such as domestic violence shelters, health-care services, and law enforcement agencies because of a lack of health insurance, language and cultural barriers, and a general distrust of formal systems. Caucasian women report less IPV than do non-Caucasians, and Asian women report significantly less IPV than do other racial groups. Peedicayil and colleagues (2004) conducted a study of 9,938 women in India and reported a 13% prevalence rate of moderate to severe violence—including slapping, beating, kicking, and use of a weapon—during pregnancy. It is important for nurses to remember that violence may be underreported as a result of cultural norms. Although cultures may differ in their perceptions and definitions of abuse, the act of inflicting harm to another is against the law.

Those who perpetrate the abuse may refuse to allow their victims to work or attend school. Women who are abused are more likely to be unemployed, suffer from health problems, and receive public assistance than are women who are not victims of abuse. Those with severe and persistent mental illness are more likely to be involved in controlling and violent relationships. In the workplace, an additional burden is frequently placed on coworkers to compensate for the IPV victim's repeated absenteeism. Another indicator of the substantial economic burden of abuse is reflected in the millions of tax dollars channeled into supporting programs created to assist IPV victims (Black et al., 2011).

Nursing Insight— Accuracy issues with reported IPV statistics

Accuracy in regard to IPV statistics is difficult to determine. During the period from 2006 to 2010, only 35% of rapes/sexual assaults were actually reported to the police (Langton, Berzofsky, Kerbs, & Smiley-McDonald, 2012). Findings from the CDC 2010 NISVS Report revealed lifetime estimates for women ranging from 25.3% to 49.1% for rape, physical violence, and/or stalking by an intimate partner; for men, lifetime estimates ranged from 17.4% to 41.2% for rape, physical violence, and/or stalking by an intimate partner (Black et al., 2011). Victims of abuse may be reluctant to report personal violence because of fear or embarrassment, the belief that the police cannot or will not do anything to help, or because those from whom they sought help did not directly ask about abuse

---

Statistically, victims of repeated violence over time sustain more serious injuries than do victims of one-time abuse incidents. Young women and economically challenged individuals are affected more often by IPV than any other population. Economic hardship is known to exacerbate IPV. Financial stress may lead to more frequent and violent abuse: Out-of-work husbands and boyfriends spend more time at home and thus have more opportunities to abuse their partners, and women are less likely to leave abusive situations for fear that they will not be able to support themselves (ACOG, 2012).

Approximately 50% of children living in homes of intimate partner violence are also victimized. Children living in households affected by maternal abuse are 57 times more likely to suffer personal harm and are at greater risk for psychiatric disorders, developmental problems, school failure, violence against others, and low self-esteem. Those who perpetrate IPV create instability within their families while causing untold physical and psychological damage (Hamby, Finkelhor, Turner, & Ormrod, 2011).

 Nursing Insight— *Recognizing social factors in violent behavior*

Violent behavior in intimate relationships is often rooted in multiple social factors. For example, the perpetrators and victims of family violence may learn about violent behavior by either witnessing or experiencing it firsthand. Other social factors include poverty and oppression, low income, unemployment, difficulty in maintaining interpersonal ties, marital instability and disruption, and single-parent families (Hamby et al., 2011).

The CDC (2013) and other researchers list multiple factors that place an individual at risk for committing intimate partner abuse and for being a victim of intimate partner abuse (Tables 1-1 and 1-2).

Now Can You— **Discuss certain facts about IPV?**

1. Define the term *intimate partner violence*?
2. Identify a national goal related to IPV and discuss how nurses can be instrumental in helping the nation to achieve this goal?
3. Explain why it is difficult to obtain accurate statistics about the prevalence of IPV?

4. List 10 risk factors for committing IPV and 10 risk factors for being a victim of IPV?

Types of Abuse

Abuse may occur in many forms, and victims may be repeatedly subjected to more than one type of abuse. Physical abuse is only one manifestation of intimate partner violence. The CDC (2012) recognizes four categories of IPV: physical violence; sexual violence; threats of physical or sexual violence; and psychological or emotional violence (Box 1-1). Other types of abuse include social abuse and economic abuse.

PHYSICAL VIOLENCE

Physical abuse may include spitting; scratching; kicking; punching; pushing; shoving; throwing; grabbing; biting; burning; choking; shaking; slapping; strangling; using a weapon; and using restraints or one's body, size, or strength against another person. The abused woman may be seen in the health clinic, doctor's office, or emergency department with vague, chronic, nonspecific complaints, and often there is a history of overuse of health services or unexplainable injuries such as bruises and fractures. Nurses should be alert to the patient's chronic issues as possible symptoms of abuse. For example, the woman may seek treatment for headaches, anxiety, stress, insomnia, or fatigue. The IPV victim's appearance may vary: She may be disheveled, dirty, and distressed or neat, well groomed, and calm. Oftentimes, abused women are subjected to unnecessary diagnostic testing to determine the cause of the chronic conditions (CDC, 2012; Ward & Wood, 2009).

Table 1-1 Risk Factors for Committing Intimate Partner Violence	
Individual Factors	**Relationship Factors**
Young age	Marital conflict—fights, tension, and other struggles
Low self-esteem	Marital instability—divorces or separations
Low income	Dominance and control of the relationship by one partner over the other
Low academic achievement	Unhealthy family relationships and interactions
Aggressive or delinquent behavior as a youth	Economic stress
Heavy alcohol and drug use	**Community Factors**
Emotional dependence and insecurity	Poverty and associated factors (e.g., overcrowding)
Unemployment	Low social capital—lack of institutions, relationships, and norms that shape a community's social interactions
Depression	Weak community sanctions against IPV (e.g., unwillingness of neighbors to intervene in situations where they witness violence)
Anger and hostility	**Societal Factors**
Antisocial personality traits	Traditional gender norms (e.g., women should stay at home, not enter workforce, and be submissive; men support the family and make the decisions)
Borderline personality traits	
Prior history of being physically abusive	
Having few friends and being isolated from other people	
Belief in strict gender roles (e.g., male dominance and aggression in relationships)	
Desire for power and control in relationships	
Perpetrating psychological aggression	
Being a victim of physical or psychological abuse (consistently one of the strongest predictors of perpetration)	
History of experiencing poor parenting as a child	
History of experiencing physical discipline as a child	

Source: CDC (2010).

Table 1-2 Risk Factors for Being a Victim of Intimate Partner Violence

Individual Factors	Relationship Factors
History of child abuse	Marital conflict
History of physical abuse	Marital instability
History of sexual abuse	Male dominance in the
Prior injury from the same partner	family
Having a verbally abusive partner	Poor family functioning
Economic stress, low income	Partner history of alcohol
Tobacco, alcohol, and illicit drug use	or drug abuse
Depression or suicide attempts	
History of sexually transmitted diseases	
Young age (less than 24 years, especially adolescents)	
Lack of high school diploma	
Unplanned pregnancies (often as a result of birth control sabotage)	

Source: CDC (2010).

Box 1-1 CDC Categories of IPV

Physical violence: The intentional use of physical force with the potential for causing death, disability, injury, or harm

Sexual violence: Includes the use of physical force to compel a person to engage in a sexual act against his or her will, whether or not the act is completed; attempted or completed sex act involving a person who is unable to understand the nature or condition of the act, to decline participation, or to communicate unwillingness to engage in the sexual act (e.g., owing to illness, disability, or the influence of alcohol or other drugs or because of intimidation or pressure); and abusive sexual contact

Threats of physical or sexual violence: The use of words, gestures, or weapons to communicate the intent to cause death, disability, injury, or physical harm

Psychological or emotional violence: Trauma to the victim caused by acts, threats of acts, or coercive tactics. Stalking, which refers to harassing or threatening behavior that an individual engages in repeatedly (e.g., following a person, appearing at a person's home or place of business, making harassing phone calls, vandalizing a person's property) is frequently included among the types of IPV.

Source: CDC (2012).

Optimizing Outcomes— Recognizing signs of intimate partner violence

By recognizing signs of IPV, nurses can be instrumental in helping to make an accurate diagnosis and in securing appropriate assistance for the abused woman. Specifically, the nurse should remain alert to the following indicators, which may be signs of IPV:

- Overuse of health services
- Vague, nonspecific complaints
- Repeated missed appointments
- Unexplained injuries
- Untreated serious injuries
- Significant delay between the injury and the presentation for care
- Injuries that do not match the patient's description of how they were incurred
- Evidence or a history of previous injuries

- Bilateral or multiple injuries in various stages of healing
- Intimate partner who refuses to leave the patient's side
- Intimate partner who insists on explaining how the injury was incurred (ACOG, 2011, 2012; Davilla et al., 2013)

Certain behavioral clues may point to abuse. For example, the intimate partner may refuse to leave the victim during the interview and physical assessment. The abuser may display extreme attentiveness toward the victim and attempt to describe to the care provider exactly how the injuries were sustained. The abuser may hover, dominate, and control the information given. The abuser may refuse to allow the victim to share private time with the health professional. The information about the circumstances surrounding the injury may not match the actual injuries. Frequently, victims suffer repeated injuries and delay medical treatment for serious injuries. Nurses and other health-care professionals should remember that medical encounters can be extremely distressing and anxiety producing for individuals who have been abused in family or intimate relationships. For example, routine procedures such as gynecological exams, blood pressure checks, and abdominal palpation can trigger intense reactions of fear, dread, and avoidance (Alpert, 2010; ACOG, 2014; Ward & Wood, 2009).

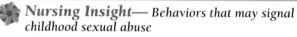 **Nursing Insight—** *Behaviors that may signal childhood sexual abuse*

During a gynecological examination, it is important to recognize certain behaviors that may signal sexual abuse during childhood. For example, the woman may display an exaggerated startle response, hostility, irritability, anger, difficulty concentrating, or disassociation. A compassionate, sensitive approach can foster trust and may allow the examination to serve as an opportunity for the nurse to help the childhood sexual victim begin to heal (Roller, 2011).

Optimizing Outcomes— Recognizing physical patterns of IPV injury

Nurses should be aware that physical injuries inflicted during intimate partner violence are likely to appear in a central pattern on the face, chest, breasts, abdomen, and neck. The patient may complain of abdominal pain upon palpation, chest pain related to rib trauma, or musculoskeletal pain accompanied by redness and swelling. Bruises may be noted on the inner aspect of the arms and/or legs, along with injuries suggestive of a defensive-type posture, such as an injury to the ulnar aspect of the forearm (Ward & Wood, 2009). The most common sites for genital injuries (e.g., lacerations, hematomas, ecchymosis, abrasions, redness, edema) are the posterior fourchette, the labia minora, the hymen, and the fossa navicularis (the boat-shaped depression between the vagina and the fourchette (Sommers, 2007).

Intimate partner violence frequently results in head, neck, and facial injuries. It is estimated that up to 90% of abused victims sustain head and neck injuries, and IPV is believed to account for between 34% and 73% of all facial injuries in women. Between 88% and 94% of IPV victims seek medical attention for injuries to the head and neck, and 56% of those have facial fractures (Arosarena, Fritsch, Hsueh, Aynehchi, & Haug, 2009; Blereau, 2009).

Arosarena and colleagues (2009) discovered that specific patterns of facial injury are more likely to be associated with IPV than with other sources of injury, such as motor vehicle crashes or even with assault by a stranger. The researchers reviewed the medical and dental records of 326 women with facial trauma treated by specialists at a university hospital. Their findings revealed that injuries around the eye or upper face were more likely to be associated with IPV, whereas mandible fractures were more likely to be caused by assault by an unknown assailant. Victims of IPV more often sustain zygomatic complex fractures, orbital blow-out fractures, and intracranial injuries than did other patients with facial trauma (Arosarena et al., 2009; Blereau, 2009; Saddki, Suhaimi, & Daud, 2010; Wu, Huff, & Bhandari, 2010).

✿ *Nursing Insight*— *IPV and patterns of facial trauma*

A woman's face is the most meaningful area on her person; it is the most conspicuous and unique part of the body that contributes to an individual's self-image and self-esteem. According to an otolaryngologist who has extensively studied injuries inflicted during IPV, the pattern of facial trauma sustained is reflective of this fact. Thus, hitting in the face figures prominently in IPV. This particular pattern may be contrasted with that typically seen in the assault of a robber, for example, whose ultimate goal is primarily to disable the victim (Blereau, 2009; Saddki et al., 2010).

Women who are strangled during IPV may or may not demonstrate physical evidence of an injury to the neck. Visible evidence such as red marks, scratches, scrapes, bruises, or rope burns may be apparent in only 15% of strangulation cases. Nurses should be alert to patient complaints such as persistent throat pain, voice changes, or difficulty swallowing, which may be indicators of neck trauma sustained during an act of violence. Chin abrasions may be present—as the victim lowers the chin in an instinctive effort to protect the neck, the skin is scraped against the abuser's hands. Victims of strangulation attempts should be evaluated for possible damage (e.g., fracture) to the hyoid bone, a small horseshoe-shaped bone in the neck that supports the tongue. Although breathing difficulty may initially appear to be mild, damage to the hyoid bone or other underlying structures may result in fatal asphyxiation up to 36 or more hours after the assault (Volochinsky, 2012).

✿ *Nursing Insight*— *Recognizing the unique problems of older women subjected to IPV*

Women of all ages are at risk for IPV. When trying to leave an abuser, older women may face challenges such as feelings of shame and worries about money. However, abused women who are 55 years and older are confronted with still another challenge. Having grown up and gotten married during a time when IPV was often ignored, older women have suffered many years of abuse and, like other victims of IPV, frequently have problems with poor self-image and guilt. Older women who

have been abused are also less likely to confide in anyone about the abuse, they may have health problems that keep them dependent on their abusive partner, feel committed to caring for their abusive and aging partners, and are fearful of being alone. Among postmenopausal women from the Women's Health Initiative study ($N = 91,749$), 11% reported abuse during the prior year, of which 2.1% was physical abuse, 89.1% was verbal abuse, and 8.8% was both physical and verbal abuse (ACOG, 2012; USDHHS, 2012).

---

⑤ Now Can You— Discuss physical injury associated with IPV?

1. Identify eight clinical red flags that may be indicative of IPV?
2. Describe behavioral characteristics of the abuser that may be indicative of IPV?
3. Explain what is meant by a "central pattern" of injury and why this is often observed in victims of IPV?

SEXUAL VIOLENCE

Sexual violence may include the abuser's use of force to carry out sexual intercourse or other sexual activities (whether or not they are completed) against the victim's will. It may include forced participation in an early initiation of sexual activity; forced participation in sexual activity viewed to be humiliating or degrading; decreased condom use or otherwise unprotected sexual intercourse; having multiple sexual partners; and trading sex for food, money, drugs, or other items. Sexual abuse may increase the likelihood of exposure to sexually transmitted diseases (STDs), including HIV and AIDS. Recurrent vaginal infections and/or an unusually high number of STDs or frequent miscarriages can be warning signs of sexual abuse. Interestingly, sexual assaults committed by strangers are more likely to be reported than are rapes and sexual assaults committed by an intimate partner (CDC, 2012; Futures Without Violence, 2013; Ward & Wood, 2009).

According to a 2013 report released by the U.S. Bureau of Justice Statistics, during the time period from 1995 to 2005, sexual violence against U.S. female residents aged 12 years or older declined 64%—from 5.0 per 1,000 females to 1.8—and remained unchanged through 2010. Sexual violence against females includes completed, attempted, or threatened rape or sexual assault. The majority of violence against females involved someone the victim knew. Approximately 38% of sexual violence was committed by a friend or acquaintance, 34% by an intimate partner (former or current spouse, girlfriend, or boyfriend), and 6% by a relative or family member. Interestingly, strangers committed approximately 22% of all sexual violence, and this percentage remained unchanged from 1994 to 2010 (Bureau of Justice Statistics, 2013).

---

⑤ **Where Research and Practice Meet:** **A Brief Nursing Intervention to Prevent STDs Among Battered Women; Sexual Risk, Safer Sex, and Partner Violence**

Laughon, Sutherland, and Parker (2011) implemented a brief nursing intervention (BNI) with 18 women in a rural health department family planning clinic who screened positive for IPV. The BNI was a 10-minute face-to-face counseling session that consisted of four previously developed components: IPV information; Danger assessment; Safety planning & operations; and Resources (McFarlane, Groff, O'Brien, & Watson, 2006). For this study, HIV/STD prevention was also addressed, following the same model as the IPV intervention. Severity and frequency of violence, IPV safety behaviors, and safer sex behaviors were measured at baseline and again at 3 months. The frequency of physical and sexual violence decreased from baseline to 3-month follow-up, and while not statistically significant, the number of safer sex behaviors reported increased from baseline to follow-up. The addition of HIV/STD information to a BNI for battered women shows promise as a strategy for women living in violent relationships who are at increased risk for STDs.

Working with a convenience sample of 179 sexually active women, Sutherland and colleagues (2012) examined sexual risk behaviors and safe sex behaviors between those who reported past year physical partner violence (n =70) and those who did not (n = 109). Women who had experienced physical violence and those who had not both reported sexual risk behaviors including multiple partners and unprotected vaginal intercourse. However, women in abusive relationships reported "significantly higher rates of coercive risk behaviors, including verbal threats and physical force to engage in oral, anal, and vaginal sex activities" (p. 720). The findings underscore the importance of screening not only for IPV but also for coercive sexual behaviors often associated with abusive relationships.

Another manifestation of sexual violence involves forcing undesired pregnancy or forcing pregnancies to occur rapidly, one after one another. Pregnancy constitutes an especially dangerous time for abused women. Physical violence during pregnancy has far-reaching effects for the infant as well as for the mother. Battery during pregnancy is associated with a greater incidence of low-birth-weight neonates, preterm birth, and neonatal death. According to the WHO (2011), the global prevalence of physical IPV in pregnancy ranges from 1% (Japan city) to as much as 40% (Africa).

In this country, approximately 324,000 pregnant women are abused each year. IPV accounts for 31% of the homicides among pregnant women and is the leading cause of traumatic death for pregnant and postpartum women in the United States. In the WHO multicountry study on women's health and domestic violence against women, the majority of women who reported physical abuse during pregnancy had also been beaten prior to getting pregnant, although about 50% of women in three sites stated that they were beaten for the first time during a pregnancy (ACOG, 2012; WHO, 2011).

🌸 *Nursing Insight— Maternal intimate partner violence: The sobering statistics*

Among pregnant women in the United States during 2008, physical abuse during the 12 months prior to becoming pregnant varied by state, from 1.8% to 6.0%, and rates for physical abuse during pregnancy ranged from 1.3% to 4.6% (USDHHS, 2012). Women who experience abuse in the year prior to and/or during a recent pregnancy are 40% to 60% more likely than nonabused women to suffer from high blood pressure, vaginal bleeding, severe nausea, and kidney or urinary tract infections during pregnancy. They are also more likely to require hospitalization during pregnancy and are 37% more likely to give birth to preterm infants. Neonates born to abused mothers are 17% more likely to be underweight at birth and are 30% more likely than other infants to require neonatal intensive care (ACOG, 2012; Records, 2011).

⊛ **Where Research and Practice Meet:**
Long-term Effects of Maternal Abuse

McFarlane and colleagues (2014) compared a group (n = 46) of abused women seeking assistance for partner abuse during pregnancy with a group (n = 22) of abused women who reported abuse only outside of pregnancy to evaluate long-term (i.e., 24 months after delivery) safety and functioning outcomes and children's behavior. The researchers found that the risk for murder remained higher for women reporting abuse during pregnancy for 8 months after delivery, depression was higher for up to 20 months after delivery, and PTSD was appreciably higher for 24 months. Children living with mothers abused during pregnancy displayed more behavioral problems (e.g., depression, anxiety) for the entire 24-month period. The study findings highlight the far-reaching adverse impacts of maternal abuse on safety and functioning for at least 24 months after delivery, and underscore the importance of universal abuse screening and appropriate intervention during the ante- and postnatal periods.

PSYCHOLOGICAL (EMOTIONAL) VIOLENCE

Psychological or emotional violence includes acts such as coercion, making threats, and stalking. The abuser may verbally abuse the victim with criticism, insults, put-downs, or name-calling. The perpetrator may use facial expressions or gestures to intimidate and instill fear. Other forms of emotional abuse include the perpetrator's use of threats of harm to children, family members, or pets. Not uncommonly, abusers destroy the victim's property, abuse their pets, or display weapons to force the victim into submission. The abuser may mislead children into viewing the victim as having "earned" the abuse by causing the perpetrator to become angry—in this situation, the children often blame the victim for the resulting violence. The perpetrator frequently places the blame on the victim—denying fault and instead claiming that any physical injury resulted from the victim's "clumsiness." Often, the victim's injuries are minimized and the abuser creates excuses for the abusive behavior. The perpetrator may also attempt to convince others that the victim is incompetent or guilty of fabrication and not to be believed or taken seriously (CDC, 2013).

⊛ Now Can You— **Discuss aspects of sexual and psychological violence?**

1. Identify four examples of sexual violence?
2. Describe maternal and neonatal problems that may stem from abuse during pregnancy?
3. Identify three characteristics of psychological violence?

SOCIAL ABUSE

Social abuse may include the abuser isolating or limiting the victim's contact and time spent with family and friends; the abuser may also require the victim to obtain permission to leave the house. The victim may be forbidden to seek outside employment or to attend school. The perpetrator may conduct "odometer checks" on the victim's car to confirm that the victim has not left home and, in some situations, the victim is required to provide a detailed account of any time spent away from the abuser. The victim may be denied access to medical services. The abuser may prevent the victim from keeping medical or other appointments, thereby creating strain on relationships with health-care providers, employers, friends, and family members (Americans Overseas Domestic Violence Crisis Center, 2014; CDC, 2013).

The abuser may harm the victim's reputation and intimidate the victim's family and friends. Not infrequently, a breakdown in the victim's interpersonal relationships occurs, removing an important source of emotional support for the victim. Social abuse may include the perpetrator stalking the victim. According to CDC's 2010 NISVS, approximately 5.2 million women were stalked in the 12 months prior to taking the survey, and of these, two-thirds were stalked by a current or former intimate partner. It has been estimated that only 50% of stalking activity against women is actually reported to the police. Stalking constitutes a serious threat, and the victim should be encouraged to report this behavior to the police (Black et al., 2011; CDC, 2013).

ECONOMIC ABUSE

Economic abuse may include the abuser controlling all aspects of the victim's finances, refusing to share money, forcing the victim to account for any money spent, and forbidding the victim to work outside of the home. For the perpetrator, these actions help to bring about the victim's emotional and financial dependency on the abuser. The abuser may force the victim to miss work repeatedly, place frequent telephone calls to the victim at the workplace, or show up at the workplace unannounced in an attempt to jeopardize the victim's work ethic and job security. According to data compiled by the American Bar Association (2008), 70% of IPV victims are employed, and greater than 70% of them admit that their abusers harass them at work, either over the telephone or in person. Also, abusers cause more than 60% of their victims to be late or absent from work or both (American Bar Association, 2008).

✿ Nursing Insight— *Use of the power and control wheel to enhance understanding*

The Power and Control Wheel (Fig. 1-1) was developed by battered women in Duluth, Minnesota. The women, all victims of IPV, were attending women's education groups sponsored by a women's shelter. The Power and Control Wheel is meant to graphically illustrate the scope of men's abusive behaviors toward women.

The Equality Wheel (Fig. 1-2), also developed by the Minnesota Domestic Abuse Intervention Project, was created to describe the changes needed for men who batter to move from being abusive to being part of a nonviolent partnership. Used together, the wheels provide a mechanism for identifying and exploring abuse and then making behavioral changes toward nonviolent behavior.

ABUSE AND NEGLECT DIRECTED TOWARD ELDERLY AND VULNERABLE ADULTS

A vulnerable adult is often defined as a person aged 18 years or older whose ability to perform the normal activities of daily living or to provide personal care or protection is impaired owing to a mental, emotional, long-term physical, or developmental disability or dysfunction, or brain damage. Elder abuse is defined as a single or repeated act or lack of appropriate actions, which causes harm, risk of harm, or distress to an individual aged 60 years or older (ACOG, 2013a). According to the CDC (2012), types of elder abuse that also apply to vulnerable adults include the following: physical abuse, emotional/psychological abuse, neglect, abandonment, financial or material exploitation, and self-neglect (Box 1-2).

Nurses should be aware that certain vulnerable individuals might be more likely to be affected by IPV. For example, women with disabilities are vulnerable to physical; sexual; and mental abuse, neglect, and exploitation. The abuse may include withholding necessary assistive devices, care, or treatment. Immigrant and refugee women are also at risk for violence and abuse because of isolation and manipulation by their partners, language and cultural differences, and a prevailing lack of awareness of their rights and legal and social resources (ACOG, 2012).

⊚ Now Can You— Discuss aspects of social and economic abuse?

1. Describe three characteristics of social abuse?
2. Describe three characteristics of economic abuse?
3. Explain how the Power and Control Wheel and the Equality Wheel may be used to enhance understanding about male-directed abusive behavior toward women and offer behavioral strategies for the transition into a nonviolent, noncontrolling relationship?
4. Identify three CDC categories of abuse/neglect toward elderly and vulnerable adults?

Phases of Abuse

Three phases of abuse have been identified: (1) tension building; (2) acute violence; and (3) a tranquil, loving period of calm and remorse, sometimes termed the *honeymoon period*. Although not all abusive relationships follow this cycle, many victims can readily recognize this pattern (Walker, 1979, 1984).

TENSION-BUILDING PHASE

The first phase is characterized as a period of increasing tension. During this time, the abuser demonstrates hostility and anger without culminating into violent outbursts. The victim senses the escalating behavior and attempts to placate the abuser. In many situations, the victim's behavior postpones rather than prevents the abuse. At some point, the victim realizes that she cannot control the violent behavior and withdraws to cope. This action only heightens the abuser's anger (Advocates to End Domestic Violence, 2014; Walker, 1979, 1984).

ACUTE-VIOLENCE PHASE

In the second phase, the abuser discharges the pent-up tension. This phase may be triggered by an internal response in the abuser or by an external crisis. Over a period of hours or days, the abuser may engage in a number of violent acts, such as biting, slapping, punching, stomping, choking, pushing, burning, or mutilating. Most injuries are directed at the face, neck, chest, breasts, buttocks, and abdomen; the hands and forearms are often damaged as the

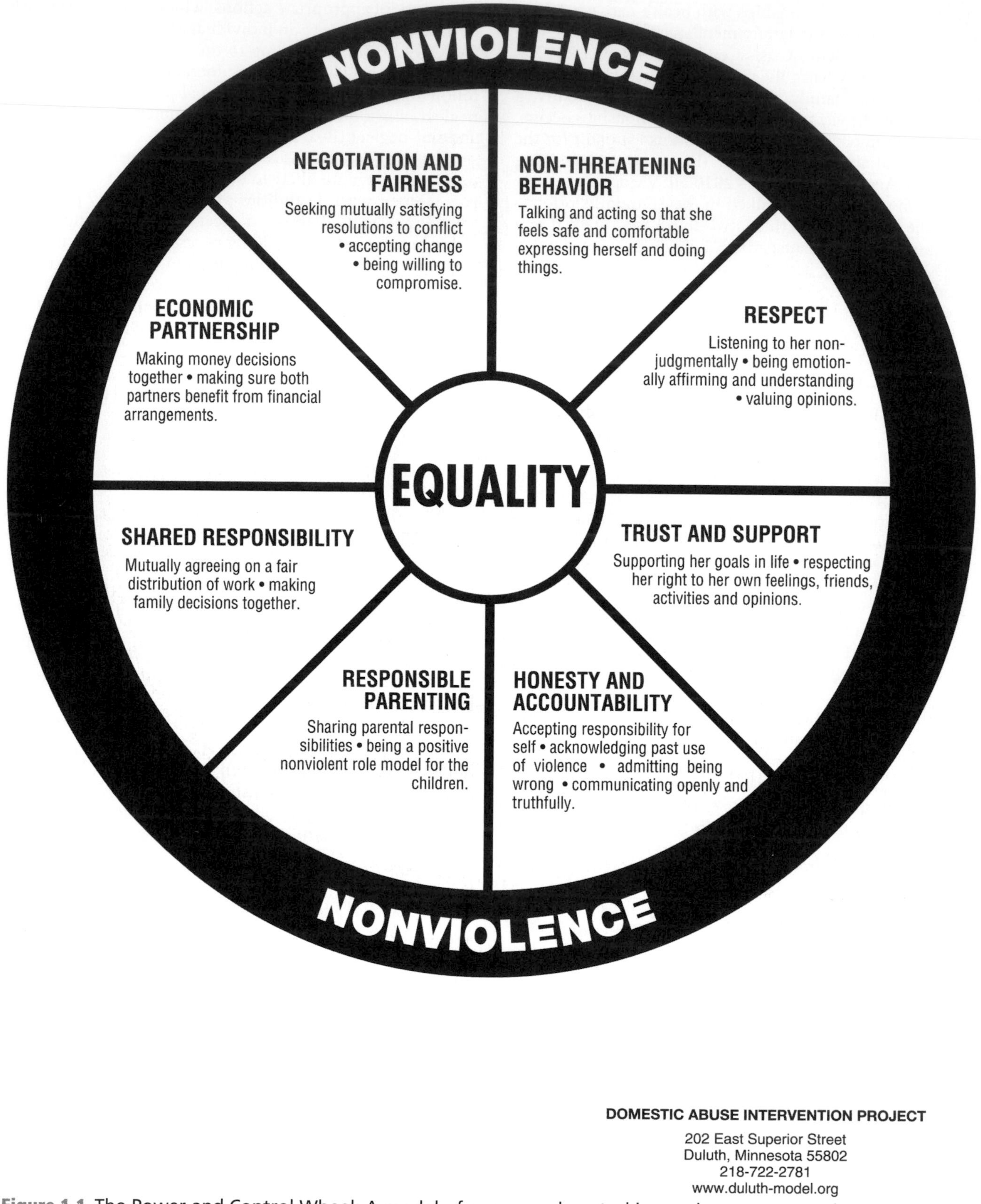

NONVIOLENCE

NEGOTIATION AND FAIRNESS
Seeking mutually satisfying resolutions to conflict • accepting change • being willing to compromise.

NON-THREATENING BEHAVIOR
Talking and acting so that she feels safe and comfortable expressing herself and doing things.

ECONOMIC PARTNERSHIP
Making money decisions together • making sure both partners benefit from financial arrangements.

RESPECT
Listening to her non-judgmentally • being emotionally affirming and understanding • valuing opinions.

EQUALITY

SHARED RESPONSIBILITY
Mutually agreeing on a fair distribution of work • making family decisions together.

TRUST AND SUPPORT
Supporting her goals in life • respecting her right to her own feelings, friends, activities and opinions.

RESPONSIBLE PARENTING
Sharing parental responsibilities • being a positive nonviolent role model for the children.

HONESTY AND ACCOUNTABILITY
Accepting responsibility for self • acknowledging past use of violence • admitting being wrong • communicating openly and truthfully.

NONVIOLENCE

DOMESTIC ABUSE INTERVENTION PROJECT
202 East Superior Street
Duluth, Minnesota 55802
218-722-2781
www.duluth-model.org

Figure 1-1 The Power and Control Wheel: A model of power and control issues that perpetuate battering. (Developed by the Duluth Domestic Abuse Intervention Project, Duluth, Minnesota.)

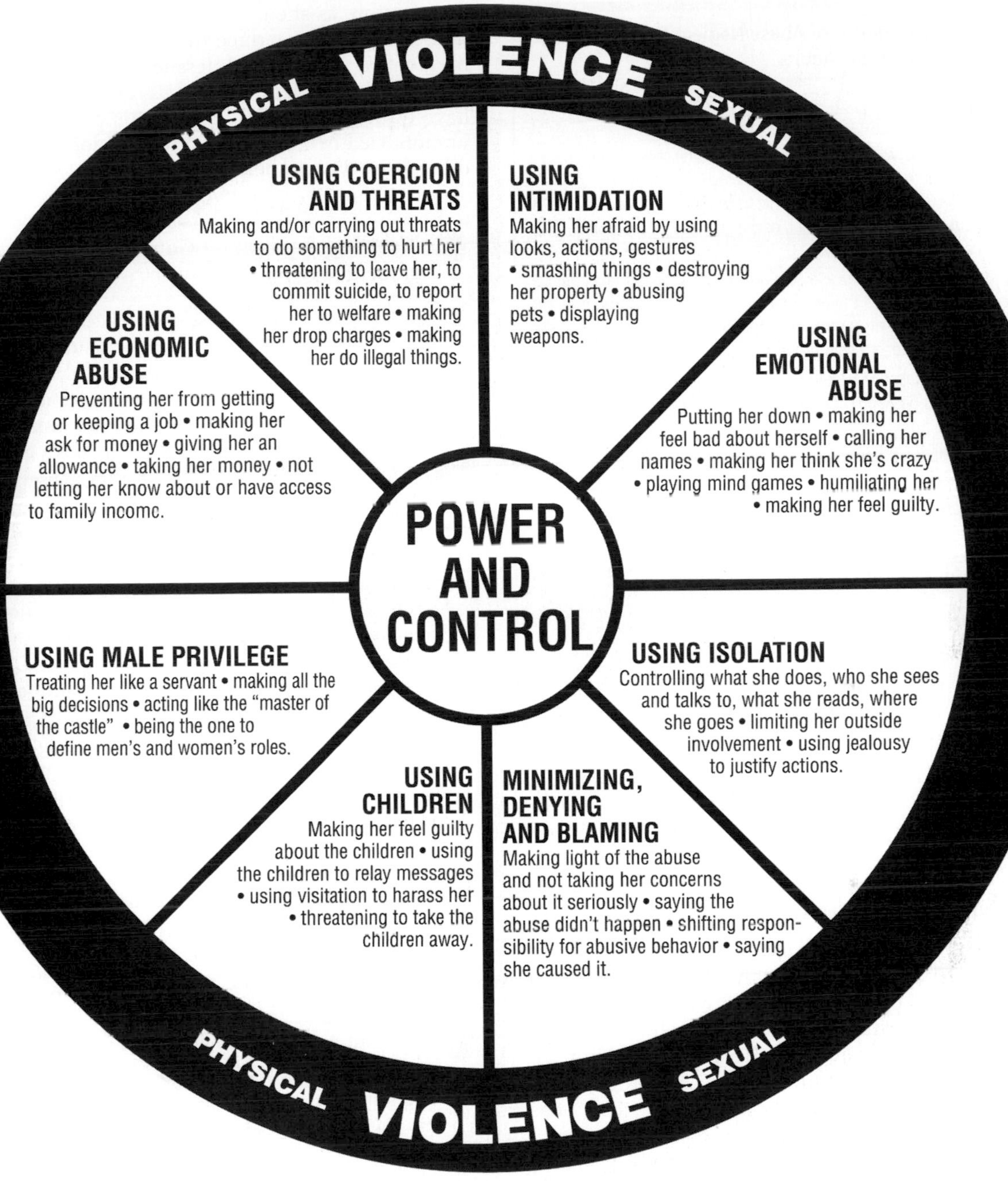

PHYSICAL VIOLENCE SEXUAL

POWER AND CONTROL

USING COERCION AND THREATS
Making and/or carrying out threats to do something to hurt her • threatening to leave her, to commit suicide, to report her to welfare • making her drop charges • making her do illegal things.

USING INTIMIDATION
Making her afraid by using looks, actions, gestures • smashing things • destroying her property • abusing pets • displaying weapons.

USING ECONOMIC ABUSE
Preventing her from getting or keeping a job • making her ask for money • giving her an allowance • taking her money • not letting her know about or have access to family income.

USING EMOTIONAL ABUSE
Putting her down • making her feel bad about herself • calling her names • making her think she's crazy • playing mind games • humiliating her • making her feel guilty.

USING MALE PRIVILEGE
Treating her like a servant • making all the big decisions • acting like the "master of the castle" • being the one to define men's and women's roles.

USING ISOLATION
Controlling what she does, who she sees and talks to, what she reads, where she goes • limiting her outside involvement • using jealousy to justify actions.

USING CHILDREN
Making her feel guilty about the children • using the children to relay messages • using visitation to harass her • threatening to take the children away.

MINIMIZING, DENYING AND BLAMING
Making light of the abuse and not taking her concerns about it seriously • saying the abuse didn't happen • shifting responsibility for abusive behavior • saying she caused it.

PHYSICAL VIOLENCE SEXUAL

DOMESTIC ABUSE INTERVENTION PROJECT

202 East Superior Street
Duluth, Minnesota 55802
218-722-2781
www.duluth-model.org

Figure 1-2 The Equality Wheel: May be used in concert with the Power and Control Wheel to help individuals see alternate ways of being in relationships with women that are free of violence and controlling behavior. (Developed by the Duluth Domestic Abuse Intervention Project, Duluth, Minnesota.)

Box 1-2 CDC Categories of Abuse/Neglect Toward Elderly and Vulnerable Adults

Physical abuse: Occurs when an individual is injured, assaulted, or threatened with a weapon, or inappropriately restrained

Sexual abuse or abusive sexual contact: Constitutes any sexual contact against an individual's will; includes acts in which the elderly person is unable to understand the act or is unable to communicate. Abusive sexual contact includes intentional touching of the genitalia, anus, groin, breast, mouth, inner thigh, or buttocks.

Psychological (emotional) abuse: Occurs when an elder experiences trauma after exposure to threatening acts or coercive tactics (e.g., humiliation, embarrassment, controlling behavior, social isolation, trivializing needs, damaging or destroying property)

Neglect: Failure or refusal of a caregiver or other responsible person to provide for an elder's basic physical, emotional, or social needs, or failure to protect an elder from harm

Abandonment: The willful desertion of an elderly person by a caregiver or other responsible person

Financial abuse/exploitation: The unauthorized or improper use of an elder's resources for monetary or personal benefit, profit, or gain (e.g., forgery, misuse or theft of money or possessions, improper use of guardianship or power of attorney)

Source: CDC (2012).

---

victim attempts to protect herself. The abuser often makes the victim feel that she has angered the abuser and thus is responsible for the abuse. Frequently, the woman minimizes the extent of injury and is reluctant to seek medical care (Advocates to End Domestic Violence, 2014; Walker, 1979, 1984).

THE HONEYMOON PHASE

During the third phase, the abuser feels remorse and apologizes profusely. He promises that the abuse will never happen again and may even believe that it will not. The abuser showers his victim with love and kindness, lulling her into forgiveness and a desire to continue the relationship. The victim desperately wants to believe her abuser and is renewed in her hope that he really will change. This phase provides the positive reinforcement for remaining in the relationship. The victim denies the reality that the abuse will recur. Unless there is some intervention at this point, this phase will end and the cycle of violence will be repeated (Advocates to End Domestic Violence, 2014; Walker, 1979, 1984).

VICTIMS' REACTIONS TO THE PHASES OF ABUSE

Victims react in various ways to each of the three phases of abuse. During the first, or tension-building, phase, the woman uses denial as a defense mechanism. If the relationship is not terminated at this point, the abuse continues to escalate in frequency and violence, and the victim indirectly "gives permission" for the abuse to continue. During the second (acute-violence) phase, the woman can no longer deny that the violence is occurring. Unfortunately, she is unable to stop the violence because she is fearful of provoking further violence. She resorts to the use of various coping mechanisms, such as dutiful obedience and

cooperation, as she conforms to the abuser's wishes in a desperate effort to reduce the violence. This behavior has been called "learned helplessness." Not surprisingly, the victim feels hopeless, powerless, and depressed and may have difficulty seeking help at this point because she is immobilized by a sense of guilt and does not believe that others may wish to help her.

> **Nursing Insight—** *Gaining an understanding of the IPV victims' behavior/recovery phases*
>
> Kearney's (2001) seminal research was designed to gain insight into why IPV victims remain with or return to their abusers. Four phases of IPV victim recovery were identified:
>
> *Enduring love/relationship obligation:* Characterized by a desire to love/be loved; belief that the relationship is "forever"; fearfulness of disclosure to family and friends; personal feelings of shame and guilt and self-blame for the abuse
>
> *The more I do, the worse I am:* Characterized by attempts to meet the abuser's needs despite the fact that the abuse now occurs routinely; feelings of self-doubt, loss of personal identity; displaying of harmful behaviors (e.g., substance abuse, alcoholism, suicide attempts) to cope with the emotional strain or coping behaviors (e.g., extreme dieting or overeating) to gain some semblance of control over their lives (CDC, 2013)
>
> *I've had enough:* Characterized by the realization that the relationship is abusive and will not be tolerated, but fear of the unknown and a lack of information about how to seek safe shelter—this point in the relationship is an opportune time for nurses to advocate for victims by providing support, education, and information about community resources
>
> *I was finding me:* Characterized by the ability to live a life separate from the abuser; may need tools (e.g., economic resources) to remain independent; requires continued support and encouragement; ongoing self-discovery/recovery; moving from the role of "victim" to one of "survivor"

> **Now Can You— Discuss the phases of abuse?**
>
> 1. Identify the three phases of abuse and describe characteristics of each phase?
> 2. Explain how victims often react to each of the three phases of abuse?
> 3. Describe how Kearney's (2001) research provides insights into IPV victims' behavior and how this information is useful to nurses?

Intimate Partner Violence Screening, Documenting, and Reporting

SCREENING FOR IPV

In 2000, the American Nurses Association (ANA) published a position statement on violence against women. This important document advocates universal screening, routine assessment, and documentation of abuse for all victims in any health-care setting. "Universal screening" means that *all* patients are assessed for IPV, regardless of the presence or absence of any abuse indicators. Routine screening can facilitate early identification of IPV when signs and symptoms may not be readily apparent and can

Sprague and colleagues (2012) conducted a systematic review to identify barriers to IPV screening and to improve the understanding of IPV barriers among various health-care providers.

Categories of IPV screening barriers included personal barriers, resource barriers, perceptions and attitudes, fears, and patient-related barriers. The most frequently reported individual barriers were personal discomfort with the issue, lack of knowledge, and time constraints. Interestingly, provider-related barriers were reported more often than patient-related barriers. To provide compassionate, holistic care, nurses must recognize potential barriers to routine IPV screening in the clinical setting. For example, time constraints, a lack of awareness of IPV or how to inquire about abuse, language and cultural differences, and a personal history of abuse may negatively impact routine IPV screening. Other researchers (Kang, Gottlieb, Raker, Aneja, & Boardman, 2010), who found that ambulatory gynecology patients were more likely to be screened for IPV when the health-care provider performed other preventive health screening using a standardized health history form, suggested that embedding inquiries about intimate partner abuse in the medical record may improve overall IPV screening rates. The investigators also concluded that one of the strongest influences on a health-care provider's screening behavior might be the tendency to perform comprehensive preventive health screening. In 2003, Chang and colleagues explored positive and negative consequences of IPV screening. Positive consequences included the following: a feeling that the practitioners cared, growing awareness that IPV is a problem, and a reduction in the victims' sense of social isolation. Negative consequences included feelings of being judged and being intruded upon, increasing anxiety, and disappointment in the practitioner's response.

mean a timely referral for appropriate services that may prevent further injury. If the screening tool suggests that the patient may be at high risk for abuse, a more detailed assessment should be performed.

In 2004, the U.S. Preventive Services Task Force (USP-STF) found insufficient evidence to recommend for or against routine screening of women for IPV. At that time, the Task Force stated that the potential harms (e.g., anxiety, fear of being stigmatized) of screening for IPV needed documentation in more rigorous studies, and noted that no studies had yet determined the validity of the screening tools designed to identify IPV.

In 2012, the USDHHS Agency for Healthcare Research and Quality initiated a systematic evidence review as an update for the prior USPSTF recommendation on screening women for IPV and elderly and vulnerable adults for abuse and neglect (Nelson, Bougatsos, & Blazina, 2012), and the updated summary of recommendations and evidence was published in January 2013. Specifically, the USPSTF recommends that clinicians screen women of childbearing age for IPV and provide or refer women who screen positive to intervention services. The recommendation applies to women who do not have signs or symptoms of abuse. The USPSTF concluded that the current evidence is insufficient to assess the balance of benefits and harms of screening all elderly or vulnerable adults for abuse and neglect (Moyer, 2013).

Health-care settings continue to provide a unique opportunity for IPV victims to confide in their care providers and to seek help. Consistent with new clinical guidelines, all women of childbearing age should be screened for abuse; the potential risk for harm resulting from IPV screening is considered "no greater than small." The updated recommendation is consistent with those of numerous medical and nursing organizations including the ACOG, the American College of Emergency Physicians, the American Academy of Pediatrics, and the Emergency Nurses Association (ACOG, 2012; Futures Without Violence, 2013; Institute of Medicine, 2012; Moyer, 2013).

"What to say" — *Conducting the IPV interview*

All interviews should take place in a private place. Children over the age of 3 years should be gently removed from the room and cared for by a staff member while the interview takes place. If language is a concern, a trained interpreter should be available to facilitate communication. The woman's partner, family members, or friend should not be used as a translator. After ensuring privacy, the nurse should maintain eye contact and begin with a statement such as, "In this office, a part of our routine care is to ask about intimate partner violence." Then, proceed with open-ended questions such as, "How are things at home? Do you feel safe at home? Do you feel safe in your community?" before asking more direct questions such as, "Do you ever feel pressured to have sex?" If the woman hesitates to answer yes or no, offer the choice of "sometimes" as a response. It is important not to pressure her to respond to the questions. If injuries are present, it is important to acknowledge them and ask how they occurred. If the patient's responses do not seem to match the mechanism of the injury, voice concern about the inconsistency, but don't push for details. Always promote trust and convey caring and let the patient know that violence is wrong and that no one deserves to be hurt. Demonstrating a nonjudgmental attitude and creating trust is an essential strategy in facilitating the patient's disclosure of abuse, especially in a busy clinical setting. Research suggests that IPV screening does not necessarily add significant time to a patient visit (Bull, 2009; Davila et al., 2013; Futures Without Violence, 2013; Moore, 2013; Records, 2011; Ward & Wood, 2009).

Once a patient discloses abuse, the nurse should facilitate an assessment to determine urgent safety needs and to guide the plan of care. If the patient is in immediate danger, an assessment for suicide and/or homicide may be indicated as well (Ward & Wood, 2009).

✿ *Nursing Insight— Finding the right words to*
facilitate understanding and disclosure of abuse

Patients may not always use the word *abuse* when describing their intimate relationships. It is important to be aware of words that suggest that abuse is occurring. For example, the patient may confide that her partner "has a temper" or "gets angry easily." Care should be taken to avoid the use of stigmatizing terms such as *rape* and instead use more neutral phrases such as *forced to have sex*. Using the same terms expressed by the patient may enhance her comfort in confiding about the full extent of the abuse (Davila et al, 2013; Records, 2011).

✦ *Across Care Settings*: Community resources share in supporting the victim of IPV

When IPV is identified, nurses and other health-care professionals share the responsibility of offering referrals to confidential victim and social support resources within the community. Referrals should be made regardless of whether the woman chooses to report the abuse to law enforcement. In the ideal situation, all health-care providers should be a part of a coordinated community response to reduce domestic violence, a response in which shelters, hospitals, health-care providers, legal advocates, and law enforcement work together to improve safety and save lives. Women should also be encouraged to consider self-defense courses, assertiveness courses, self-help groups, and courses designed for educational or skills development (Association of Women's Health, Obstetric and Neonatal Nurses [AWHONN], 2007; Davila et al., 2013; Records, 2011).

A number of screening tools have been developed to assess for intimate partner violence. Those with the highest levels of sensitivity and specificity are the Woman Abuse Screening Tool/Woman Abuse Screening Tool-Short Form (WAST/WAST-SF); the Hurt, Insult, Threaten, and Scream (HITS); the Slapped, Threatened, and Throw (STaT); Humiliation, Afraid, Rape, Kick (HARK); Modified Childhood Trauma Questionnaire-Short Form (CTQ-SF); and the Ongoing Abuse Screen/Ongoing Violence Assessment Tool (OAS/OVAT) (Kottenstette & Stulberg, 2013). The Abuse Assessment Screen (AAS) is a brief, easy-to-use validated tool that contains five simple questions along with a body map to provide visual reference for physical injury (Fig. 1-3). If the woman has disclosed IPV, the nurse must document that a risk assessment was completed.

❝What to say❞ — *Providing essential preexamination information to a sexual assault victim*

If a sexual assault victim contacts her health-care provider prior to undergoing a physical examination, it is essential that the nurse offer the following suggestions:

- Report immediately to the medical care facility.
- Do not bathe or change your clothes.
- Do not rinse out your mouth.
- Do not douche, urinate, or defecate.
- Do not clean your fingernails.
- Do not smoke, eat, or drink.

⬡ **Where Research and Practice Meet:** Adolescent Women and IPV Reporting

Hanson (2010) analyzed data from the 2001 Youth Risk Behavior Survey to determine the similarities and differences between adolescent women reporting IPV and/or forced sexual intercourse (FSI) and those not reporting those experiences on a series of health-enhancing and health-compromising behaviors. Of the 1,608 female high school students included, 450 reported no IPV or FSI, 457 reported IPV, 473 reported FSI, and 228 reported experiencing IPV and FSI. The groups of adolescent women experiencing IPV and FSI were more likely to participate in health-compromising behaviors (e.g., alcohol, drug, and tobacco use; risky sexual and violence-related behaviors; physical inactivity) and less likely to participate in health-enhancing behaviors such as annual health and dental visits, responsible sexual behaviors, sun protection, and physical activity and sports participation. Nurses who care for adolescent women should create trusting environments conducive to disclosure of health-compromising behaviors, IPV and FSI, routinely screen for IPV/FSI, and educate students about IPV and its associated health consequences (Hanson, 2010).

DOCUMENTING IPV

Accurate documentation is essential, as it provides a record of the abuse, facilitates communication among the various professionals who are dealing with the case, and provides a record of previous episodes of abuse. Because documentation provides evidence of abuse escalation, it can be beneficial in helping the patient to recognize and acknowledge the abuse (Ward & Wood, 2009).

⬡ **legal alert**— Obtain patient consent before IPV information disclosure

Nurses are aware that careful documentation of IPV-related information is essential in supporting the victim's assertions and charges. Proper documentation enables the woman to obtain protection and assistance, which may range from obtaining a restraining order to receiving victim compensation. However, nurses must remember that disclosure of confidential information may take place only with the explicit consent of the patient (ACOG, 2014; Ward & Woods, 2009).

In addition to obtaining the past health history, social history, and sexual history, the nurse documents subjective data related to the current IPV incident. Information recorded includes a description of the incident in the patient's own words. If the victim names the abuser, the name should be documented as well. All subjective information provided by the patient is recorded in quotation marks to indicate that the statements represent exactly what the patient said. It is important to record the time that the patient reports that the incident occurred, as well as the time that the patient's descriptive statements were made. The nurse also notes the date and location of the incident (Futures Without Violence, 2013; Ward & Wood, 2009).

The patient's general appearance and demeanor are recorded, and additional subjective information, such as reported threats and psychological abuse perpetrated by the abuser, is documented as well. Findings from the physical examination are carefully documented. It is important to remember that *rape* and *sexual assault* are legal terms that should not be used in medical records. Body maps are useful in accurately pinpointing the areas of injury, including the location, size, and age. Once the patient's signed consent has been obtained, photographs may be taken. Photographs provide an excellent visual record of the injuries. Additional information including the results of laboratory and diagnostic tests, radiography, and all referrals (e.g., other health-care professionals, local shelters) are recorded on the patient's health record (ACOG, 2014; Ward & Wood, 2009).

1) Have you ever been emotionally or physically abused by your partner or someone important to you?

Yes ☐   No ☐

If yes by whom? _____

Total number of times _____

2) Within the last year, have you been hit, slapped, kicked or otherwise physically hurt by someone?

Yes ☐   No ☐

If yes by whom? _____

Total number of times _____

3) Since you've been pregnant, have you been hit, slapped, kicked, or otherwise physically hurt by someone?

Yes ☐   No ☐

If yes by whom? _____

Total number of times _____

4) Within the last year, has anyone forced you to have sexual activities?

Yes ☐   No ☐

If yes by whom? _____

Total number of times _____

5) Are you afraid of your partner or anyone you listed above?

Yes ☐   No ☐

MARK THE AREA OF INJURY ON A BODY MAP AND SCORE EACH INCIDENT ACCORDING TO THE FOLLOWING SCALE.

If any of the descriptions for the higher number apply, use the higher number.

1 = Threats of abuse including use of a weapon

2 = Slapping, pushing; no injuries and/or lasting pain

3 = Punching, kicking, bruises, cuts, and/or continuing pain

4 = Beating up, severe contusions, burns, broken bones

5 = Head injury, internal injury, permanent injury

6 = Use of weapon; wound from weapon

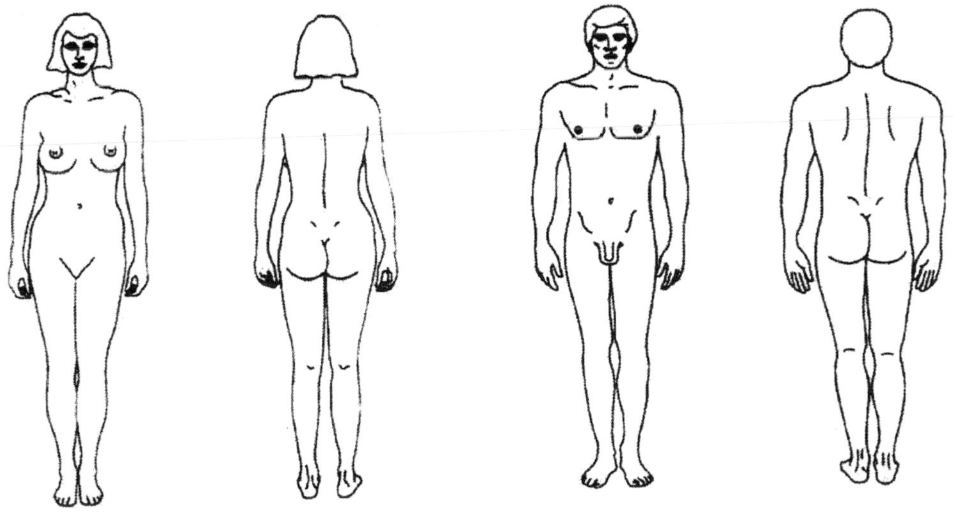

Figure 1-3 Abuse Assessment Screen. (Produced by Futures Without Violence [formerly the Family Violence Prevention Fund], 383 Rhode Island St., Ste. 304, San Francisco, CA, 94103-5133, [415] 252-8900, TTY: [800] 595-4889, www.endabuse.org.)

The CDC (2010) recommends testing for *Chlamydia trachomatis* and gonorrhea, along with a wet mount to assess for bacterial vaginosis, trichomoniasis, and candidiasis, especially if the patient has symptoms. Hepatitis B vaccination should be initiated if the woman hasn't been vaccinated previously; the repeat hepatitis B vaccination should be given at 1 to 2 months and 4 to 6 months after the assault. There are no recommendations either for or against HIV postexposure prophylaxis. Emergency contraception should be provided as needed. Laws in all 50 states and the District of Columbia strictly limit the evidentiary use of a survivor's previous sexual history, including evidence of previously acquired STDs, as part of an effort to undermine the credibility of the survivor's testimony, and evidentiary privilege against revealing any aspect of the examination or treatment also is enforced in most states (ACOG, 2014; CDC, 2010).

Optimizing Outcomes— With photographs of the injuries

A minimum of three photographs should be taken of each injury: a full-body photograph of the victim to establish identity, an injury photo taken a medium distance from the body, and a close-up photo of each individual injury. All photographs are clearly labeled with the patient's name, date, time that they were taken, and the photographer's name. Ideally, a blue background, which shows the depth and defines the clarity of an injury, is used. Additional photographs can be taken at the follow-up visit (2 to 4 days) to provide additional documentation of the progression of the injuries (Constantino, Crane, & Young, 2012; Hammer, Moynihan, & Pagliaro, 2011; Ward & Wood, 2009).

REPORTING IPV

It is important for nurses to be knowledgeable about IPV reporting guidelines for their particular practice state. Proponents of mandatory IPV reporting describe the following benefits associated with mandatory IPV reporting:

- Facilitates the prosecution of perpetrators
- Helps to identify victims; promotes interventions
- Improves data collection (Thomas, 2009; Ward & Wood, 2009)

legal alert— Be knowledgeable of state laws regarding reporting of IPV

Nurses must be familiar with laws on the mandatory reporting of IPV; requirements vary from state to state. Certain states mandate that injuries resulting from criminal conduct (which encompasses IPV) be reported. Also, some states require medical personnel to report specific types of injuries (i.e., burns, firearms, stab or knife wounds, and injuries resulting from a deadly weapon) to law enforcement, no matter the statement of the victim. Forty-four states require the reporting of any wounds caused by firearms; 25 states mandate that nonaccidental or stab wounds caused by a sharp pointed object or a knife be reported; and the District of Columbia, Michigan, Minnesota, New York, and Utah have laws directing that any injuries caused by a weapon be reported to law enforcement personnel. All 50 states and the District of Columbia have laws in effect authorizing the provision of adult protective services in cases of elder abuse or the abuse of individuals with disabilities. A synopsis of current state statutes and reporting guidelines is available at http://www.aaos.org/about/abuse/ststatut.asp. AWHONN supports health-care professionals reporting IPV with the informed consent of the abused woman. However, the organization recognizes that health-care providers must abide by state law (ACOG, 2012; AWHONN, 2007).

However, it must be pointed out that mandatory reporting violates the framework on which the ethical codes of nursing are based. The ANA Code of Ethics for Nurses, provision 3, states, "The nurse promotes, advocates for, and strives to protect the health, safety, and rights of the patient" (ANA, 2005). Mandatory reporting of IPV may place victims in danger and violates the victim's right to make personal choices. Furthermore, mandatory reporting laws place the responsibility of the victim's safety on health-care professionals, who, in turn, must rely on law enforcement and the courts to provide safety for the victim. This process may not necessarily be a desirable alternative, considering that in many situations the abuser is incarcerated for only a brief period of time (Smith, Rainey, Smith, Alamares, & Grogg, 2008; Ward & Wood, 2009).

Collaboration in Caring— *The sexual assault nurse examiner*

A sexual assault nurse examiner (SANE) is a registered nurse who has received specialized training in providing medical-forensic examinations for victims of sexual assault. The mission of the SANE program is to "meet the needs of the sexual assault victim by providing immediate, compassionate, culturally sensitive, and comprehensive evaluation and treatment by trained, professional nurse experts within the parameters of the individual's State Nurse Practice Act, the SANE standards of the International Association of Forensic Nurses, and the individual agency policies" (Ledray, n.d., p. 8). In most situations, SANE programs provide 24/7 nursing care to sexual assault survivors in emergency departments and clinics throughout the country. The sexual assault evidence collection kits (rape kits) are more thoroughly completed by SANE than by non-SANE clinicians, and it is important for women to understand that according to federal law, they cannot be required to pay out of pocket for a forensic sexual assault exam. Also, when a victim has an exam completed by a SANE, she is not required to file charges or even speak with anyone in law enforcement. If she wishes, she may have the evidence collected in the event she decides to press charges at a later date, although there is a time limit that varies according to individual state law (Wadsworth & Van Order, 2012).

Now Can You— Discuss IPV screening, documenting, and reporting?

1. Explain the nurse's role in conducting screening for IPV?
2. Describe how to document IPV and identify when the patient's informed consent must be obtained?
3. Identify the IPV reporting requirements of your practice state?

Nursing Interventions

EDUCATION AND COUNSELING

Education and counseling constitute an essential nursing role in IPV care. The nurse should inquire about violence and family conflict, listen to the woman's story, and provide information and referrals. Nurses should reassure their patients that they will provide help regardless of whether they choose to remain in the relationship. Nurses must assist victims of violence by informing them of available options and by providing support in making decisions. Allowing the woman to break the cycle of abuse restores her power and enables her to regain control of her life (Davila et al., 2013; Ward & Wood, 2009). Nursing diagnoses may be related to physical injuries, emotional trauma, and the need for seeking help (Box 1-3). In addition, abused women may be

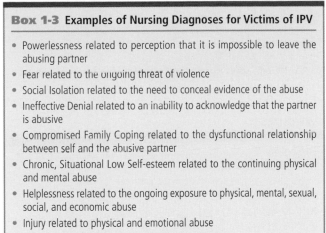

Box 1-3 Examples of Nursing Diagnoses for Victims of IPV

- Powerlessness related to perception that it is impossible to leave the abusing partner
- Fear related to the ongoing threat of violence
- Social Isolation related to the need to conceal evidence of the abuse
- Ineffective Denial related to an inability to acknowledge that the partner is abusive
- Compromised Family Coping related to the dysfunctional relationship between self and the abusive partner
- Chronic, Situational Low Self-esteem related to the continuing physical and mental abuse
- Helplessness related to the ongoing exposure to physical, mental, sexual, social, and economic abuse
- Injury related to physical and emotional abuse
- Knowledge Deficit related to the cycle of violence
- Knowledge Deficit related to available resources

formally diagnosed as having PTSD if their symptoms meet the explicit criteria outlined in the *Diagnostic and Statistical Manual of Mental Disorders* (5th ed.) (American Psychiatric Association, 2013).

Collaboration in Caring— *Safety cards to facilitate IPV screening and education*

Futures Without Violence (http://www.futureswithoutviolence.org/) has developed small, easy-to-conceal, wallet-sized safety cards in both English and Spanish that have been cobranded by the ACOG. The safety cards provide information about unhealthy relationships and include self-administered questions for IPV and reproductive and sexual coercion along with safety planning strategies and tips on obtaining help and other resources. Health-care providers can use the safety cards to facilitate IPV screening and education; use of the cards provides a brief, evidence-based intervention that can be reviewed with the patient in less than 1 minute (ACOG, 2013b; Miller et al., 2011).

Nurses can educate their patients about strategies to protect themselves from harm in their home environment. When physical abuse appears to be imminent, women should be taught to remove themselves from the kitchen where there are weapons such as knives that may be used to inflict harm. Victims should also be taught to stay out of bathrooms, closets, or small spaces in which the abuser can trap the victim. If possible, the woman should leave the home or go to a room with a door she can lock the abuser outside of or window from which she can escape. Women should be encouraged to call 911 in an emergency and go to their health-care provider or nearest emergency room for care when their injuries require medical attention. Victims may go to a local women's shelter or crisis center for housing and counseling. It has been estimated that 50% of all homeless women and children in the United States are fleeing IPV. They may also call the National Domestic Violence Hotline (1-800-799-SAFE [7233]) for additional information and assistance. Women should also be encouraged to learn self-defense skills through enrollment in a course, if possible, and to seek education from an IPV program (Futures Without Violence, 2013).

The woman may also be encouraged to prepare a packed bag with essential items that will be needed if she needs to make a hasty escape from her abuser. Hiding the bag in a handy, safe place or leaving it with a neighbor helps to ensure that the "ready escape bag" will be available if needed. Necessary items include certain documents that will be needed to establish stability, such as housing and financial assistance (Davila et al., 2013).

Optimizing Outcomes— **With a ready escape bag containing important items**

Nurses can teach IPV victims how to assemble a ready escape bag to facilitate a hasty departure from an unsafe home situation. The bag should contain money, an extra set of car keys, birth certificates, lists of medications and doses, medical records (for self and children), passports, court papers, Social Security card, car title, insurance card, and immigration papers (Davila et al., 2013; Ward & Wood, 2009).

It is important to ensure that the woman keep all information about her safety plan stored in a safe place away from her abuser. Danger to the victim is heightened if the abuser believes that the victim may leave or report the abuse to the police (Futures Without Violence, 2013).

If the abuser has moved out of the home, the woman should be advised to change the locks on the doors and secure locks for the windows. She may ask neighbors to call the police if they observe the abuser at the victim's house, and the victim and neighbor(s) may develop a system of signals to alert the neighbor when to call the police. The nurse should counsel the woman to obtain an unlisted phone number, block caller ID, and use an answering machine to screen phone calls. Rather than use a personal home computer, it may be wise to use a friend's or library computer, as the abuser may be able to monitor the woman's computer activities or have access to the e-mail addresses of the victim's family members and friends. The woman should also be encouraged to change her online passwords and create a new e-mail account to avoid the abuser's harassment (Davila et al., 2013). Additional safety strategies are listed in Box 1-4.

Box 1-4 Safety Strategies for Victims of IPV

Nurses can teach women to do the following:

- Remain aware of surroundings at all times.
- Identify trusted others who can check on your safety.
- Keep the car parked pointing out, the gas tank filled, and readily accessible extra keys.
- Create and rehearse a safety plan with the children and teach them how to dial 911.
- Shop and bank at different places, especially if being stalked.
- Use different routes for driving to work, or try to receive rides from different persons.
- Obtain a protection order.
- Refrain from lunching alone.
- Cancel all joint credit card and bank accounts.
- Ask for workplace escorts to the car or public transportation.
- Determine whether an immediate danger exists; if so, go to a preestablished safe place and call 911 (Davila et al., 2013).

Optimizing Outcomes— Using the ABCDES to provide sensitive care for the IPV victim

Nurses should remember the ABCDES of Caring (Campbell & Furniss, 2002) to provide appropriate, sensitive care for victims of IPV:

A—Reassuring the woman that she is not **alone**

B—Expressing the **belief** that violence directed against the woman is unacceptable and not her fault

C—**Confidentiality** of the shared information will be maintained (explain the mandatory reporting laws of the practice state, when applicable)

D—**Documentation**—descriptive documentation includes quoted statements, accurate descriptions of all injuries, and photographs (with the woman's written consent)

E—**Education** about the cycle of violence and community and national resources

S—**Safety**—always the most important component of the intervention, especially because one of the most dangerous times for the victim is the point at which she decides to leave her abuser

---

TREATMENT AND FOLLOW-UP

In the clinic, office, or hospital setting, nurses should carefully document all injuries in great detail and use body maps to enhance clarification. For example, terms such as *strangulation* should be used in place of *choked*. By definition, strangulation is an assault with malicious intent that causes harm to the victim, while choking occurs when a foreign object has been lodged in the patient's trachea or esophagus. Treatment interventions and discharge information must be clearly noted on the chart, along with a description of all referrals and follow-up options that were provided to the patient. Nurses can offer immediate contact with an IPV counselor either in person or by phone, and referral to a mental health provider may also be appropriate (Ward & Wood, 2009).

Nurses must ensure that an adequate referral system is in place for victims of IPV. A number of resources are available to assist nurses in providing appropriate, sensitive care in a timely manner and to take action against IPV perpetrators (Box 1-5). Establishing a professional relationship with the local domestic violence center empowers the nurse with a variety of resources to better help the victim of abuse (Ward & Wood, 2009).

IPV centers offer services that frequently include a 24-hour hotline, advocacy with community systems, and temporary shelter for victims who cannot return home because of safety concerns for themselves and their children. Advocacy with community systems includes referral for services such as legal aid, housing, mental health, substance abuse, and dental referral resources. In most situations, IPV centers also assist victims in accessing local and state government programs (Ward & Wood, 2009).

Nurses who deal with victims of IPV should also be familiar with the local sexual assault center. Women who have been sexually assaulted can benefit from the specialized services (e.g., individualized counseling, support groups) provided by these centers. Nurses can also advocate for IPV awareness and assistance by placing information about local resources in various public and private

---

Box 1-5   Additional IPV Resources

HOTLINES
- National Domestic Violence Hotline
  1-800-799-SAFE (7233)
- Rape Abuse & Incest National Network (RAINN)
  1-800-656-HOPE (4673)

WEB SITES
- Futures Without Violence (formerly known as Family Violence Prevention Fund)
  www.futureswithoutviolence.org
- National Coalition Against Domestic Violence
  www.ncadv.org
- National Network to End Domestic Violence
  www.nnedv.org
- National Resource Center on Domestic Violence
  www.nrcdv.org
- Office on Violence Against Women
  www.usdoj.gov/ovw

---

locations throughout the clinic or office (e.g., waiting area, restroom, examination room) where patients can have ready access to them. Many clinics distribute business-size IPV cards that contain essential information such as strategies for self-protection and protection of children and the National Domestic Violence Hotline phone number. The business-size card is particularly useful as it can be easily concealed (Ward & Wood, 2009).

Nurses must also recognize the victim's need for legal information. For those with access to a computer, the Web site WomensLaw.org (http://www.womenslaw.org) contains an abundance of easy-to-understand information for women living with or escaping IPV. The Web site offers suggestions for obtaining restraining orders, court forms, and other legal documents, and provides locations for various law enforcement offices. Women who have no access to a computer may receive assistance by dialing the toll-free phone number for the National Domestic Violence Hotline (1-800-799-SAFE [7233]).

Excellent IPV resources are available for nurses and other health-care professionals. The Minnesota Center Against Violence and Abuse (http://www.mincava.umn.edu) offers educational resources for training on violence of any type, including IPV, teen violence, and dating violence.

Optimizing Outcomes— With an IPV tool designed especially for health-care professionals

"A Medical Provider's Guide to Managing the Care of Domestic Violence Patients Within a Cultural Context" is a training and reference guide specifically developed for health-care professionals. The tool is designed to help reduce cultural, linguistic, and systemic barriers that keep IPV victims, particularly immigrant women and women of color, from reporting abuse to their care providers. The guide is available at http://www.nyc.gov/html/ocdv/downloads/pdf/providers_dv_guide.pdf

---

Once a patient leaves the health-care setting, a lack of personal contact does not mean that interventions cannot occur. McFarland and colleagues (2004) used telephone interviews to conduct a longitudinal study on abused women. After an initial personal contact with abused women to ask about inclusion in the study and to obtain informed consent, researchers contacted the women with either six intervention and four follow-up calls (experimental group) or four follow-up calls only (control group). During the phone calls, the interviewers asked women in the experimental group to answer yes or no to a series of safety-promoting behaviors. These behaviors included such actions as hiding money; hiding house and car keys; removing weapons from the house; asking neighbors to call police if violence begins; establishing a code with family and friends; and obtaining items such as birth certificates, important phone numbers, identification cards, and rent and utility receipts. The research findings indicated that women in the intervention group (those who received six additional phone calls) practiced more safety-promoting behaviors than did those in the control group and that the required nursing time was minimal. Such research findings are significant in supporting the important role that nurses and other members of the health-care team can have in helping victims of domestic violence take control of their environments and practice positive behaviors that can break the cycle of abuse.

Now Can You— **Discuss the nurse's role when caring for victims of IPV?**

1. Formulate five nursing diagnoses that may be appropriate for victims of IPV?
2. Describe three ways that IPV victims can enhance personal safety at home and items that they should include in a "ready escape bag"?

? Global Health Case Study Selena G.

Intimate Partner Violence

Selina G. is a single 19-year-old Hispanic woman who is visiting the Family Planning Clinic for her annual exam. During the interview, she tells the nurse about an incident that occurred two nights ago when her estranged boyfriend forced his way into her home and demanded that she have sex with him. She acquiesced because she knew that he had been drinking and was afraid he would hurt her if she refused. Selena has been trying to break off the relationship because her ex-boyfriend is controlling and abusive, but she is afraid to go to the police for fear of retaliation.

critical thinking questions

1. How should the nurse respond?
2. What other resources may the nurse provide?

Summary Points

- *Intimate partner violence* (IPV) is defined as physical, sexual, or psychological harm or social isolation perpetrated by a current or former partner in an intimate or dating relationship.
- The abuser's actions are intended to instill fear and to intimidate and control the victim.

- Intimate partner violence reaches across all strata of society and affects persons regardless of economic status, ethnic background, educational level, or religious status.
- Women who are abused are more likely to be unemployed, suffer from health problems, and receive public assistance than are women who are not victims of abuse.
- Routine screening can facilitate early identification of IPV when signs and symptoms may not be readily apparent.
- Accurate documentation of abuse is essential, and nurses must be knowledgeable about IPV reporting guidelines for their particular practice state.
- Nurses must assist victims of violence by informing them of available options and by providing support in making decisions.

Review Questions

Multiple Choice

1. Nurses should be alert to signs of IPV, which may include
   A. Overuse of health services
   B. Injuries consistent with the patient's explanation as to cause
   C. Consistency in keeping health-care appointments
   D. Reporting specific, descriptive complaints

2. Potential barriers to routine IPV screening in the clinical setting may include
   A. Having an awareness of IPV
   B. Sharing the patient's language and cultural values
   C. Understanding how to inquire about abuse
   D. Having a personal history of abuse

3. When physical abuse is imminent, a home safety strategy that the nurse can teach the patient is to
   A. Hide in the bathroom
   B. Seek shelter in a closet
   C. Remove herself from the kitchen
   D. Confront the abuser in an assertive way

4. The nurse can encourage the woman to develop a plan to facilitate safety from the abuser. A safety strategy is to
   A. Pack a ready escape bag containing essential items
   B. Leave a "good-bye" note for the abuser
   C. Maintain usual habits for banking and shopping
   D. Keep computer e-mail accounts and online passwords as originally set up

5. IPV is an abusive relationship characterized by the abuser's desire to have
   A. The victim's sympathy
   B. Power and control in the relationship
   C. A sense of intimacy
   D. Financial security

REFERENCES

Advocates To End Domestic Violence. (2014). *Domestic violence facts.* Retrieved from http://www.aedv.org/index.php/domestic-violence-facts

Alpert, E.J. (2010). *Intimate partner violence: The clinician's guide to identification, assessment, intervention, and prevention* (5th ed.). Waltham, MA: Massachusetts Medical Society.

American Bar Association. (2008). *Survey of recent statistics.* Commission on Domestic & Sexual Violence. Retrieved from http://www.americanbar.org/groups/domestic_violence/resources/statistics.html

American College of Obstetricians and Gynecologists (ACOG). (2011). Adult manifestations of childhood sexual abuse. Committee Opinion No. 498. *Obstetrics & Gynecology, 118*(2), 392–395.

American College of Obstetricians and Gynecologists (ACOG). (2012). Intimate partner violence. Committee Opinion No. 518. *Obstetrics & Gynecology, 119*(2), 412–417.

American College of Obstetricians and Gynecologists (ACOG). (2013a). Elder abuse and women's health. Committee Opinion No. 568. *Obstetrics & Gynecology, 122*(1), 187–191.

American College of Obstetricians and Gynecologists (ACOG). (2013b). Reproductive and sexual coercion. Committee Opinion No. 554. *Obstetrics & Gynecology, 121*(2), 411–415.

American College of Obstetricians and Gynecologists (ACOG). (2014). Sexual assault. Committee Opinion No. 592. *Obstetrics & Gynecology, 123*(4), 905–908.

American Nurses Association (ANA). (2000). *Violence against women* (Position statement). Retrieved from http://www.nursingworld.org/MainMenu Categories/Policy-Advocacy/Positions-and-Resolutions/ANAPositionStatements/Position-Statements-Alphabetically/Violence-Against-Women.html

American Nurses Association (ANA). (2005). *Code of ethics for nurses with interpretive statements.* Retrieved from http://www.nursingworld.org /MainMenuCategories/EthicsStandards/CodeofEthicsforNurses/Code-of-Ethics.pdf

American Psychiatric Association. (2013). *Diagnostic and statistical manual of mental disorders* (5th ed.). Washington, DC: American Psychiatric Publishing.

Americans Overseas Domestic Violence Crisis Center. (2014). *Types of abuse.* Retrieved from http://www.866uswomen.org/Types-of-Abuse .aspx

Arosarena, O.A., Fritsch, T.A., Hsueh, Y., Aynehchi, B., & Haug, R. (2009). Maxillofacial injuries and violence against women. *Archives of Facial Plastic Surgery, 11*(1), 48–52.

Association of Women's Health, Obstetric and Neonatal Nurses (AWHONN). (2007). *Mandatory reporting of intimate partner violence* (Position paper). Washington, DC: Author. Retrieved from https:// www.awhonn.org/awhonn/content.do?name=07_PressRoom/07_ PositionStatements.htm

Black, M.C., Basile, K.C., Breiding, M.J., Smith, S.G., Walters, M.L., Merrick, M.T., . . . Stevens, M.R. (2011). *The National Intimate Partner and Sexual Violence Survey (NISVS): 2010 summary report.* Atlanta, GA: National Center for Injury Prevention and Control, Centers for Disease Control and Prevention.

Blereau, R.P. (2009). Woman with multiple head and neck injuries. *Consultant, 49*(9), 565–568.

Breiding, M.J., Chen, J., & Black, M.C. (2014). *Intimate partner violence in the United States – 2010.* Atlanta, GA: National Center for Injury Prevention and Control, Centers for Disease Control and Prevention.

Brown, J., Lent, B., Schmidt, G., & Sas, G. (2000). Application of the Women Abuse Screening Tool (WAST) and WAST-Short in the family practice setting. *Journal of Family Practice, 49*(10), 896–903.

Bulechek, G.M., Butcher, H.K., & Dochterman, J.M. (2013). *Nursing interventions classification (NIC)* (6th ed.). St. Louis, MO: Elsevier Mosby.

Bull, A. (2009). Screening for intimate partner violence: Offering the tissue box. *Journal for Nurse Practitioners, 5*(8), 620–621.

Bureau of Justice Statistics. (2013). Over 60 percent decline in sexual violence against females from 1995 to 2010. Retrieved from http://www.bjs.gov/content/pub/press/fvsv9410pr.cfm

Campbell, J. (1986). Nursing assessment for risk of homicide with battered women. *Advances in Nursing Science, 8*(4), 36–51.

Campbell, J., & Furniss, K. (2002). *Violence against women: Identification, screening, and management of intimate partner violence.* Washington, DC: Association of Women's Health, Obstetric and Neonatal Nurses.

Catalano, S.M. (2007). *Intimate partner violence in the United States.* U.S. Department of Justice, Bureau of Justice Statistics. Retrieved from http://bjs.ojp.usdoj.gov/index.cfm?ty=pbdetail&iid=1000

Catalano, S.M., Smith, E., Snyder, H., & Rand, M. (2009). *Female victims of violence.* U.S. Department of Justice, Bureau of Justice Statistics. Retrieved from http://bjs.ojp.usdoj.gov/content/pub/pdf/fvv.pdf

Centers for Disease Control and Prevention (CDC). (2010). *Sexual assault and STDs: 2010.* Retrieved from http://www.cdc.gov/std/treatment /2010/sexual-assault.htms

Centers for Disease Control and Prevention (CDC). (2012). *Understanding intimate partner violence: Fact sheet.* Retrieved from http://www.cdc .gov/violenceprevention/pdf/ipv_factsheet-a.pdf

Centers for Disease Control and Prevention (CDC). AU21> (2013). *Intimate partner violence: Risk and protective factors.* Retrieved from http://www.cdc.gov/violenceprevention/intimatepartnerviolence/riskp rotectivefactors.html

Centers for Disease Control and Prevention (CDC), National Center for Injury Prevention and Control. (2003). *Costs of intimate partner violence against women in the United States.* Retrieved from http://www .cdc.gov/violenceprevention/pub/IPV_cost.html

Chang, J.C., Decker, M., Moracco, K.E., Martin, S.L., Petersen, R., & Frasier, P.Y. (2003). What happens when health care providers ask about intimate partner violence? A description of consequences from the perspectives of female survivors. *Journal of the American Medical Women's Association, 58*(2), 76–81.

Constantino, R., Crane, P., & Young, S. (2012). *Forensic nursing: Evidence-based principles and practice.* Philadelphia, PA: F.A. Davis.

Davila, Y.R., Mendias, E.P., & Juneau, C. (2013). Under the RADAR: Assessing and intervening for intimate partner violence. *The Journal for Nurse Practitioners—JNP, 9*(9), 594–599. doi:org/10.1016/j.nurpra .2013.05.022

Federal Bureau of Investigation (FBI). (2013). Summary reporting system (SRS) user manual version. Criminal Justice Information Services (CJIS) Division, Uniform Crime Reporting (UCR) Program. Washington, DC: Author. Retrieved from http://www.fbi.gov/about-us/cjis/ucr/nibrs /summary-reporting-system-srs-user-manual

Futures Without Violence. (2013). *Facts and information on domestic violence.* Retrieved from http://www.futureswithoutviolence.org/

Gerber, M.R., Fried, L.E., Pineles, S.L., Shipherd, J.C., & Bernstein, C.A. (2012). Posttraumatic stress disorder and intimate partner violence in a women's headache center. *Women & Health, 52*(5), 454–471.

Hamby, S., Finkelhor, D., Turner, H., & Ormrod, R. (2011). *Children's exposure to intimate partner violence and other family violence* (Bulletin No. NCJ 232272). Atlanta, GA: U.S. Department of Justice, Office of Juvenile Justice and Delinquency Prevention.

Hammer, R., Moynihan, B., & Pagliaro, E. (2011). *Forensic nursing* (2nd ed.). Sudbury, MA: Jones & Bartlett Learning.

Hanson, M.J. (2010). Health behavior in adolescent women reporting and not reporting intimate partner violence. *Journal of Obstetric, Gynecologic & Neonatal Nursing, 39*(3), 263–276. doi:10.1111/j.1552-6909 .2010.01138.x

Institute of Medicine (IOM). (2011). *Clinical preventive services for women: Closing the gaps.* Consensus report. Retrieved from http://www.iom .edu/Reports/2011/Clinical-Preventive-Services-for-Women-Closing-the-Gaps.aspx

Kang, J.A., Gottlieb, A.S., Raker, C.A., Aneja, S.S., & Boardman, L.A. (2010). Interpersonal violence screening for ambulatory gynecology patients. *Obstetrics & Gynecology, 115*(6), 1159–1166.

Kearney, M. (2001). Enduring love: A formal theory of women's experience of domestic violence. *Research in Nursing and Health, 24*(3), 270–282.

Kottenstette, J.B., & Stulberg, D. (2013). Time to screen routinely for intimate partner violence? *Clinician Reviews, 23*(3), 15–17.

Langton, L., Berzofsky, M., Krebs, C., & Smiley-McDonald, H. (2012). U.S. Department of Justice. National Crime Victimization Survey. *Victimizations not reported to the police,* Retrieved from http://www.bjs .gov/content/pub/pdf/vnrp0610.pdf

Laughon, K., Sutherland, M.A., & Parker, B.J. (2011). A brief intervention for prevention of sexually transmitted infections among battered women. *Journal of Obstetric, Gynecologic & Neonatal Nursing, 40*(6), 702-708. doi:10.1111/j.1552-6909.2011.01305.x

Ledray, L.E. (n.d.). Sexual assault nurse examiner SANE development and operation guide. Retrieved from http://www.ojp.usdoj.gov/ovc /publications/infores/sane/saneguide.pdf

McFarlane, J., Christoffel, K., Bateman, L., Miller, V., & Bullock, L. (1991). Assessing for abuse: Self-report versus nurse interview. *Public Health Nursing, 8*(4), 245–250.

McFarlane, J., Groff, J.Y., O'Brien, J.A., & Watson, K. (2006). Secondary prevention of intimate partner violence: A randomized controlled trial. *Nursing Research, 55,* 52–64. doi:00006199-2006010000-00007

McFarlane, J., Maddoux, J., Cesario, S., Koci, A., Liu, F., Gilroy, H., & Bianchi, A. (2014). Effect of abuse during pregnancy on maternal and child safety and functioning for 24 months after delivery. *Obstetrics & Gynecology, 123*(4), 839–847. doi:10.1097/AOG.0000000000000183

McFarland, J., Malecha, A., Gist, J., Watson, K., Batten, E., Hall, I., & Smith, S. (2004). Original research: Increasing the safety promoting behaviors of abused women. *American Journal of Nursing, 104*(3), 40–51.

Miller, E., Decker, M.R., McCauley, H.L., Tancredi, D.J., Levenson, R.R., Waldman, J., . . . Silverman, J.G. (2011). A family planning clinic partner violence intervention to reduce risk associated with reproductive coercion. *Contraception, 88*(3), 274–280. doi:10.1016/j.contraception .2010.07.013

Moore, V. (2013). Annual exams in women before age 21. *The Journal for Nurse Practitioners—JNP, 9*(9), 615–616. doi:org/10.1016/j.nurpra.2013.05.022

Moorhead, S., Johnson, M., Maas, M.L., & Swanson, E. (2013). *Nursing outcomes classification (NOC)* (5th ed.). St. Louis, MO: Elsevier Mosby.

Moyer, V.A. (2013). Screening for intimate partner violence and abuse of elderly and vulnerable adults: U.S. Preventive Services Task Force Recommendation Statement. *Annals of Internal Medicine, 158*(6), 478-486. doi: 10.7326/0003-4819-158-6-2013190-00588

Nelson, H.D., Bougatsos, C., & Blazina, I. (2012). *Screening women for intimate partner violence and elderly and vulnerable adults for abuse: Systematic review to update the 2004 U.S. Preventive Services Task Force Recommendation* (Evidence Syntheses, No. 92). Rockville, MD: Agency for Healthcare Research and Quality.

Parker, B., & McFarlane, J. (1991). Nursing assessment of the battered pregnant woman. *American Journal of Maternal Child Nursing, 16*(6), 161–164.

Peedicayil, A., Sadowski, L.S., Jeyaseelan, L., Shankar, V., Jain, D., Suresh, S., & Bangdiwala, S.I. (2004). Spousal physical violence against women during pregnancy. *British Journal of Obstetrics and Gynaecology, 111*(7), 682–687.

Peterlin, B.L., Rosso, A.L., & Merikangas, K.R. (2011). Post-traumatic stress disorder, drug abuse and migraine: New findings from the National Comorbidity Survey Replication (NCS-R). *Cephalagia, 31*(2), 235–244.

Records, K. (2011). Intimate partner violence. In S. Mattson & J. Smith (Eds.), *Core curriculum for maternal-child nursing* (4th ed., pp 417–431). Philadelphia, PA: W.B. Saunders.

Roller, C. (2011). Determining my sexual being: A framework for clinical practice with adult survivors of childhood sexual abuse. *Women's Health Care: A Practical Journal for Nurse Practitioners, 10*(5), 10–16.

Saddki, N., Suhaimi, A.A., & Daud, R. (2010). Maxillofacial injuries associated with intimate partner violence in women. *BMC Public Health, 10*, 269–272. doi:10.1186/1471-2458-10-268

Smith, J., Rainey, S., Smith, K., Alamares, C., & Grogg, D. (2008). Barriers to the mandatory reporting of domestic violence encountered by nursing professionals. *Journal of Trauma Nursing, 15*(1), 9–11.

Sommers, M.S. (2007). Defining patterns of genital injury from sexual assault. *Trauma, Violence, & Abuse, 8*(3), 270–280.

Sprague, S., Madden, K., Simunovic, N., Godin, K., Pham, N., Bhandari, M., & Goslings, J. (2012). Barriers to screening for intimate partner violence. *Women & Health, 52*(6), 587–605. doi:10.1080/03630242.2012.690840

Stringer, M. (2011). Healthy women lead to healthy cities. *Journal of Obstetric, Gynecologic & Neonatal Nursing, 40*(3), 667-668. doi:10.1111/j.1552-6909.2011.011301.x

Sutherland, M.A., Fantasia, H.C., Fontenot, H., & Harris, A.L. (2012). Safer sex and partner violence in a sample of women. *The Journal for Nurse Practitioners—JNP, 8*(9), 717–724. doi:10.1016/j.nurpra.2012.03.016

Thomas, I. (2009). Against the mandatory reporting of intimate partner violence. *Virtual Mentor, 11*(2), 137–140.

Tjaden, P., & Thoennes, N. (2000). *Full report of the prevalence, incidence, and consequences of violence against women: Findings from the National Violence Against Women Survey, 2000.* Retrieved from http://www.ncjrs.gov/pdffiles1/nij/183781.pdf

U.S. Department of Health and Human Services (USDHHS). (2012). *Screening women for intimate partner violence and elderly and vulnerable adults for abuse: Systematic review to update the 2004 U.S. Preventive Services Task Force Recommendation* (AHRQ Publication No. 12-05167-EF-1). Rockville, MD: Agency for Healthcare Research and Quality.

U.S. Department of Health and Human Services (USDHHS). (2011). *Healthy People 2020.* Retrieved from http://www.healthypeople.gov/2020/topicsobjectives2020/default.aspx

U.S. Preventive Services Task Force. (2004). Screening for family and intimate partner violence. *Annals of Internal Medicine, 140*(8), 382–386.

Volochinsky, B.P. (2012). Obtaining justice for victims of strangulation in domestic violence: Evidence-based prosecution and strangulation—specific training. *Student Pulse, 4*(10). Retrieved from http://www.studentpulse.com/a?id=706

Wadsworth, P., & Van Order, P. (2012). Care of the sexually assaulted woman. *The Journal for Nurse Practitioners—JNP, 8*(6), 433–440. doi:org/10.1016/j.nurpra.2011.10.007

Walker, L. (1979). *The battered woman.* New York, NY: Harper & Row.

Walker, L. (1984). *The battered woman syndrome* (Vol. 6). New York, NY: Springer.

Ward, C., & Wood, A. (2009). Intimate partner violence: NP role in assessment. *American Journal for Nurse Practitioners, 13*(10), 9–15.

World Health Organization. (2011). *Intimate partner violence during pregnancy.* Geneva, Switzerland: Author. Retrieved from http://whqlibdoc.who.int/hq/2011/WHO_RHR_11.35_eng.pdf?ua=1

World Health Organization. (2013). *Women's health.* Geneva, Switzerland: Author. Retrieved from http://who.int/topics/womens_health/en/

World Health Organization & United Nations Human Settlement Programme. (2010). *Hidden cities: Unmasking and overcoming health inequities in urban settings.* Geneva, Switzerland: Author. Retrieved from http://www.hiddencities.org/downloads/WHO_UN-HABITAT_Hidden_Cities_Web.pdf

Wu, V., Huff, H., & Bhandari, M. (2010). Pattern of physical injury associated with intimate partner violence in women presenting to the emergency department: A systematic review and meta-analysis. *Trauma, Violence, & Abuse, 11*(2), 71–82. doi:10.1177/1524838010367503

DavisPlus | For more information, go to **http://www.davisplus.fadavis.com/.**

CONCEPT MAP

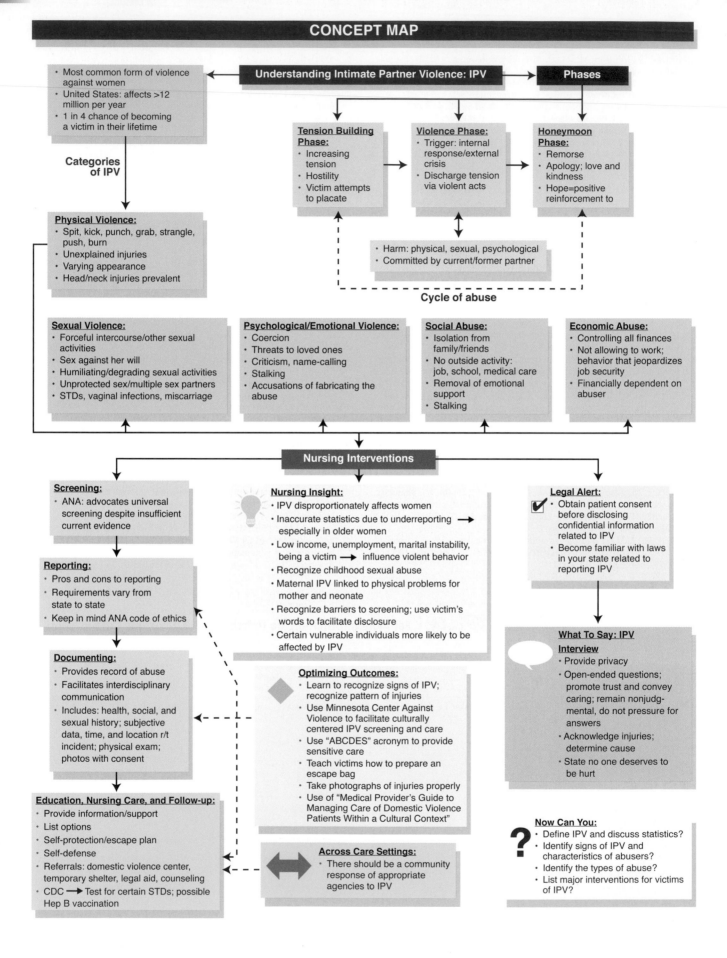

Understanding Intimate Partner Violence: IPV

- Most common form of violence against women
- United States: affects >12 million per year
- 1 in 4 chance of becoming a victim in their lifetime

Phases

Tension Building Phase:
- Increasing tension
- Hostility
- Victim attempts to placate

Violence Phase:
- Trigger: internal response/external crisis
- Discharge tension via violent acts

Honeymoon Phase:
- Remorse
- Apology; love and kindness
- Hope=positive reinforcement to

Categories of IPV

- Harm: physical, sexual, psychological
- Committed by current/former partner

Cycle of abuse

Physical Violence:
- Spit, kick, punch, grab, strangle, push, burn
- Unexplained injuries
- Varying appearance
- Head/neck injuries prevalent

Sexual Violence:
- Forceful intercourse/other sexual activities
- Sex against her will
- Humiliating/degrading sexual activities
- Unprotected sex/multiple sex partners
- STDs, vaginal infections, miscarriage

Psychological/Emotional Violence:
- Coercion
- Threats to loved ones
- Criticism, name-calling
- Stalking
- Accusations of fabricating the abuse

Social Abuse:
- Isolation from family/friends
- No outside activity: job, school, medical care
- Removal of emotional support
- Stalking

Economic Abuse:
- Controlling all finances
- Not allowing to work; behavior that jeopardizes job security
- Financially dependent on abuser

Nursing Interventions

Screening:
- ANA: advocates universal screening despite insufficient current evidence

Reporting:
- Pros and cons to reporting
- Requirements vary from state to state
- Keep in mind ANA code of ethics

Documenting:
- Provides record of abuse
- Facilitates interdisciplinary communication
- Includes: health, social, and sexual history; subjective data, time, and location r/t incident; physical exam; photos with consent

Education, Nursing Care, and Follow-up:
- Provide information/support
- List options
- Self-protection/escape plan
- Self-defense
- Referrals: domestic violence center, temporary shelter, legal aid, counseling
- CDC → Test for certain STDs; possible Hep B vaccination

Nursing Insight:
- IPV disproportionately affects women
- Inaccurate statistics due to underreporting especially in older women
- Low income, unemployment, marital instability, being a victim → influence violent behavior
- Recognize childhood sexual abuse
- Maternal IPV linked to physical problems for mother and neonate
- Recognize barriers to screening; use victim's words to facilitate disclosure
- Certain vulnerable individuals more likely to be affected by IPV

Optimizing Outcomes:
- Learn to recognize signs of IPV; recognize pattern of injuries
- Use Minnesota Center Against Violence to facilitate culturally centered IPV screening and care
- Use "ABCDES" acronym to provide sensitive care
- Teach victims how to prepare an escape bag
- Take photographs of injuries properly
- Use of "Medical Provider's Guide to Managing Care of Domestic Violence Patients Within a Cultural Context"

Across Care Settings:
- There should be a community response of appropriate agencies to IPV

Legal Alert:
- Obtain patient consent before disclosing confidential information related to IPV
- Become familiar with laws in your state related to reporting IPV

What To Say: IPV Interview
- Provide privacy
- Open-ended questions; promote trust and convey caring; remain nonjudgmental, do not pressure for answers
- Acknowledge injuries; determine cause
- State no one deserves to be hurt

Now Can You:
- Define IPV and discuss statistics?
- Identify signs of IPV and characteristics of abusers?
- Identify the types of abuse?
- List major interventions for victims of IPV?

Promoting Reproductive Health Through an Understanding of Premenstrual Syndrome

Live your life while you have it.
Life is a splendid gift—there is nothing small about it.

—Florence Nightingale

LEARNING TARGETS *At the completion of this chapter, the student will be able to:*

◆ Identify diagnostic criteria for premenstrual syndrome.

◆ Discuss the unique characteristics of symptoms that accompany premenstrual syndrome.

◆ Describe nonpharmacological and pharmacological approaches to care for women who experience premenstrual syndrome.

◆ Discuss the nurse's role when caring for a patient with a premenstrual disorder.

PICO(T) Questions

The intent of Evidence-Based Practice (EBP) is to provide nursing care that integrates the best available evidence. An initial step in EBP is to write a PICO(T) question that effectively guides the research. A PICOT question is an acronym that stands for population (P), intervention or issue (I), comparison of interest (C), outcome (O), and timeframe (T). Depending on the question, all or some of the question components are used in the research process.

Use these PICO(T) questions to spark your thinking as you read the chapter.

1. Do (P) women with Premenstrual Syndrome (PMS) report (I) affective symptoms as being (O) more troublesome (C) than physical symptoms?

2. What (I) nursing interventions do (P) women with premenstrual dysphoric disorder (PMDD) report as being (O) most helpful?

Evidence-Based Practice

Sassoon, S.A., Colrain, I.M., & Baker, F.C. (2011). Personality disorders in women with severe premenstrual syndrome. *Archives of Women's Mental Health, 14,* 257–264.

The purpose of this study was to examine the relationship between premenstrual syndrome (PMS) and personality disorders and traits as defined by the *Diagnostic and Statistical Manual of Mental Disorders* (4th ed.) (DSM-IV). The investigators hypothesized that women with PMS would have a higher incidence of personality disorder traits than women without PMS and that obsessive-compulsive and avoidant disorders would be the most common personality disorder traits identified.

Premenstrual syndrome and premenstrual dysphoric disorder (PMDD) affect 5% to 18% of childbearing-age women. Of these,

approximately 3% to 8% of women suffer from a lifetime of impairment with PMDD, the most severe form of PMS. PMS encompasses a variety of physical, behavioral, and affective symptoms. Components that differentiate PMS from PMDD include symptom severity and timing as well as the impact on the individual's level of functioning. Previous research has attempted to demonstrate a relationship between PMDD and personality disorders but findings have been inconsistent. Personality disorders or traits identified in women with PMS and PMDD include avoidant personality disorder, obsessive-compulsive disorder, borderline personality

(continued)

Evidence-Based Practice (continued)

disorder, hysterical personality types, and schizoid and schizotypal disorders.

For this study, participants were recruited through flyers, announcements, word of mouth, and physician referrals. One hundred eighty-seven (187) women participated in an initial phone interview. Of these, 129 reported severe PMS symptoms and 58 reported minimal or no PMS symptoms. The Premenstrual Symptoms Screening Tool (PSST) is a self-report tool used to assess severity and impairment on 11 separate PMDD symptoms, and results from the PSST were used to determine study inclusion. The following inclusion criteria were applied: regular menstrual cycles, regular sleep-wake schedules, good health, and no regular medications in the past 3 months. Exclusion criteria included a history of schizophrenia, eating disorders, bipolar disorder, substance use disorders, and/or a current Axis I psychopathology. A total of 33 women with severe PMS symptoms and 26 asymptomatic women were included in the study.

Data were gathered through the use of two reliable and valid standard interview forms: the Structured Clinical Interview for DSM-IV-TR Axis I Disorders, and the Structured Interview for DSM-IV Personality Disorders. In addition, the participants were questioned about premenstrual symptoms based on the DSM-IV-TR

Data Group	Severe PMS Symptoms Group	Asymptomatic Group
Mean age	30.6	28.9
Average years of education	16.3	16.3
Average body mass index	23.3	22.3
Average age of menarche	12.5	12.5
Average length of the menstrual cycle	29 days	28.2 days
Average length of menses	5 days	4.8 days
Prevalence of personality disorders	27%	0%

criteria for a diagnosis of PMDD. All participants assigned to the severe PMS symptom group met the criteria, which included the presence of at least five of 11 PMDD symptoms and included at least one symptom of depressed mood; anxiety/ tension; irritability or affective lability; and impairment in work, school, usual daily activities, or personal relationships. Participants also received a Daily Symptom Rating (SDR) diary to evaluate the severity and duration of their premenstrual symptoms throughout two menstrual cycles. This tool lists 17 common symptoms, which are rated on a five-point scale, where 0 = none and 4 = extreme. A diagnosis of severe PMS requires a score of 80 or more. A summary of the participant data groups is presented in the following table.

Data analysis revealed that women with severe PMS symptoms had a higher prevalence (27%) of personality disorders than did women classified as asymptomatic (0%). According to the investigators, this figure, nearly twice that of the general population prevalence (14.8%), demonstrates a significant relationship between psychological pathology and severe PMS. Those classified with a higher prevalence of personality disorders were more likely to have odd-eccentric, dramatic-erratic, and anxious-fearful personality disorder traits. Obsessive-compulsive personality disorder, the most common personality disorder identified, was noted in 18% ($n = 6$) of participants in the severe PMS symptoms group and in none in the asymptomatic group. Avoidant personality disorder was identified in 3% ($n = 2$) of the severe PMS symptom participants, but this finding was not significant. Twenty-three (23) of 33 severe PMS symptom participants completed the Daily Symptom Rating diary; of these, 14 met the criteria for PMDD and 9 met the criteria for severe PMS. All of the asymptomatic participants returned the diaries and reported no or only mild PMS symptoms.

The researchers concluded that personality disorder traits were more common in women with severe PMS. Although obsessive-compulsive personality disorders were more prevalent in women with severe PMS and associated with poorer life functioning, they were not necessarily associated with more severe PMS.

1. How is this information useful to clinical nursing practice?

2. Based on these findings, what are the implications for further research?

See Suggested Responses for Evidence-Based Practice on Davis*Plus*.

Introduction

This chapter explores premenstrual syndrome (PMS), a common women's health problem during the childbearing years. In the past, many in the medical profession viewed symptoms of PMS to be wholly attributable to the woman's emotional state and without any physiological basis. PMS-related research was infrequently conducted and consisted mostly of anecdotal experiences. As the women's movement grew in strength and the public's awareness about women's health issues increased, views began to shift. At the same time, a growing body of medical information began to identify various physiological imbalances and theories were proposed to explain the causes of PMS. Today, PMS is viewed as a complex interplay of genetic influences and various hormonal imbalances that can adversely affect a woman's physical, mental, and emotional health. Various nonpharmacological and pharmacological therapies have been shown to be effective in reducing PMS symptoms. Nurses have traditionally played an important role in promoting women's reproductive health. They can be instrumental in helping women to deal with premenstrual disorders by offering ongoing education and support. These interventions empower women to seek and embrace strategies to help them gain control over their lives and, ideally, to enjoy life more fully.

Scope of the Problem

Premenstrual disorders affect many women during the reproductive years. PMS is defined as the presence of emotional and physical symptoms and behavioral changes that occur during the second half, or luteal phase, of the menstrual cycle and cease at or within a few days after the onset of menses. The timing of the symptoms in relation to the menstrual cycle, rather than the symptoms themselves, constitutes the unique element in this disorder.

A & P review   Phases of the Uterine (Endometrial) Cycle

Following menstruation (the "menstrual phase"), follicle-stimulating hormone (FSH) stimulates the growth and development of the ovarian graafian follicle, which secretes estrogen. The first phase of the menstrual cycle is termed the *follicular* or *proliferative* phase; this phase lasts from the end of menses through ovulation (approximately days 7 to 14). When estrogen production reaches a peak, the pituitary

gland releases luteinizing hormone (LH), which triggers ovulation. The "luteal phase" of the ovarian cycle begins at ovulation and ends with the onset of menses. The corpus luteum produces some estrogen but mainly produces progesterone. Eighty percent of all the progesterone secreted during the entire menstrual cycle is secreted during the first 8 days after ovulation. In the absence of fertilization, the life span of the corpus luteum is 14 days. Thus, the luteal phase of the uterine cycle is 14 days in length. As the end of the luteal phase nears, low levels of FSH and LH cause degeneration of the corpus luteum, which is associated with declining levels of estrogen and progesterone. The decreased hormonal levels trigger degeneration of the endometrium and the onset of menses (the *menstrual phase*) (Fig. 2-1). ◆

Major Characteristics of PMS

The following three criteria constitute the major characteristics of PMS:

- The woman's symptoms occur in a cyclical pattern.
- The symptoms are not caused by any underlying physical or mental condition.
- The symptoms greatly disrupt one or more areas of the woman's life.

Since 1987, PMS has been recognized as a mental disorder. More than 150 symptoms, which can affect almost

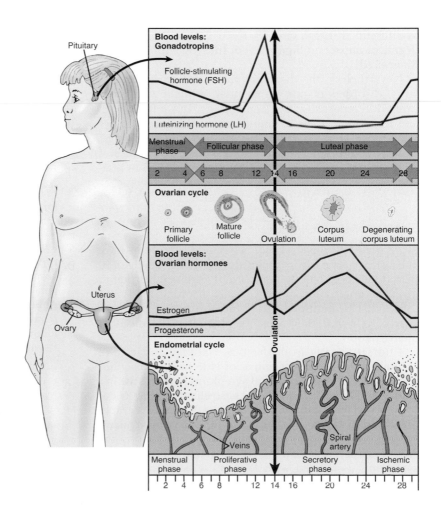

Figure 2-1 The female reproductive cycle. Levels of the hormones secreted from the anterior pituitary are shown relative to one another and throughout the cycle. Changes in the ovarian follicle are depicted. The relative thickness of the endometrium is also shown.

every organ system in various combinations and intensity, have been identified (American College of Obstetricians & Gynecologists [ACOG], 2000; American Psychiatric Association [APA], 2000; Association of Women's Health, Obstetrical and Neonatal Nurses, 2003).

🌸 Nursing Insight— *PMS and PMT*

Premenstrual syndrome is sometimes referred to as *premenstrual tension syndrome* (PMT). When first described in 1931, premenstrual tension centered on women's symptoms of tension, self-deprecation, and severe depression during the 7 to 10 days preceding menstruation. By the 1950s, the spectrum of reported symptoms had dramatically increased, and there was a growing realization that the previously described "tension" was just one aspect of the problem. A medical report published in 1953 introduced the term *premenstrual syndrome* to encompass the extensive list of symptoms, and this is the name most often used today.

Prevalence and Economic Impact

Sources vary in estimates of the number of women who experience symptoms of PMS. It has been estimated that more than 80% of childbearing-age women experience various emotional and physical changes during the premenstrual period. However, according to experts, most patients who self-diagnose do not actually have PMS. Of the women with premenstrual symptoms, approximately 20% to 40% regard the emotional and physical changes as difficult, although only 5% to 10% report a significant degree of impact on their work or lifestyle (ACOG, 2000; Raines, 2010).

Nevertheless, the disability associated with premenstrual disorders is quite substantial. Women who suffer from PMS reportedly have higher absenteeism from work and make more visits to ambulatory health-care facilities than those who do not experience PMS. On average, women with premenstrual disorders have an increase of $59 in direct annual health-care costs and $4,333 in indirect costs (Heinemann, Minh, Heinemann, Lindemann, & Filonenko, 2012; Whyte & Peraud, 2009).

SYMPTOMS OF PMS

More than 100 physical and behavioral symptoms have been experienced by women during the premenstrual period (see Box 2-1). It is important to remember that to meet the criteria for a premenstrual disorder, the symptoms must be confined to the luteal phase of the menstrual cycle and they must resolve after the onset of menstruation.

Clinical criteria from the U.S. National Institute of Mental Health for the diagnosis of PMS include a significant change in the intensity of symptoms between the follicular and late luteal phases. These changes must occur for at least two consecutive cycles (Whyte & Peraud, 2009). Other definitions, such as symptom intensity, have been developed for research purposes. According to the ACOG (2000), at least one of the affective and/or somatic symptoms associated with PMS must be present—and

---

Box 2-1   **Selected Premenstrual Symptoms Reported by Women**

LISTED IN ALPHABETICAL ORDER

• Anxiety	• Hostility
• Asthma	• Hot flashes
• Backache	• Increased appetite
• Bloating	• Insomnia
• Breast swelling	• Irritability
• Breast tenderness	• Joint pain
• Cold sweats	• Joint swelling
• Constipation	• Lack of coordination
• Cramps	• Migraine
• Depression	• Mood swings
• Diarrhea	• Nausea
• Dizziness	• Palpitations
• Easy bruising	• Shakiness
• Fainting	• Sore throat
• Fatigue	• Sugar cravings
• Hay fever	• Water retention
• Headaches	• Weight gain
• Hives	

---

appropriately timed with the menstrual cycle—to meet the diagnostic criteria. Fritz and Speroff (2010) proposed a simple, commonsense definition of PMS: "The cyclic appearance of one or more of a large constellation of symptoms just prior to menses, occurring to such a degree that lifestyle or work is affected, followed by a period of time entirely free of symptoms" (p. 289).

It has been noted that PMS symptoms commonly occur in clusters, with some women reporting as many as 10 symptoms at one time. Those who experience severe symptoms may be prone to extremes of behavior, with an increased likelihood of accidents, alcohol abuse, and suicide attempts. For others, PMS symptoms may be described as annoying but mild.

❝What to say❞ — *Nonpharmacological measures for menstrual migraines*

During the late luteal and early follicular phases of the menstrual cycle, estrogen levels sharply decline, triggering the onset of menses. In susceptible women, the decrease in estrogen is probably related to the increase in migraine headaches that often occurs premenstrually. Although pharmacological interventions are usually required to treat migraine, the nurse can offer the following suggestions that may serve as adjunct therapy (Dixon & Bergstrom, 2011):

- For nonpain symptoms, try ice, heat, and peppermint oil (for nausea and vomiting).

- Certain lifestyle changes may alleviate or prevent migraine headaches. Be sure to get sufficient sleep and exercise and drink plenty of water. Avoid caffeine, chocolate, and alcohol, and keep a diary of possible "triggers" for your headaches.

⊘ Now Can You— Discuss certain broad aspects of PMS?

1. Explain why the timing of symptoms is an essential component of premenstrual syndrome?
2. Identify three major characteristics of PMS?
3. Identify at least 20 symptoms that may be associated with PMS?

Premenstrual Dysphoric Disorder (PMDD)

Premenstrual dysphoric disorder (PMDD) is a diagnostic term for the most severe form of PMS. It is estimated that nearly 5 million American women have PMDD. PMDD pertains to women with PMS who suffer from more severe and disabling emotional symptoms. PMS and PMDD may be viewed as a spectrum of premenstrual disorders that begins with mild emotional and/or physical symptoms that are cyclical but not debilitating and proceeds through PMS to PMDD. Women with PMDD most frequently report the following symptoms: abdominal bloating, anxiety, tension, breast tenderness, crying episodes, depression, fatigue and a lack of energy, irritability, difficulty concentrating, appetite changes, thirst, and swelling of the extremities (Fritz & Speroff, 2010; Kelderhouse & Taylor, 2013; van den Akker, 2012).

⊛ **Collaboration in Caring**— *Facilitating appropriate referrals*

When evaluating a patient with PMS/PMDD symptoms, the nurse must always take any report of suicidal thoughts or other indicators of extreme mood change most seriously. The woman will need appropriate medications, close follow-up, and referral to a qualified mental health professional. In the ideal situation, mental examinations are timed to occur during both the luteal and follicular phases of the menstrual cycle. If the patient experiences significant mood symptoms (e.g., suicidal ideation) during both the luteal and follicular phases, referral to a psychiatrist is indicated. Once she is stable, various interventions such as lifestyle changes, dietary alterations, and conventional and complementary care approaches can be initiated that will become an important part of her long-term health promotion and maintenance (Whyte & Peraud, 2009).

Women who seek care for symptoms associated with premenstrual disorders should be given a complete physical examination and thorough clinical evaluation to rule out illness that may be the source of the symptoms. A detailed health history is the cornerstone in the accurate diagnosis of PMS/PMDD. Nurses should inquire about risk factors such as emotional stress, poor nutritional habits, side effects noted when taking combined hormonal contraceptives (if indicated), increased intake of alcohol, salt, and caffeine, tobacco use (women who smoke cigarettes are more than twice as likely to have more severe symptoms), personal history of depression, preeclampsia, or eclampsia, and family history of PMS (Raines, 2010).

When taking the menstrual history, it is crucial that careful attention be paid to the cyclical timing of symptoms. For most women with PMS, symptoms develop from 2 to 12 days prior to menstruation and resolve within 24 hours following the onset of menses. Women who have symptoms that primarily occur during the menstrual flow or during the first 2 weeks of the menstrual cycle do not have PMS as defined in the literature (Fritz & Speroff, 2010; Whyte & Peraud, 2009).

⊛ *Nursing Insight*— *Identifying populations most likely to experience PMS*

Although all age groups are affected, women in their late 20s to late 40s most frequently report symptoms of premenstrual disorders; symptoms often worsen as the woman approaches the menopausal transition. Also, women with a body mass index of 30 or above, those who have at least one child, those with a personal or family history of major depression, and those with a history of postpartum depression or an affective mood disorder are most often affected. It is important to note that premenstrual disorders:

* Occur only in ovulatory women
* Occur only during the luteal phase of the menstrual cycle
* Resolve within 4 days following the onset of menses

The occurrence of premenstrual disorders is not dependent on the presence of monthly menses. Interestingly, women who have had a hysterectomy without bilateral salpingo-oophorectomy (removal of both ovaries) can still have cyclical PMS symptoms (Nelson & Baldwin, 2011).

Causes of Premenstrual Disorders

Clinical research has not yet determined the exact cause of premenstrual disorders. Variations in the cyclical fluctuation of estrogen and progesterone may well account for symptoms in certain individuals. However, the cause is believed to be multifactorial—that is, a genetic predisposition and multiple biological, psychosocial, and sociocultural factors most likely play a role in the development of premenstrual disorders (Nelson & Baldwin, 2011; Taylor, Schuiling, & Sharp, 2011).

Although it was once believed that low levels of progesterone were the primary cause of PMS, research has failed to find a significant difference between PMS sufferers and non-PMS sufferers in levels of various hormones, including progesterone, estradiol, FSH, LH, prolactin, sex hormone-binding globulin (SHBG), and testosterone. It has been proposed, however, that women with PMS may have a greater biological vulnerability to the normal fluctuations in hormone levels than do women without PMS. There appears to be a genetic component to the development of PMS. Women who have a genetic predisposition to the development of PMS are believed to have a heightened sensitivity to various cyclical hormonal changes or a varied response to naturally occurring neurotransmitters (e.g., serotonin). Interestingly, a genetic predisposition to PMS is also known to be associated with a predisposition to other psychiatric disorders

(Biggs & Demuth, 2011; Gingnell, Comasco, Oreland, Fredrikson, & Sundstrom-Poromaa, 2010; Nelson & Baldwin, 2011).

It has been demonstrated that levels of the gonadal steroids (i.e., androgens, estrogens, progestogens) are the same in patients with and without PMS. However, the responses to fluctuating levels of the hormones are different in women with PMS. Another area of research has explored the role of the neurotransmitters serotonin and gamma-aminobutyric acid (GABA) in the etiology of premenstrual disorders. It has been suggested that a dysregulation in serotonin in particular is linked to many of the psychological symptoms in PMS, such as tension, irritability, and dysphoria (an emotional state characterized by anxiety, depression, or unease) (Gingnell et al., 2010; Nelson & Baldwin, 2011).

Optimizing Outcomes— Teaching women about the serotonin-stress relationship

Nurses can empower women with information about the normal workings of their bodies and how certain lifestyle changes may promote an enhanced sense of well-being and diminish PMS symptoms. For example, explaining the relationship between cyclical estrogen fluctuation and changes in serotonin levels may be beneficial in promoting an understanding about serotonin, one of the natural brain chemicals that assists one in coping with life's normal stressors.

Other clinical investigations have focused on the renin–angiotensin–aldosterone system. It has long been noted that many premenstrual symptoms, such as bloating, breast swelling, and weight gain, are caused by fluid retention. Estrogen increases the production of the serum globulin angiotensinogen (a precursor for angiotensin), which leads to increased aldosterone and fluid levels. Under normal circumstances, progesterone competes with aldosterone and prevents excessive fluid retention. However, in the late luteal phase of the menstrual cycle, declining progesterone levels give rise to an increase in the effect of estrogen (Nelson & Baldwin, 2011; Whyte & Peraud, 2009).

Now Can You— Discuss possible causes of premenstrual disorders?

1. Describe premenstrual dysphoric disorder?
2. List three characteristics common to premenstrual disorders?
3. Describe three possible causes of premenstrual disorders?

Diagnosis

In general, the diagnostic work-up for PMS/PMDD consists of four components:

1. A detailed history with a focus on the medical, psychosocial, psychosexual, and substance abuse histories (the gynecological history must include the timing of the symptoms and the regularity of the menstrual cycle)
2. A complete physical examination

3. Laboratory tests (as appropriate to rule out other disorders such as hypothyroidism)
4. A record of the woman's symptoms over a 2- or 3-month period

Nursing Insight— Hormonal testing unnecessary in PMS diagnosis

Laboratory testing of the sex steroid hormonal levels is not necessary for the diagnosis of PMS. Depending on the history and clinical findings, appropriate serum testing may include a chemistry profile, a complete blood cell count, or measurement of the thyroid-stimulating hormone level (Whyte & Peraud, 2009).

Optimizing Outcomes— Recognizing other conditions that may masquerade as premenstrual disorder

When interviewing patients with premenstrual disorder symptomatology, it is essential to obtain a detailed history. Dysmenorrhea, hypothyroidism, depressive disorders, pain disorders, and generalized anxiety disorders are other conditions that may produce similar symptoms. Hypothyroidism, for example, may be associated with fatigue, bloating, irritability, and depression. Breast disease (breast tenderness) or anemia (fatigue) may be responsible for other common symptoms. Various gynecological disorders such as polycystic ovary syndrome or endometriosis may also cause symptoms that can be confused with PMS (Whyte & Peraud, 2009).

THE SYMPTOM DIARY

The patient must be instructed to record her symptom types, timing, and severity each day. Maintaining a prospective symptom diary for at least two to three consecutive menstrual cycles is an essential element in the diagnostic work-up for premenstrual disorders. Because many medical disorders are exacerbated during the luteal phase, the symptom diary is instrumental in determining the severity and the timing of the symptoms (Nelson & Baldwin, 2011).

Several symptom inventories are available. The use of a standardized form such as the Daily Record of Severity of Problems (DRSP) was designed to diagnose PMDD. This tool has shown high test/retest reliability and is available from the Madison Institute of Medicine. Other symptom diaries designed to track premenstrual symptoms include the Calendar of Premenstrual Experiences (COPE), the Penn Daily Symptom Report (DSR), the Prospective Record of the Impact and Severity of Menstruation (PRISM), and the Premenstrual Symptoms Screening Tool (PSST).

Optimizing Outcomes— A daily calendar alternative for tracking PMS symptoms

The nurse may teach the patient how to record her symptoms by taking notes on a regular calendar each day, as an alternative method to using a commercially available symptom inventory form. The woman is taught to write down the symptoms experienced each day, note their severity (using a numeric scoring system where 1 = mild, 2 = moderate, 3 = severe), and record the dates of her menstrual period. If the number of symptoms is excessive or overwhelming, the patient may record only the three to five symptoms that most profoundly bother her. Under ideal circumstances, the patient's weight, basal body temperature, or home ovulation test results are also documented (Nelson & Baldwin, 2011).

The daily symptom records are useful in that they often heighten the patient's awareness of her symptoms, allow her to gain insights into her problem, and empower her to become more involved in her diagnostic work-up and treatment plan. A discussion of cyclical hormonal changes and PMS may be of benefit in heightening an understanding of premenstrual disorders and in promoting a greater sense of control over the situation. If the woman is reluctant to track her daily symptoms, her partner or a family member can be taught to assist with the data collection. It is helpful to ask the patient to continue her charting after therapy has been initiated so that she can identify which interventions improve her symptoms (Nelson & Baldwin, 2011; Whyte & Peraud, 2009).

After the patient has been instructed in the use of a daily symptom diary, she should return in 2 or 3 months for an evaluation of her symptom pattern. Symptoms do not need to recur with equal intensity in each cycle. In fact, the patient may experience different symptoms during different cycles. It is important to recognize, however, that the diagnosis of PMS/PMDD hinges on the timing of symptoms: They must peak in the luteal phase and disappear with the onset of menses (Nelson & Baldwin, 2011).

DIAGNOSTIC CRITERIA FOR PMS AND PMDD

According to the ACOG (2000), to meet the diagnostic criteria for premenstrual syndrome, at least one of the following symptoms must be present, occur during the luteal phase of the menstrual cycle, and resolve within 4 days of the onset of menses. Also, the symptoms must not represent an exacerbation of another disorder, and the symptoms should be bothersome but not necessarily debilitating.

PMS Affective Symptoms
- Angry outbursts
- Irritability
- Mild psychological discomfort
- Confusion
- Poor concentration
- Depression
- Sleep disturbances
- Social withdrawal

PMS Somatic Symptoms
- Abdominal bloating
- Headache
- Aches and pains
- Swelling of the extremities
- Breast tenderness
- Weight gain
- Change in appetite

Diagnostic criteria for PMDD defined by the APA include four major symptom categories and seven additional symptoms. To meet the criteria, the woman must report that her symptoms interfere with her usual activities; the symptoms must not represent an exacerbation of another disorder; at least five symptoms must be present for 1 to 2 weeks premenstrually, with relief by the fourth day of menses; and the criteria must be confirmed by prospective daily ratings for at least two cycles (APA, 2000; Nelson & Baldwin, 2011).

PMDD Major Symptom Categories (at least one must be present)
- Anger or irritability
- Anxiety, edginess, nervousness
- Depressed mood
- Moodiness

Other, Additional PMDD Symptoms (at least five must be present)
- Appetite changes or cravings
- Decreased interest in usual activities
- Difficulty concentrating
- Fatigue
- Feelings of being overwhelmed or out of control
- Insomnia or hypersomnia
- Physical symptoms (listed in the PMS diagnostic criteria)

Now Can You— **Discuss aspects of the PMS/PMDD diagnostic work-up?**

1. Discuss four components of a diagnostic work-up for premenstrual disorders?
2. Teach a patient how to keep a symptom diary?
3. Identify the three components of diagnostic criteria for premenstrual disorders as defined by the ACOG?

Patient Care and Management of PMS Symptoms

Women with mild to moderate symptoms of PMS often respond well to reassurance, emotional support, and simple health promotion strategies. Education constitutes a central component in the care of women with PMS. Nurses can teach women about self-help modalities intended to reduce symptoms and enhance coping with various discomforts.

Nonpharmacological therapies are often initiated during the initial visit; patients can then implement them as they complete their daily symptom charting and discuss helpful and unhelpful approaches at the follow-up visit. The first step in treatment centers on validating the woman's experience and acknowledging that the symptoms are real and have a physiological base. For many women, the simple act of validation brings relief and opens the door to healing. Nursing diagnoses such as Anxiety, Fear, Knowledge Deficit, and Related Discomforts are developed to address the patient's specific symptoms:

- Anxiety related to anticipation of cyclical discomfort
- Fear related to the medical diagnosis
- Depression related to cyclical hormonal changes
- Excess Fluid Volume related to cyclical hormonal changes

Where Research and Practice Meet:
Promoting School-Based PMS
Education Programs

Delara and colleagues (2012) conducted a cross-sectional study to evaluate health-related quality of life in 602 Iranian adolescent students with premenstrual disorders (PMS and PMDD). Findings from their investigation revealed that PMS is a common health problem among adolescent students, and those with PMDD (*n* = 224) reported a poor health-related quality of life, especially as related to role emotional, role physical, social functioning, and bodily pain (subscales included in the Short Form Health Survey, used to assess quality of life). Based on their findings, the researchers identified a need for school-based reproductive health education programs designed to enhance understanding of PMS-related health disorders and to empower students with information for coping with PMS/PMDD and strategies for improving their overall quality of life.

- Deficient knowledge related to limited information regarding premenstrual syndrome
- Pain related to cyclical breast changes

"What to say" — *Teaching patients about strategies to cope with PMS symptoms*

Nurses can suggest strategies to help women cope with specific PMS symptoms. For example, a fitted support or sports bra may ease the discomfort associated with breast tenderness. Abdominal pain and backache are often relieved with the local application of heat; some women benefit from performing stretching exercises, and NSAIDs are useful in reducing the production of pain-producing prostaglandins. Others may be interested in exploring the possibility of using extended cycle hormonal contraceptives to prevent ovulation. The nurse can also encourage the patient to engage in relaxation techniques and, if available, participate in a PMS support group to help reduce premenstrual tension and anxiety. Support groups provide a forum for the sharing of feelings and concerns and offer an opportunity for learning new strategies for self-care.

PHYSICAL ACTIVITY

Various lifestyle changes have been shown to improve PMS symptoms for many women. These include physical activity, aerobic exercise, stress reduction, and relaxation techniques such as yoga and meditation. Nurses should encourage patients with PMS, as well as all women, to regularly engage in physical activity such as brisk walking, swimming, cycling, or other aerobic activity. Vigorous aerobic exercise may lift the mood, reduce stress, and diminish certain physical symptoms in PMS. The 2008 *Physical Activity Guidelines for Americans*, which are included in the *Healthy People 2020* national initiative, recommend that adults engage in at least 150 minutes per week of moderate-intensity, or 75 minutes a week of vigorous-intensity, aerobic physical activity or an equivalent combination of moderate- and vigorous-intensity aerobic activity (U.S. Department of Health and Human Services [USDHHS], 2008, 2012).

DIETARY ALTERATIONS, VITAMINS, AND MINERALS

Dietary alterations may play a role in reducing certain premenstrual disorder symptoms, although various clinical investigations have not conclusively determined that modification of specific substances, including caffeine, sugar, fat, soy, and complex carbohydrates, ameliorates premenstrual symptoms. Drinking an increased amount of water beginning around 7 to 10 days before menstruation may help to decrease fluid retention. Nurses can provide written information that lists foods to avoid (e.g., cola, coffee, hot dogs, potato chips, canned goods) and foods to encourage (e.g., fruits, vegetables, milk, complex carbohydrates, high-fiber foods, low-fat meals) to assist patients in making appropriate food choices for a healthy lifestyle. Also, eating four to six smaller meals per day (rather than three large meals) during the premenstrual period may be beneficial in reducing symptoms of food cravings.

 Complementary Care: *Enhancing comfort with water and other natural diuretics*

Nurses can encourage women with PMS symptoms related to excessive fluid retention to reduce their sodium intake and consume increased amounts of water during the days preceding the expected menses. The water may serve as a natural diuretic and help reduce edema. Foods that may promote a natural diuresis include peaches, parsley, watermelon, asparagus, and cranberry juice.

Vitamins and minerals have also been prescribed to reduce PMS symptoms. Pyridoxine (vitamin B_6), which plays a role in the biosynthesis of neurotransmitters, may be useful in diminishing premenstrual breast pain and depression. Supplementation with vitamin E (alpha-tocopherol) or magnesium (especially in combination with vitamin B_6) may be beneficial in reducing certain PMS symptoms, although stronger evidence exists for the supplementation of calcium and vitamin D. Calcium may be of benefit in reducing PMS symptoms through its interaction with estrogen and parathyroid hormone (Fathizadeh, Ebrahimi, Valiani, Tavakoli, & Yar, 2010; Nelson & Baldwin, 2011). High dietary intake of vitamin D may reduce the risk of PMS by affecting calcium levels, cyclical sex steroid hormone fluctuations, and/or neurotransmitter function (Bertone-Johnson, Chocano-Bedoya, Zagarins, Micka, & Ronnenberg, 2010).

Critical Nursing Action Counseling About Vitamin Supplements

When counseling about vitamin supplements for premenstrual disorders, the nurse must ensure that women understand the dangers of vitamin overdose. Dosages of vitamin B_6 must remain lower than 100 mg/day, as excessive amounts may lead to peripheral neuropathy. Vitamin E supplements should never exceed 400 IU per day; higher amounts are associated with a number of side effects, including diarrhea, flatulence, bloating, weakness, headache, fatigue, abdominal pain, blurred vision, and an increased risk of bleeding.

HERBAL SUPPLEMENTS AND OTHER COMPLEMENTARY AND ALTERNATIVE MEDICINE MODALITIES

Chasteberry (*Vitex agnus-castus*) has been used throughout the ages to treat a variety of conditions. The fruit of the shrublike chasteberry is also known as "vitex" and "monk's pepper." Today, this herb is used widely in Europe for a variety of gynecological disorders, including PMS, dysfunctional uterine bleeding, and menstrual cycle irregularities. Native to central Asia and the Mediterranean region, chasteberry is now grown in the southeastern United States. It can be prepared as a medicinal tea and is also available as a tincture and in capsule form. A low dose of chasteberry increases prolactin and progesterone levels and decreases estrogen levels. Chasteberry is well tolerated; reported adverse effects are infrequent and include gastrointestinal complaints, dizziness, and dry mouth. Women who take medications that impact dopamine (e.g., certain antipsychotic medications and Parkinson's disease medications) should not take chasteberry; also, this supplement may affect the function of hormonal medications such as oral contraceptives and menopausal hormone therapy (National Center for Alternative and Complementary Medicine [NCCAM], 2012).

Evening primrose oil (*Oenothera biennis*) has been recommended for relief of PMS-related breast tenderness; however, to date, clinical trials of this omega-6 essential fatty acid–rich supplement have failed to demonstrate statistically or clinically significant results.

For many women, various nonpharmacological approaches may diminish PMS symptoms. Trials of cognitive behavioral therapy, group therapy, and relaxation therapy have demonstrated improvement in physical and/or psychological symptoms of PMS, although few studies have randomized patients. For some women, other modalities such as massage, yoga, aromatherapy, biofeedback and guided imagery, acupuncture, self-hypnosis, reflexology, chiropractic, and bright-light therapy (used daily for 30 minutes) may have a beneficial effect on PMS symptoms.

 Where Research and Practice Meet:
Chasteberry and Saffron for Moderate to Severe PMS

Ma, Lin, Chen, and Wang (2010) investigated the efficacy of the extract of *Vitex agnus-castus* (VAC) in the treatment of Chinese women suffering from moderate to severe premenstrual syndrome. The 67 study participants, who were randomly assigned to the experimental (VAC) and control (placebo) groups, were followed for three treatment cycles. The premenstrual syndrome diary (PMSD) sum scores decreased significantly in the experimental group and all four-symptom factor scores were significantly reduced by the third treatment cycle. The investigators concluded that based on their findings, VAC was effective in treating moderate to severe PMS in Chinese women, especially in symptoms of negative affect and fluid retention. Other researchers (Doll, 2009; He et al., 2009; Zamani, Neghab, & Torabian, 2012) found similar results and a 2012 systematic review of clinical trials using *Vitex agnus-castus* extracts for various female reproductive disorders (van Die, Burger, Teede, & Bone, 2013) concluded that the results suggest benefits for VAC extracts in the treatment of PMS, PMDD, and latent hyperprolactinemia.

Saffron, an expensive herb that is extracted from the dried stigma of the crocus flower, is used as a spice, dye, and medicinal plant. Saffron contains more than 50% of the U.S. Department of Agriculture's recommended daily allowance of vitamin C, iron, and magnesium, and more than 30% of the recommended daily phosphorus and potassium. Health benefits for saffron are most likely derived from crocetin, a potent antioxidant and carotenoid. In 2008, Agha-Hosseini and colleagues conducted a randomized, double-blind trial of 50 women with diagnoses of consecutive, cyclical PMS to determine the efficacy of saffron versus placebo in alleviating PMS symptoms. Nineteen of the 25 women in the saffron group showed a 50% or greater reduction in severity of symptoms, as compared with just two women in the placebo group. Considered a safe supplement when administered in doses of 25 to 30 mg per day, saffron may be useful in relieving the emotional and physical symptoms of premenstrual disorders (Sego, 2012).

 Nursing Insight— *Asian medicine and PMS*

Nurses should recognize that the fundamental healing approach offered in Asian medicine may well be of benefit in diminishing symptoms of PMS. With the Asian perspective, premenstrual syndrome is viewed as an energetic imbalance, a blockage and stagnation of vital energy (called "qi" or "chi"), which normally flows through the body and enlivens it. When an individual's vital energy is blocked in the pelvic region, it can be manifest in many of the symptoms associated with PMS. Asian healing approaches are designed to restore and balance the body energies, thereby allowing the hormonal and nervous systems to return to a harmonious equilibrium.

PHARMACOLOGICAL INTERVENTIONS

If the nonpharmacological approaches fail to provide satisfactory symptom relief in 2 to 3 months, medication is often initiated.

Ovulation suppressants may be beneficial in the treatment of PMS. Although oral contraceptive pills have been used to treat premenstrual symptoms, most clinical trials have not demonstrated any efficacy in this approach. For some women, however, extended-cycle dosing of continuous combined oral contraceptives, vaginal contraceptive rings, and regular administration of Depo-Provera may be useful in providing symptom relief by suppressing ovulation and by reducing the number of withdrawal bleeding episodes (and associated symptoms) (Nelson & Baldwin, 2011).

 Where Research and Practice Meet:
Acupuncture to Reduce Symptoms of PMS

Acupuncture is an ancient alternative medicine methodology of treating patients through the manipulation of thin, solid needles inserted into various acupuncture points in the skin. According to traditional Chinese medicine, stimulation of the acupuncture points can correct imbalances in the flow of qi through channels known as meridians (energy pathways). Cho and Kim (2010) conducted a systematic review to investigate the efficacy of acupuncture in the treatment of

PMS symptoms. The review included nine randomized controlled trials and evaluated all forms of acupuncture techniques including classical (the insertion and manipulation of needles into 74 meridians, or energy pathways), electroacupuncture (a small electric current is passed between pairs of acupuncture needles), laser acupuncture (low-energy laser beams, rather than traditional acupuncture needles, are used), and acupoint injection (liquid medicine is injected into acupuncture points). Six of the trials reported superior results of acupuncture therapy, as compared with the controls (included pharmacological and herbal medications). Limitations included the small number of trials and methodology flaws that may have exaggerated the positive effects of acupuncture. Although this systematic review cannot conclude that acupuncture is an effective treatment for PMS above other modalities, the findings show promise and suggest a need for additional research in this field (Robinson & Wiczyk, 2011).

Spironolactone (Aldactone), a potassium-sparing diuretic, is a nonhormonal medication that has been shown to be beneficial in the treatment of PMS. Administered in a dosage of 25 mg two to four times a day during the luteal phase, this agent reduces bloating, weight fluctuations, and mastalgia and improves mood in many patients. However, it should be noted that use in PMS management is considered off-label (Nelson & Baldwin, 2011).

For PMDD, there are two major pharmacological strategies to treatment. One targets the central nervous system processes that are believed to contribute to premenstrual mood symptoms; the other approach centers on eliminating the hormonal cyclicity by suppressing ovulation. Pharmacological therapy is reserved for women who qualify as having PMDD or severe manifestations of PMS. The U.S. Food and Drug Administration (FDA) has approved two classes of medications to treat the physical and emotional symptoms of PMDD: a class of antidepressant drugs known as selective serotonin reuptake inhibitors (SSRIs) and a monophasic oral contraceptive that contains the progestin drospirenone (Nelson & Baldwin, 2011).

FDA-approved SSRIs for the treatment of PMDD include fluoxetine (Prozac, Sarafem), sertraline (Zoloft), paroxetine (Paxil), and escitalopram oxalate (Lexapro). Currently, these medications constitute the mainstay of medical treatment. They have been studied extensively for the treatment of PMDD symptoms, and dosing may be administered on a continuous or intermittent schedule. Luteal-phase dosing should be initiated about 14 days before menses and continued until the onset of menstruation. Use of any of the central nervous system agents for treatment of PMS/PMDD does not contraindicate the use of any hormonal or nonhormonal contraceptive method to prevent pregnancy (Nelson & Baldwin, 2011; O'Brien, Rapkin, Dennerstein, & Nevatte, 2011).

 legal alert— Teach about potential adverse effects associated with SSRIs

Although most patients tolerate SSRIs without difficulty, nurses must make certain that the patient is aware of the following side effects associated with these medications: nausea, nervousness, anxiety, headache, drowsiness, dizziness,

Where Research and Practice Meet:
Sertraline and Psychological Symptom Improvement

Freeman, Sammel, Lin, Rickels, and Sondheimer. (2010) conducted a secondary data analysis to examine the response of 447 women to treatment with sertraline (a first-line SSRI therapy) for PMS and PMDD. The results revealed that all psychological symptoms (i.e., mood swings, irritability, anxiety/tension, out-of-control/overwhelmed sensation, sad/depressed state, hopelessness, difficulty concentrating) improved significantly with sertraline relative to placebo. However, while the prevalent PMS symptoms of breast tenderness and swelling or bloating improved with sertraline, most physical symptoms (e.g., appetite changes, poor coordination, fatigue, headache, cramps, aches, sleep disturbances) did not. Based on their findings, the investigators emphasize the importance of careful evaluation of women's individual symptoms prior to the initiation of SSRI therapy, which may not be beneficial in the treatment of certain physical manifestations of premenstrual disorders.

impaired concentration, decreased libido, and insomnia. The risk of side effects is dose related—lower doses, which often suffice for the symptoms of PMS, are associated with fewer side effects. Limiting dosing days to the luteal phase of the cycle has also been shown to be effective in PMS/PMDD. Teaching women about their specific medications is an important step in helping them to understand their diagnosis and the rationale for the prescribed pharmacological treatment (Nelson & Baldwin, 2011; Vallerand & Sanoski, 2013).

The other FDA-approved therapy for the treatment of PMDD is the monophasic oral contraceptive with active pills that contain ethinyl estradiol and drospirenone, a novel progestin. Clinical trials with this formulation have demonstrated significant improvement in physical, psychological, and behavioral symptoms of PMDD (Mayhew, 2010; Nelson & Baldwin, 2011).

Other medications have been prescribed off-label for the treatment of PMDD. Buspirone may be prescribed for women who are unable to tolerate SSRIs but who would benefit from psychotropic medication, and the anxiolytic medication alprazolam has shown efficacy in the treatment of PMDD. However, anxiolytic medications are habit forming and have the potential for abuse. Women with histories of alcoholism or other substance abuse are not appropriate candidates (Nelson & Baldwin, 2011).

? **Global Health Case Study** Abha S.

Premenstrual Syndrome

Abha S. is a 29-year-old Asian nulligravida who has lived in the United States for the past 6 years. She visits the women's health clinic for an evaluation of increasingly bothersome premenstrual symptoms. At present, Abha is not sexually active, but she has a diaphragm for birth control and is pleased with her contraceptive method. Her menstrual periods are regular, occur every 28 to 30 days, are moderate in flow, and last 6 to 7 days. Abha tells the nurse that each month beginning approximately 1 week before the onset of menstrual flow, she experiences painful, tender, swollen breasts; bloating; weight gain; and feelings of "being down" and irritable.

critical thinking questions

1. What additional information is needed to help confirm the diagnosis of PMS?

2. What can the nurse teach Abha about PMS and self-care strategies that may help to minimize her symptoms?

◆ See Suggested Answers to Case Studies on DavisPlus.

Now Can You— **Discuss nursing care for patients with premenstrual disorders?**

1. Describe the nurse's major role when caring for a patient with a premenstrual disorder?
2. Discuss various nonpharmacological therapies for premenstrual disorders?
3. Discuss various pharmacological therapies for premenstrual disorders?

Summary Points

◆ Premenstrual syndrome may be viewed as a complex constellation of genetic influences and hormonal imbalances that adversely affects a woman's physical, mental, and emotional health.

◆ Women have reported more than 100 different physical and behavioral symptoms during the premenstrual period.

◆ The cause of PMS is believed to be multifactorial.

◆ To meet the criteria for PMS, the woman's symptoms must occur cyclically, be unrelated to any physical or mental condition, and greatly disrupt one or more areas of the woman's life

◆ The diagnostic work-up for a premenstrual disorder includes the patient history, a physical examination, appropriate laboratory tests, and review of the daily symptom diary.

◆ Management of premenstrual syndrome may include nonpharmacological and pharmacological approaches.

◆ Nurses are instrumental in helping women to deal with premenstrual disorders by offering ongoing education and support.

Review Questions

Multiple Choice

1. In earlier times, premenstrual syndrome was believed to be related to:
   A. The patient's emotional makeup
   B. Pregnancy
   C. Insanity
   D. Tobacco use

2. One of the criteria for the diagnosis of premenstrual syndrome is that the symptoms:
   A. Occur during the menstrual phase of the uterine cycle
   B. Persist for 25 or more days
   C. Are not caused by any underlying physical or mental condition
   D. Occur during the proliferative phase of the uterine cycle

3. Most women with PMS experience relief of symptoms:
   A. During the luteal phase of the uterine cycle
   B. Within 24 hours following the onset of menstrual flow
   C. Around the time of ovulation
   D. Following removal of the uterus (hysterectomy)

4. An important component in the diagnostic work-up for PMS involves:
   A. Obtaining serum levels of iron and prolactin
   B. Evaluating the basal body temperature
   C. Assessing the urine for glucose, protein, and ketones
   D. Evaluating the daily symptom diary

5. When teaching a woman with PMS about self-help strategies to help diminish symptoms, the nurse may suggest:
   A. Decreasing physical activity approximately 1 week before expected menses
   B. Decreasing the intake of water approximately 5 to 7 days before menstruation
   C. Taking evening primrose oil during the menstrual period
   D. Engaging in relaxation techniques and stress-relief therapies such as massage and yoga

REFERENCES

Agha-Hosseini, M., Kashani, L., Aleyaseen, A., Ghoreishi, A., Rahmanpour, H., Zarrinara, A.R., & Akhondzadeh, S. (2008). *Crocus sativus L.* (saffron) in the treatment of premenstrual syndrome: A double-blind, randomized and placebo-controlled trial. *British Journal of Obstetrics and Gynecology, 115*(4), 515–519. doi:10.1111/j.1471-0528.2007.01652.x

American College of Obstetricians and Gynecologists (ACOG). (2000). *Premenstrual syndrome* (ACOG Practice Bulletin No. 15). Washington, DC: Author

American Psychiatric Association. (2000). *Diagnostic and statistical manual of mental disorders* (4th ed., text rev.). Washington, DC: Author.

Association of Women's Health, Obstetrical and Neonatal Nurses. (2003). *Evidence-based practice guideline: Nursing management for cyclic perimenstrual pain and discomfort.* Washington, DC: Author.

Bertone-Johnson, E.R., Chocano-Bedoya, P.O., Zagarins, S.E., Micka, A.E., & Ronnenberg, A.G. (2011). Dietary vitamin D intake, 25-hydroxyvitamin D$_3$ levels and premenstrual syndrome in a college-aged population. *Journal of Steroid Biochemistry and Molecular Biology, 121*(1–2), 434–437.

Biggs, W.S., & Demuth, R.H. (2011). Premenstrual syndrome and premenstrual dysphoric disorder. *American Family Physician, 84*(8), 918–924.

Bulechek, G.M., Butcher, H.K., Dochterman, J.M., & Wagner, C. (2013). *Nursing interventions classification (NIC)* (6th ed.). St. Louis, MO: Elsevier Mosby.

Cho, S.H., & Kim, J. (2010). Efficacy of acupuncture in management of premenstrual syndrome. A systematic review. *Complementary Therapies in Medicine, 18*(2), 104–111. doi:10.1016/j.ctim.2009.12.001

Delara, M., Ghofranipour, F., Azadfallah, P., Tavafian, S.S., Kazemnejad, A., & Montazeri, A. (2012). Health related quality of life among adolescents with premenstrual disorders: A cross sectional study. *Health and Quality of Life Outcomes, 10*(1), 65–25. doi:10.1186/1477-7525-10-1

Dixon, P.C., & Bergstrom, L. (2011). Menstrual migraine: Current strategies for diagnosis and management. *The Journal for Nurse Practitioners—JNP, 7*(6), 469–478.

Doll, M. (2009). The premenstrual syndrome: Effectiveness of *Vitex agnus-castus*. *Medizinische Monatsschrift für Pharmazeuten, 32*(5), 186–191.

Fathizadeh, N., Ebrahimi, E., Valiani, M., Tavakoli, N., & Yar, M.H. (2010). Evaluating the effect of magnesium and magnesium plus vitamin B_6 supplement on the severity of premenstrual syndrome. *Iranian Journal of Nursing and Midwifery Research, 15*(Suppl. 1), 401–405.

Ford, O., Lethaby, A., Roberts, H., & Mol, B.W.J. (2012). Progesterone for premenstrual syndrome. *Cochrane Database of Systematic Reviews 2012,* Issue 3. Art. No.: CD003415. doi:10.1002/14651858.CD003415.pub4

Freeman, E.W., DeRubeis, R.J., & Rickels, K. (1996). Reliability and validity of a daily diary for premenstrual syndrome. *Psychiatry Research, 65*(2), 97–106.

Freeman, E.W., Sammel, M.D., Lin, H., Rickels, K., & Sondheimer, S.J. (2011). Clinical subtypes of premenstrual syndrome and responses to sertraline treatment. *Obstetrics & Gynecology, 118*(6), 1293–1300. doi:10.1097/AOG.0b013e318236edf2

Fritz, M.A., & Speroff, L. (2010). *Clinical gynecologic endocrinology and infertility* (8th ed.). Philadelphia, PA: Lippincott Williams & Wilkins.

Gingnell, M., Comasco, E., Oreland, L., Fredrikson, M., & Sundstrom-Poromaa, I. (2010). Neuroticism-related traits are related to symptom severity in patients with premenstrual dysphoric disorder and to the serotonin transporter gene-linked polymorphism 5-HTTPLPR. *Archives of Women's Mental Health, 13*(4), 417–423. doi:10.1007/s00737-101-0164-4

He, Z., Chen, R., Zhou, Y., Geng, L., Zhang, Z., Chen, S., . . . & Lin, S. (2009). Treatment for premenstrual syndrome with *Vitex agnus-castus*: A prospective, randomized multi-center placebo controlled study in China. *Maturitas, 63*(1), 99–103.

Hinemann, L.A., Minh, T.D., Heinemann, K., Lindemann, M., & Filonenko, A. (2012). Intercountry assessment of the impact of severe premenstrual syndrome. *Health Care for Women International, 33*(2), 109–124. doi:10.1080/07399332.2011.610530

Kelderhouse, K., & Taylor, J.S. (2013). A review of treatment and management modalities for premenstrual dysphoric disorder. *Nursing for Women's Health, 17*(4), 294–305. doi:10.1111/1751-486X.12048

Lentz, G.M. (2012). Primary and secondary dysmenorrhea, premenstrual syndrome, and premenstrual dysphoric disorder: Etiology, diagnosis, management. In G.M. Lentz, R.A. Lobo, D.M. Gershenson, & V.L. Katz (Eds.), *Comprehensive gynecology* (6th ed., pp 791–804). Philadelphia, PA: Mosby.

Ma, L., Lin, S., Chen, R., & Wang, X. (2010). Treatment of moderate to severe premenstrual syndrome with *Vitex agnus-castus* (BNO 1095) in Chinese women. *Australia New Zealand Journal of Obstetrics and Gynaecology, 50*(2), 189–193.

Mayhew, M.S. (2010). Tailoring contraceptive use to patient needs. *The Journal for Nurse Practitioners—JNP, 6*(6), 471–472.

Moorhead, S., Johnson, M., Maas, M. L., & Swanson, E. (2013). *Nursing outcomes classification (NOC)* (5th ed.). St. Louis, MO: Elsevier Mosby.

National Center for Alternative and Complementary Medicine (NCCAM). (2012). Chasteberry. Retrieved from http://nccam.nih.gov/health/chasteberry

Nelson, A.L., & Baldwin, S. (2011). Menstrual disorders. In R.A. Hatcher, J. Trussell, A.L Nelson, W. Cates, D. Kowal, & M.S. Policar, (Eds.), *Contraceptive technology* (20th rev. ed., pp. 533–570). Decatur, GA: Bridging the Gap Communications.

O'Brien, S., Rapkin, A., Dennerstein, L., & Nevatte, T. (2011). Diagnosis and management of premenstrual disorders. *British Medical Journal, 342*(6), 222–231. doi:http://dx.doi.org/10.1136/bmj.d2994

Raines, K. (2010). Diagnosing premenstrual syndrome. *The Journal for Nurse Practitioners—JNP, 6*(3), 224–225.

Robinson, C., & Wiczyk, H. (2011). Treating common gynecologic conditions with acupuncture. *The Female Patient, 36*(5), 32–38.

Sassoon, S.A., Colrain, I.M., & Baker, F.C. (2011). Personality disorders in women with severe premenstrual syndrome. *Archives of Women's Mental Health, 14,* 257–264.

Sego, S. (2012). Saffron. *The Clinical Advisor, 15*(4), 94–96.

Speroff, L., & Fritz, M.A. (2010). *Clinical gynecologic endocrinology and infertility* (8th ed.). Philadelphia, PA: Lippincott Williams & Wilkins.

Taylor, D., Schuiling, K., & Sharp, B. (2011). Menstrual cycle pain and discomforts. In K. Schuiling & F. Liskis (Eds.), *Women's gynecologic health* (2nd ed., pp. 573–608). Sudbury, MA: Jones & Bartlett.

U.S. Department of Health and Human Services (USDHHS). (2008). *Physical activity guidelines for Americans: 2008 activity guidelines for Americans summary.* Retrieved from http://www.health.gov/paguidelines/guidelines/summary.aspx

U.S. Department of Health & Human Services (USDHHS). (2012). Introducing *Healthy People 2020.* Retrieved from http://www.healthypeople.gov/2020/about/default.aspx

Vallerand, A.H., & Sanoski, C.A. (2013). *Davis's drug guide for nurses* (13th ed.). Philadelphia, PA: F.A. Davis.

van Die, M.D., Burger, H.G., Teede, H.J., & Bone, K.M. (2013). *Vitex agnus-castus* extracts for female reproductive disorders: A systematic review of clinical trials. *Planta Medica. 79*(7). 562-575. doi: 10.1055/s-0032-1327831.

van den Akker, O.B.A. (2012). Premenstrual dysphoric disorder. In O.B.A. van den Akker, *Reproductive health psychology* (pp. 79–89). Chichester, England: Wiley-Blackwell.

Whyte, J., & Peraud, P. (2009). Premenstrual disorders: A primary care primer. *Consultant, 49*(1), 15–24.

Zamani, M., Neghab, N., & Torabian, S. (2012). Therapeutic effect of *Vitex agnus-castus* in patients with premenstrual syndrome. *Acta Medica Iranica, 50*(2), 101–106.

CONCEPT MAP

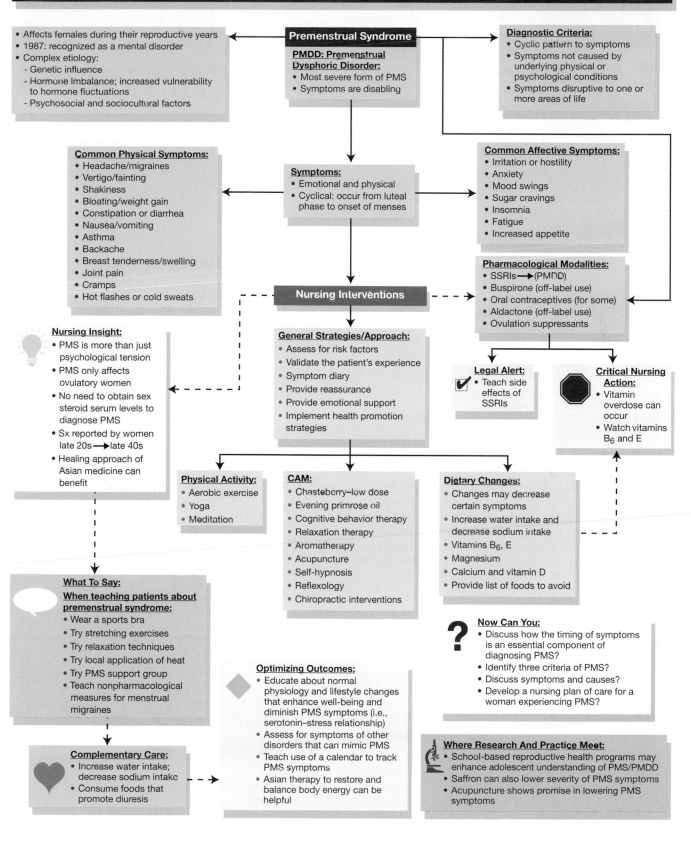

Premenstrual Syndrome

PMDD: Premenstrual Dysphoric Disorder:
• Most severe form of PMS
• Symptoms are disabling

• Affects females during their reproductive years
• 1987: recognized as a mental disorder
• Complex etiology:
  - Genetic influence
  - Hormone Imbalance; increased vulnerability to hormone fluctuations
  - Psychosocial and sociocultural factors

Diagnostic Criteria:
• Cyclic pattern to symptoms
• Symptoms not caused by underlying physical or psychological conditions
• Symptoms disruptive to one or more areas of life

Symptoms:
• Emotional and physical
• Cyclical: occur from luteal phase to onset of menses

Common Physical Symptoms:
• Headache/migraines
• Vertigo/fainting
• Shakiness
• Bloating/weight gain
• Constipation or diarrhea
• Nausea/vomiting
• Asthma
• Backache
• Breast tenderness/swelling
• Joint pain
• Cramps
• Hot flashes or cold sweats

Common Affective Symptoms:
• Irritation or hostility
• Anxiety
• Mood swings
• Sugar cravings
• Insomnia
• Fatigue
• Increased appetite

Pharmacological Modalities:
• SSRIs → (PMDD)
• Buspirone (off-label use)
• Oral contraceptives (for some)
• Aldactone (off-label use)
• Ovulation suppressants

Nursing Interventions

Nursing Insight:
• PMS is more than just psychological tension
• PMS only affects ovulatory women
• No need to obtain sex steroid serum levels to diagnose PMS
• Sx reported by women late 20s → late 40s
• Healing approach of Asian medicine can benefit

General Strategies/Approach:
• Assess for risk factors
• Validate the patient's experience
• Symptom diary
• Provide reassurance
• Provide emotional support
• Implement health promotion strategies

Legal Alert:
☑ • Teach side effects of SSRIs

Critical Nursing Action:
• Vitamin overdose can occur
• Watch vitamins B₆ and E

Physical Activity:
• Aerobic exercise
• Yoga
• Meditation

CAM:
• Chasteberry–low dose
• Evening primrose oil
• Cognitive behavior therapy
• Relaxation therapy
• Aromatherapy
• Acupuncture
• Self-hypnosis
• Reflexology
• Chiropractic interventions

Dietary Changes:
• Changes may decrease certain symptoms
• Increase water intake and decrease sodium intake
• Vitamins B₆, E
• Magnesium
• Calcium and vitamin D
• Provide list of foods to avoid

What To Say:
When teaching patients about premenstrual syndrome:
• Wear a sports bra
• Try stretching exercises
• Try relaxation techniques
• Try local application of heat
• Try PMS support group
• Teach nonpharmacological measures for menstrual migraines

Now Can You:
• Discuss how the timing of symptoms is an essential component of diagnosing PMS?
• Identify three criteria of PMS?
• Discuss symptoms and causes?
• Develop a nursing plan of care for a woman experiencing PMS?

Optimizing Outcomes:
• Educate about normal physiology and lifestyle changes that enhance well-being and diminish PMS symptoms (i.e., serotonin–stress relationship)
• Assess for symptoms of other disorders that can mimic PMS
• Teach use of a calendar to track PMS symptoms
• Asian therapy to restore and balance body energy can be helpful

Complementary Care:
• Increase water intake; decrease sodium intake
• Consume foods that promote diuresis

Where Research And Practice Meet:
• School-based reproductive health programs may enhance adolescent understanding of PMS/PMDD
• Saffron can also lower severity of PMS symptoms
• Acupuncture shows promise in lowering PMS symptoms

Promoting Breast Health

> **L**ife begins each morning . . .
> Each morning is the open door to a new world—new vistas, new aims, new tryings.
> —Leigh Hodges

LEARNING TARGETS *At the completion of this chapter, the student will be able to:*

◆ Describe normal breast anatomy.

◆ Teach a patient how to perform breast self-examination.

◆ Differentiate among various breast abnormalities.

◆ Discuss diagnostic modalities and treatment options for breast cancer.

◆ Describe the nurse's role in promoting breast health.

PICO(T) Questions

The intent of Evidence-Based Practice (EBP) is to provide nursing care that integrates the best available evidence. An initial step in EBP is to write a PICO(T) question that effectively guides the research. A PICO(T) question is an acronym that stands for population (P), intervention or issue (I), comparison of interest (C), outcome (O), and time frame (T). Depending on the question, all or some of the question components are used in the research process. Use these PICO(T) questions to spark your thinking as you read the chapter.

1. For (P) women under age 40, is (I) obesity a greater risk factor in (O) developing breast cancer than (C) alcohol intake of more than two drinks per day?

2. What (I) complementary and alternative medicine strategies are reported as (O) most beneficial in (P) women over 50 who have undergone mastectomy with breast reconstruction?

Evidence-Based Practice

Phillips, J., & Cohen, M.Z. (2011). The meaning of breast cancer risk for African American women. *Journal of Nursing Scholarship, 43*(3), 239–247.

The purpose of this study was to explore meanings and experiences of African American (AA) women considered high risk (i.e., family history, personal history, genetic mutation) for breast cancer. There is a dearth of available research that examines perceptions and behaviors among African American women, and the meaning of breast cancer risks among AA women aged 40 or younger. To promote healthy lifestyles and early detection among this population, it is important to understand the meaning of breast cancer risk.

The study participants, who were recruited from a major medical center and from referrals and various community-based settings, included 20 high-risk African American women between the ages of 23 and 40, with the following documented risk factors: family history, genetic mutations, or a personal history of breast cancer.

The study design was qualitative and used hermeneutic phenomenological methodology. Hermeneutic phenomenology is a formal qualitative research method used to uncover and interpret the lived meaning of an experience. The same researcher, who is African American, conducted all interviews in the participant's setting of choice (i.e., private home or researcher's office). The initial interviews were taped and lasted from 30 to 60 minutes. During

Evidence-Based Practice (continued)

a second interview, the participant was asked to verify, correct misconceptions, and add to what had been transcribed from the first interview. Demographic information was also collected and the participants were paid $50 for completion of both interviews.

Once all of the interviews were completed, five themes were identified. Four participants were asked to review the information, validate the themes, and confirm the researcher's interpretations. The identified themes included the following: (1) "life-changing experience"; (2) "relationships: fears, support, and concerns"; (3) the health-care experience; (4) raising "awareness"; and (5) "strong faith." Twelve of the participants had a personal history of breast cancer diagnosed between the ages of 20 and 37; eight had a first-degree relative with a history of breast cancer; seven had two or more first-degree relatives with a history of breast cancer; and two had three or more first-degree relatives with a history of breast cancer.

Based on their findings, the investigators concluded that young women at risk for breast cancer have unique emotional and support needs; these are shaped by stage in life, relationships with significant others, and interactions with the health-care delivery system. Many of the participants expressed concern that their providers didn't take their apprehension with symptoms seriously and were often reluctant to perform diagnostic tests. The participants also reported that their providers were insensitive when informing them of their cancer diagnosis.

1. How is this information useful to clinical nursing practice?

2. Based on these findings, what are implications for further research?

See Suggested Responses for Evidence-Based Practice on Davis*Plus.*

Introduction

This chapter discusses the promotion of breast health in women. Most concerns about breast care and problems are first voiced in the primary care setting. Nurses who work with women are in an ideal position to educate about the importance of breast health awareness and suggest strategies to promote the early identification of benign and malignant breast disease. As is true with other types of cancers, early detection is key in the successful treatment of breast cancer. Most experts agree that breast cancer is not a singular disease. Instead, it is believed that malignancies of the breast stem from many types of diseases, each with distinct histological, biological, and immunological characteristics. A myriad of dietary, socioeconomic, and environmental factors most likely serve as causative or contributing influences in the development of breast cancer. Breast health is an important issue for women; maintaining breast health is an essential strategy for maintaining optimal physical and psychological health.

Optimizing Outcomes— A holistic approach to breast care

Owing to the likelihood that multiple factors play a role in the development of breast cancer, nurses can embrace a holistic approach to women's health care that is centered on health promotion. This strategy focuses on individualized patient education and counseling concerning diet, lifestyle habits, and environmental exposure—all aspects of health over which individuals have control. The general health benefits of these types of changes have been proved in terms of improved quality of life. Prevention strategies such as these, when combined with early detection, empower women with knowledge and heightened awareness of the normal workings of their bodies and equips them with tools for self-care. The nurse's involvement in patient education and awareness of breast health constitutes an essential action for helping the nation to achieve an extremely important *Healthy People 2020* goal: Reduce the female breast cancer death rate to no more than 20.6 deaths per 100,000

females (U.S. Department of Health and Human Services [USDHHS], 2011).

Benign and Malignant Breast Diseases: The Scope of the Problem

Fibrocystic breast changes, also known as benign breast disease (BBD), are believed to occur in more than 50% of women. Benign breast conditions include cysts, tumors, masses, nipple discharge, infection, and inflammation of the ducts. Although these conditions are not malignant, the discovery of a benign breast mass may evoke feelings of fear, anxiety, and vulnerability and trigger worry about the future. And women have cause for concern, as research has shown that some types of BBD are an important risk factor for the later development of breast cancer (Pearlman & Griffin, 2010).

Breast cancer is the most common cancer in women in the United States, except for skin cancer, and it is the second leading cause of cancer deaths in women (American Cancer Society [ACS], 2013). The American Cancer Society predicts that in 2013, an estimated 232,340 new cases of invasive breast cancer will be diagnosed, and about 39,620 women will die from breast cancer. At present, the chance of a woman developing invasive breast cancer at some time during her life is approximately 1 in 8 (12%). The chance of dying from breast cancer is around 1 in 36 (3%). Women who live in North America have the highest rate of breast cancer in the world. To gain a perspective on the magnitude of the problem, nurses can reflect on the fact that there are more than 2.9 million breast cancer survivors living in the United States today (ACS, 2013).

Nursing Insight— *Breast cancer among American women*

Besides skin cancer, breast cancer is the most commonly diagnosed cancer among women in the United States. More than 1 in 4 cancers are breast cancer. From 1999 to 2005, the incidence of breast cancer in this country decreased by about

2% per year. The decrease occurred only in women aged 50 and older. One theory regarding this decrease centers on the reduced use of hormone therapy by women after the results of the Women's Health Initiative were published in 2002. These results suggest a correlation between hormone therapy and increased breast cancer risk (ACS, 2013; BreastCancer.org, 2012). Women of different ages have different risks of breast cancer. A woman's risk increases with age until she reaches menopause; breast cancer risk then increases more slowly with the advancing years.

Anatomy of the Breast

To enhance an understanding of the breast, it is helpful to review normal breast anatomy. The female breasts, or mammary glands, are considered to be accessory organs of the reproductive system. The two breasts lie over the pectoral and anterior serratus muscles. Breast tissue, which consists primarily of glandular, fibrous, and adipose tissue suspended within the conical-shaped breasts by Cooper's ligaments, is richly supplied with a dense network of blood vessels and lymph vessels (Fig. 3-1).

A & P review **Components of the Breast**

The glandular tissue contains 15 to 24 lobes that are separated by fibrous and adipose tissue. Each lobe contains several lobules composed of numerous alveoli clustered around tiny ducts that are layered with secretory cuboidal epithelia called alveoli or acini (Fig. 3-2).

The epithelial lining of the ducts secretes various components of milk. The ducts from several lobules come together to form the lactiferous ducts, which are larger ducts that open on the surface of the nipple. The lymphatic vessels carry lymph, an alkaline, clear, colorless tissue fluid, away from the breast. Most of the lymph vessels of the breast lead to the nodes in the axillae. The lymph nodes are small, kidney-shaped organs of lymphoid tissue (Fig. 3-3). An increase in the size of the node (lymphadenopathy) indicates a high level of activity (e.g., infection or cancer). ◆

Outer parts of the breasts include the nipples, areolae, and Montgomery tubercles. The nipples contain several

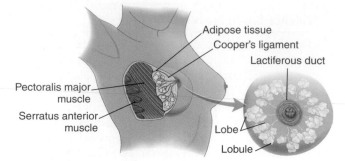

Figure 3-2 Cross section of breast; note lobe and lobule shown in detailed area.

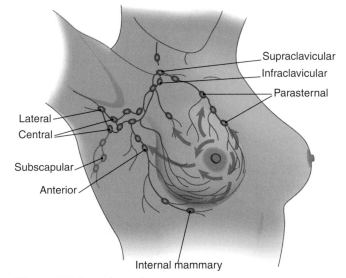

Figure 3-3 Lymph nodes.

pores that secrete colostrum (breast fluid that precedes breast milk) and breast milk during lactation. The nipples consist primarily of erectile tissue to assist with infant latch-on during suckling. The areola is a more deeply pigmented area that surrounds the nipple. Its diameter ranges from 1 to 3.9 inches (2.5 to 10 cm). The Montgomery tubercles are papillae located on the surface of the nipple and the areola; they secrete a fatty substance that lubricates and protects the nipple and areola during breastfeeding.

The primary function of the breasts is to provide nutrition to offspring through the process known as lactation. In American culture, the breasts are also closely linked with "womanhood." Many equate large breasts with increased sexiness and eroticism. Because the breasts serve as a source of sensual pleasure for both men and women, injury to or the loss of a breast can trigger major psychological distress for both genders.

The Nurse's Role in Teaching About Breast Health

The promotion of breast health encompasses several areas, including cancer screening, optimal nutrition, and physical activity. In a position statement on Breast Cancer Screening" (2010), the Association of Women's Health, Obstetric

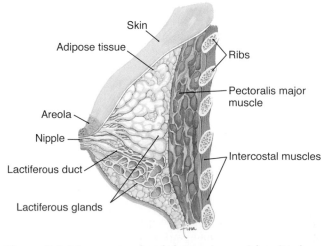

Figure 3-1 Mammary gland shown in a midsagittal section.

and Neonatal Nurses (AWHONN) strongly encouraged all women to take an active role in monitoring their own breast health. An important role for nurses centers on educating women throughout the life span about strategies for promoting breast health. Personal awareness of the normal appearance and feel of the breasts constitutes an essential first step in promoting and maintaining breast health. Nurses working with women in a variety of settings are perfectly situated to offer evidence-based information about strategies for promoting breast health and, for those who wish to do so, performing self-examinations. By providing information in a nonthreatening, therapeutic environment, nurses can help to allay women's fears and present breast self-awareness, and, when desired, breast self-examination, as a positive, empowering experience.

66 What to say 99 — *Teaching about breast health*

During a discussion about breast health, the nurse may wish to include the following information.

- As you age, your breasts experience loss of milk glands and shrinkage of collagen. This causes an increase in the fat tissue and loosening of the breast tissue. Instead of getting larger with the increase in fat tissue, however, the breast tissue begins to sag, causing the breasts to drop.

- Breast tissue weighs less than most people think: An A-cup weighs 1/4 lb, a B-cup weighs 1/2 lb, a C-cup weighs 3/4 lb, and a D-cup weighs about 1 lb.

- The skin covering the breasts stretches as you grow, causing the skin to become thinner than the skin on other parts of the body.

- It is not uncommon for women to have some degree of hair surrounding their nipples. The darker the skin, the more hair there is likely to be.

- A woman's nipples may be different sizes and may be placed in slightly different locations on each breast. This may cause the nipples to point in different directions, which is considered a normal finding.

- Fluctuating hormone levels during the monthly cycle cause changes in breast tissue. Following menstruation, when hormone levels are at their lowest, the breast tissue is smooth and nontender. As estrogen levels increase at midcycle, the breasts may become more sensitive. Also, just before menstruation, when progesterone is elevated, many women's breasts become swollen and tender, with palpable nodules.

- Ideally, your health-care provider should perform your clinical breast examination 1 week following menstruation, when the breast tissue is nontender and smooth.

- Breast implants still pose health risks, including deflation, leakage, and wrinkling. In addition, capsular contraction can occur, causing the scar tissue surrounding the implant to tighten and the breast to become hard. Cosmetic breast implants also hamper detection of breast malignancy.

- The area between the breasts has several oil and sweat glands, creating an atmosphere conducive to the growth of bacteria.

- Sleeping on your side, with a pillow to support your breasts, provides the best position for maintaining breast shape and contour over time.

- Regular exercise can strengthen the pectoral muscles, reducing sagging over time and creating a natural lift.

- It is not uncommon to have a third nipple, stemming from breast buds that form during early fetal development. These extra nipples, however, rarely contain milk glands.

- Pregnancy darkens the color of the nipple, which is an enhancement for the breastfeeding baby. This darker color does not disappear after pregnancy.

- The left breast is usually larger than the right breast.

- Breasts do not reach their full size until the early 20s.

LIFESTYLE CHOICES AND BREAST HEALTH

Lifestyle choices, including moderate alcohol consumption, weight maintenance, and avoidance of smoking can affect breast health as well. Alcohol consumption is known to be associated with an increased risk of breast cancer. The American Cancer Society (2013) recommends limiting alcohol intake to one drink per day; compared with nondrinkers, women who consume one alcoholic drink a day have a very small increase in risk. The risk of breast cancer is increased 1.5 times in women who consume two to five drinks per day.

Routine exercise, which helps to maintain a healthy weight, is associated with a decreased risk of breast cancer. Maintenance of a healthy weight is recommended for optimal breast health. Obesity is associated with an increased risk of breast cancer, particularly in postmenopausal women. Following menopause, estrogen is produced in the fat cells. In combination with dietary fat, estrogen significantly increases the likelihood of breast cancer development. Smoking is associated with an increased risk of breast cancer, lung cancer, and heart disease in women.

Now Can You— **Discuss breast health promotion?**

1. Describe normal breast anatomy?
2. Discuss the nurse's role in teaching about breast health?
3. Develop an educational program that includes essential information about the breasts?

Breast Self-Awareness and Cancer Screening

Breast self-awareness, breast self-examination (BSE), clinical breast exams, and mammography (x-ray filming of the breasts) can assist in early detection and early treatment (Fig. 3-4). The initiation and frequency of mammography depend on the woman's age and risk factors. Magnetic resonance imaging (MRI) (a noninvasive nuclear procedure for imaging tissues with high fat and water content) appears to be especially useful in detecting tumors in women with an inherited susceptibility to breast cancer, and recent findings suggest that this diagnostic method can detect cancer in the contralateral breast that was missed by mammography in women with recently diagnosed breast cancer. As a screening tool, MRI may be useful for women with breast implants in whom mammography is difficult or to determine the integrity of the implants. It has been demonstrated that breast MRI is most effective for identifying tissue with

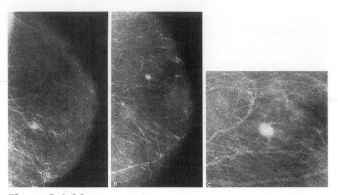

Figure 3-4 Mammogram.

increased blood flow, such as neoplastic tumors. However, breast MRI is not a substitute for a mammogram and it should not be used for routine screening of the average-risk woman. Limitations associated with this diagnostic modality include the expense, the limited specificity, and false-positive results (ACS, 2013; Aliotta & Schaeffer, 2011; Griffin & Pearlman, 2010).

Optimizing Outcomes— **Screening for breast cancer**

Best outcome: Breast self-awareness along with monthly BSE (if the woman so chooses), annual clinical breast examinations, and routine mammography allow women and their health-care providers to detect potentially cancerous tumors at the earliest stage possible. This multipronged screening approach facilitates early diagnosis and early treatment, providing the best outcome possible.

Cultural Diversity: Breast Cancer and Screening Practices

There are notable differences in breast cancer screening practices among women of different ethnic backgrounds. Although African American women are at a lower risk for developing breast cancer than Caucasian women, they are more likely to die from breast cancer owing to late diagnosis. In women under 45 years of age, breast cancer is more common in African American women (ACS, 2013).

Asian American and Pacific Islander women have very low rates of breast cancer screening. Factors responsible for the low screening rates include lack of health insurance, low income, and lack of a primary-care provider. Statistically, Hawaiians have the highest death rate from breast cancer than any racial/ethnic group in the United States (Centers for Disease Control and Prevention [CDC], Office of Minority Health & Health Disparities, 2010).

Owing to an extraordinarily low rate of preventive care, breast cancer constitutes the leading cause of death in Filipino women. Wu and Bancroft (2006) found that women were more likely to follow recommended screenings if there was support from physicians and family members, and if they had insurance. In addition, the presence of physical symptoms, family history of breast cancer, and health literacy promote adherence to recommendations. However, these women continue to be diagnosed with breast cancer at later stages and their tumors are larger at the time of diagnosis than the tumors of Caucasian

women at diagnosis. Most Filipino women refrain from professional breast examinations because they do not wish to be examined by a man, they are uncomfortable being touched by a stranger, and they have concerns about excessive radiation. Also, they are fearful of pain associated with mammography and associate the procedure with pain and cancer (Ho, Muraoka, Cuaresma, Guerrero, & Agbayani, 2010).

BREAST SELF-EXAMINATION

Familiarization with one's breasts facilitates the early detection of problems and allows for prompt evaluation. Breast self-examination (BSE), an option for women starting in the 20s, is a way for women to learn how their breasts normally feel. Routinely performing BSE is an approach that focuses on the importance of self-awareness and helps women to notice changes in breast tissue (ACS, 2013). When teaching women about breast self-examination, the nurse can display pictures of breast tissue and discuss the normal irregular contours of breasts. Breast models are also helpful and allow women to feel both normal and abnormal masses; these teaching aides may be beneficial in diminishing women's fears about checking their own breasts. Because menstruating women often experience increased discomfort and lumpiness in their breasts during the second half of the menstrual cycle, the ideal time to perform BSE is during the week after menstruation.

Routinely performing BSE helps women to perfect their technique and become familiar with the contours and tissue characteristics unique to their own breasts. Then, if they detect changes that are worrisome to them or that persist, they can schedule an evaluation. Nurses can be instrumental in facilitating women's awareness of and comfort with detecting changes in their breasts. Women should be told about the benefits and limitations of BSE, and those who choose to perform BSE should have their BSE technique reviewed during their physical exam by a health-care professional. Women who choose not to perform BSE should still be aware of how their breasts look and feel and report changes promptly (ACS, 2013).

 Where Research and Practice Meet:
Breast Cancer in Pacific Islander Women

Mounga and Maughan (2012) conducted an extensive literature review to identify the health beliefs and practices that affect breast cancer screening and care among Pacific Islander (P.I.) women (i.e., native Hawaiian, Samoan, and Tongan women living in the continental United States) and provide suggestions for how nurses can address these issues. Themes that emerged in the literature focused on culture, language, health beliefs, and health-care access. Based on their findings, the researchers concluded that nurses have a unique opportunity to significantly reduce breast cancer mortality rates among Pacific Islander women. Providing culturally sensitive counseling to women and their families, offering language-appropriate materials, partnering with local leaders, and training lay health workers to provide information to the community are strategies to enhance health screening in this population. Nurses can also assist their P.I. patients to navigate services, resources, and treatment options and partner with various community resources to offer health fairs and other free opportunities for breast cancer screening.

Family Teaching Guidelines...

TOPIC: Breast Self-Examination (ACS, 2013)

1. Lie down on your back and place your right arm behind your head. Remember, this step is done while lying down. In this position, the breast tissue spreads evenly over your chest wall and is as thin as possible. This makes it much easier to feel all of the breast tissue.

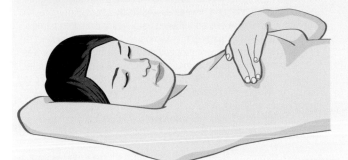

2. Use the pads of your three middle fingers on the left hand to feel for lumps in the right breast. Use overlapping dime-sized circular motions of the finger pads to feel all of the breast tissue.

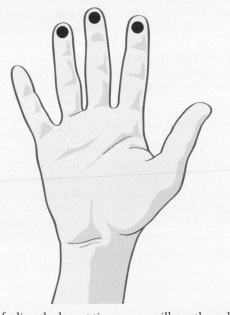

3. When feeling the breast tissue, you will use three different levels of pressure. *Light* pressure is needed to feel the tissue closest to the skin. *Medium* pressure allows you to feel a little deeper, and *firm* pressure allows you to feel the tissue closest to your chest and ribs. Remember, it is normal to feel a firm ridge in the lower curve of each breast. If you feel anything else out of the ordinary, be sure to tell your health-care practitioner. It is important to use each pressure level to feel all of the breast tissue before you move on to the next spot.

4. Move around the breast in an up-and-down pattern, starting at an imaginary line drawn straight down your side from the underarm and moving across the breast to the middle of the chest bone (sternum, breastbone). Make sure that you check the entire breast area going down until you feel only your ribs and then up to the neck or collarbone (clavicle). Using the up-and-down, or vertical, pattern is probably the most effective way to examine the entire breast without missing any breast tissue.

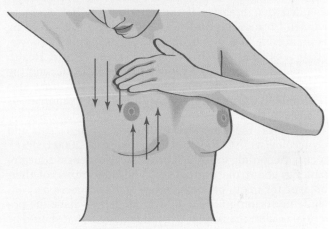

5. Repeat step 4 on your left breast, putting your left arm behind your head and using the finger pads of your right hand to do the exam.

6. Stand before a mirror, place your hands on your hips, and press down firmly. In the mirror, look at your breasts for any changes of size, shape, contour, dimpling, or redness or scaliness of the nipple or breast skin. (Pressing down on your hips contracts the muscles of the chest wall and enhances any breast changes.)

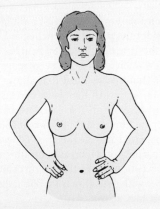

7. Sit or stand with your arm only slightly raised so that you can easily feel the underarm area. Do this on each side, feeling for lumps or thickened areas. (Raising the arm straight up causes a tightening of the tissue and makes it more difficult to examine.)

Breast self-examination is a simple yet powerful self-help behavior that can save lives. More than 75% of breast cancers are discovered by women themselves. The current procedure for performing BSE differs from previous recommendations endorsed by the American Cancer Society. The changes in technique represent an extensive review of the medical literature and input from an expert medical advisory group. Although BSE was once promoted heavily as a means of detecting cancer at a more curable stage, large randomized, controlled studies found that it was not as effective in preventing death and could actually cause harm through unnecessary biopsies and surgery. In 2009, the U.S. Preventive Services Task Force (USPSTF) recommended that breast self-examination not be taught to women because the evidence indicates this self-screening is ineffective in reducing breast cancer mortality (Lowe, 2010; USPSTF, 2009b). At present, the World Health Organization, the U.S. National Cancer Institute, and the Canadian Task Force on Preventative Health Care also recommend against the use of breast self-examinations (Nelson et al., 2009).

However, the American College of Obstetricians and Gynecologists (ACOG) does not support the 2009 USPSTF report. According to ACOG, breast self-awareness educates patients about the normal feel and appearance of their breasts; for many patients, breast self-awareness may include performing BSE, and both modalities have the potential to alert the patient to breast changes that should be reported immediately to the health-care provider and may lead to an earlier detection of breast cancer. Instruction in BSE technique should be considered for high-risk patients and is optional for women aged 20 years and older (ACOG, 2012b).

Nursing Insight— *Considering the potential benefits and harms of BSE*

When sharing information about breast awareness and BSE, it is useful to consider the potential benefits and harms that are associated with this practice. Potential benefits of BSE include empowerment (women gain a sense of control over their health); comfort (noninvasive test that allows women to become more comfortable with their own breasts); and enlightenment (women develop an increased awareness of breast changes, can palpate lumps, and may detect cancer). Potential harms include increased anxiety (heightened fear of cancer that may require counseling) and increased health-care visits, costs, and invasive interventions. Also, there is no change in mortality from breast cancer with detection from BSE (Allen, Van Gronigen, Barksdale, & McCarthy, 2010).

The American Cancer Society endorses "breast awareness." Breast awareness, or being aware of how the breasts normally look and feel, and the way they will change throughout life, may be achieved by feeling the breasts for changes or by using a step-by-step approach (BSE) on a specific schedule (e.g., after menses when the breasts are not tender or swollen). All women should report any changes in their breasts to their health-care providers (ACS, 2013; Mark, Temkin, & Terplan, 2014; Pearlman, 2014).

Where Research and Practice Meet: African American Women's Beliefs About BSE

Registe and Porterfield (2012) conducted a descriptive, correlative study to examine the relationship between health beliefs, knowledge, and attitude and the performance of BSE among 131 African American women aged 20 to 65. The Breast Cancer Screening Beliefs Instrument (Champion & Scott, 1997) was used to measure the concepts of susceptibility (to breast cancer), seriousness (of the threat of breast cancer), benefits of BSE, barriers to BSE, confidence (in performing BSE), and health motivation. Data analysis revealed a significant positive correlation between susceptibility and BSE practice; no significant correlation existed between perceived seriousness, barriers, and confidence. Most participants agreed on the beneficial aspect of BSE, but their confidence in properly performing the procedure was low. Based on their findings, the investigators suggested that an increased awareness and understanding of facilitators and barriers to breast cancer screening can assist health-care providers in addressing these issues and in guiding the development of culturally sensitive and appropriate educational interventions specifically tailored for African American women.

Nursing Insight— *Breast implants and BSE*

If they choose to do so, women with breast implants may perform BSE. Following surgery, it may be helpful for the surgeon to guide BSE teaching by identifying the edges of the implant to enhance the patient's understanding of the new contours of her breasts. For some, the increased prominence of the breast tissue following implant surgery may make it easier to perform the examination. Women who are pregnant or breastfeeding may also choose to examine their breasts regularly (ACS, 2013).

CLINICAL BREAST EXAMINATIONS

Annual clinical breast examinations (CBEs) performed by a trained health-care professional are an important tool in the early detection of breast cancer. Inflammatory breast cancer, a rare and aggressive type that may cause swelling and redness, often does not show up on mammography. Also, the clinical breast examination provides an opportunity for the clinician to reinforce a woman's self-examination technique, discuss concerns, and emphasize the value in becoming intimately familiar with the contour of one's own breasts.

Optimizing Outcomes— **The clinical breast examination**

The breast examination begins with the patient (disrobed from the waist up) in a seated position. Facing the woman, the examiner visually assesses the breasts for symmetry, skin changes such as dimpling, puckering, retraction, or lesions, and changes in upper extremity mobility. Inspection of the area beneath the breasts for the presence of yeast infections and skin nodules is performed as well. The woman is then assisted to a supine position and gentle palpation is followed by deeper palpation using a vertical stripping method (beginning at the clavicle, adjacent to the axilla, the fingers are moved up and down in "vertical strips" over the breast). The underlying ribs and costal cartilage are assessed as well (ACS, 2013; Flynn & Tipton, 2011).

Recommendations for clinical breast examination (CBE) vary depending on the organization. According to the American Cancer Society (2013), the clinical breast examination serves as a complement to mammography, and there may be some benefit in having the CBE performed shortly before the mammogram. Susan G. Komen (2013), the American College of Obstetricians and Gynecologists (2011), the National Comprehensive Cancer Network (2013), and the ACS (2013) recommend that the CBE be performed at least every 3 years for women aged 20 to 39, and every year after age 40. The American College of Radiology and the American Medical Association recommend starting the CBE at age 40 and annually thereafter, and the USPSTF states there is a lack of evidence to support CBE. The American Academy of Family Physicians follows the recommendations of the USPSTF, indicating that there is insufficient evidence to support CBE. It is important for nurses to provide information about the benefits and limitations of the CBE, as well as BSE (ACOG, 2011; ACS, 2013; Allen et al., 2010; Gulian, 2012).

MAMMOGRAPHY

A mammography examination is used to aid in the early diagnosis of breast cancer (Fig. 3-5). The examination, which requires exposure to small doses of ionizing radiation, allows for identification of small breast tissue abnormalities that may require further investigation. In recent times, two enhancements have been made to traditional mammography techniques: digital mammography and computer-aided detection (CAD). Digital mammography, also called full-field digital mammography (FFDM), converts the x-rays to electrical signals, similar to those found in digital cameras. These signals produce images that can be viewed on a computer screen or printed on special film. The images are stored for future comparison. Digital mammography provides improved screening for women determined to be at high risk for developing breast cancer. This latest technology is enhanced with the use of computer software that highlights areas of increased density, masses, and calcifications. The computer-aided detection systems provide an additional feature similar to a computer's spell-check function—they identify visible patterns in images that could represent cancer (Griffin & Pearlman, 2010).

In 2012, the U.S. Food and Drug Administration (FDA) approved the first ultrasound device (somo-v Automated Breast Ultrasound System, or ABUS) for use in combination with a standard mammography in women with dense breast tissue who have a negative mammogram and no symptoms of cancer. Mammograms of dense breasts can be difficult to interpret because there is a higher percentage of fibroglandular tissue present in dense breasts, as compared with less dense breasts. Owing to the fact that fibroglandular tissue and tumors both appear as a solid white area on a mammogram, fibroglandular tissue can obscure smaller tumors. The somo-v ABUS, which consists of a specially shaped transducer that can automatically scan the entire breast in about 1 minute to produce several images for review, is approved for use in women who have not had previous clinical breast intervention (e.g., surgery, biopsy), because these interventions may alter the appearance of breast tissue in an ultrasound image (U.S. Food and Drug Administration, 2012).

Optimizing Outcomes— Counseling women with dense breasts

It is estimated that 40% of women have dense breast tissue, which can mask cancer. A radiologist determines the density of a woman's breasts by examining her mammogram. At present, some states mandate that each mammography report provided to a patient include information about breast density and require insurance coverage for comprehensive ultrasound screening of the breasts if mammography demonstrates heterogeneous or dense breast tissue based on the Breast Imaging Reporting and Data System (BIRADS) established by the American College of Radiology. Two BIRADS scales are used to standardize mammography reporting: One scale categorizes breast density; the other scale categorizes the findings that are seen on the mammogram, and most mammography reports reference this scale (Table 3-1). Nurses can counsel women whose mammography reveals breast density to ask their health-care provider which category of breast density they have (based on the BIRADS scale), and use this information to guide care. To determine insurance laws in each state, patients can visit http://Areyoudenseadvocacy.org/ (Are You Dense Advocacy, 2014).

In a 2014 Committee Opinion, the American College of Obstetricians and Gynecologists acknowledged that women with dense breasts have a moderately increased risk of breast cancer and experience reduced sensitivity of mammography to detect breast cancer, but concluded that evidence is lacking to advocate for additional testing until there are clinically validated data that indicate improved screening outcomes. According to ACOG, screening mammography remains the most useful tool for breast cancer detection, and the routine use of alternative or adjunctive tests to screening mammography in women with dense breasts who are asymptomatic and have no additional risk factors is not recommended. However, health-care providers should comply with state laws that may require disclosure to women of their breast density as recorded in a mammogram report (ACOG, 2014).

Nursing Insight— Calcium deposits within breast tissue

Calcifications (calcium deposits) detected on mammography may be identified as *macrocalcifications* or as *microcalcifications*. Macrocalcifications, degenerative changes resulting from old trauma, inflammation, or aging of the breast arteries, occur in approximately one-half of women in the United States who are over

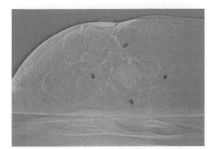

Figure 3-5 Mammography showing breast cancer.

Table 3-1	American College of Radiologists Breast Imaging Reporting and Data Systems (BIRADS)
Categorizes Breast Density	
1	Almost entirely fatty (mammogram very effective)
2	Scattered fibroglandular tissue (minor decrease in sensitivity)
3	Heterogeneously dense tissue present (moderate decrease in sensitivity)
4	Extremely dense tissue present (marked decrease in sensitivity)
Categorizes Findings Seen on Mammogram	
0	Need additional imaging evaluation or prior mammograms for comparison
1	Negative
2	Benign findings
3	Probably benign findings; short interval follow-up recommended
4	Suspicious abnormality; consider biopsy
5	Highly suggestive of malignancy; appropriate action should be taken
6	Known biopsy—proven malignancy

Sources: ACOG (2014); Are You Dense Advocacy (2014).

age 50 and are usually not related to malignancy. Microcalcifications are small specks of calcium that may be present as "residue" in areas of rapidly dividing cells (e.g., a neoplasm). A cluster of microcalcifications may be indicative of a small cancer.

Screening mammography is beneficial as routine breast surveillance for the asymptomatic woman. Clinical detection through the use of BSE (in women who wish to engage in this practice) generally does not occur until the tumor approximates the size of a walnut. By the time a palpable mass or lump is detected, the tumor most likely has been growing for some time. Hence, routine screening mammograms provide a much earlier, high-sensitivity study of developing tumors at the lowest possible cost. In addition, a screening mammogram enables the radiologist to identify changes such as calcifications that may point to malignancy.

Nursing Insight— *Differentiating between screening mammography and diagnostic mammography*

Screening mammograms are performed to check for breast cancer in women who have no signs or symptoms of the disease. They usually involve two x-rays of each breast. Diagnostic mammograms are performed to check for breast cancer after a lump or other sign or symptom of breast cancer has been detected. They may also be used to evaluate changes discovered during a screening mammogram or to view breast tissue when it is difficult to obtain a screening mammogram because of special circumstances, such as the presence of breast implants. Diagnostic mammography takes longer to perform because more x-rays are taken to obtain views of the breast from several angles (National Cancer Institute [NCI], 2012).

The value of routine screening mammography for women aged 50 and older has been well established. Recommendations for mammography screening in women aged 40 to 49 have been met with some controversy. Analysis of the major studies of women in this age group has shown a marginal benefit in decreasing the death rate from breast cancer. However, the following should be noted:

• Findings from older studies may be flawed because mammography was much cruder 30 years ago.
• Breast cancer in women aged 40 to 49 occurs with less frequency.
• Mammography in premenopausal women historically has not been as accurate owing to the density of breast tissue in women in this age group, as compared with breast tissue in postmenopausal women. Mammography may miss as many as 25% of invasive cancers in women aged 40 to 49 years, as compared with 10% in women aged 50 years and older.
• Certain tumors, even when detected early, are not curable. In general, younger women tend to have more rapidly growing tumors than do older women. This finding may be related to the higher levels of estrogen in the blood and tissues of premenopausal women that can stimulate tumor growth or a genetic predisposition that becomes expressed in this age group.

In late 2009, the USPSTF issued updated breast cancer screening recommendations for the general population. Based on evidence review, the current guidelines recommend against routine mammography screening for women before age 50 years, suggest that screening end at age 75 years, and recommend changing the screening interval from 1 year to 2 years. In December 2009, the task force amended those recommendations, clarifying that regular screening mammography before the age of 50 should be an individual decision based on the patient's needs, values, and preferences (USPSTF, 2009a). The guidelines were based on conclusions from evidence reviews of the literature and statistical analysis. It should be noted that the rationale for the change in screening recommendations applies only to women with average risk for developing breast cancer. When considering the benefits of screening women beginning at age 40, it is important to note that the benefit is smaller in women in their 40s as compared with older women, the group for whom breast cancer is more common. Younger women are more likely to have false-positive results, which lead to additional and often unnecessary testing (repeat mammography, ultrasound, biopsy), as well as financial burdens, anxiety, and possible overdiagnosis (Cibulka, 2011; Yankaskas et al., 2010).

The current USPSTF screening guidelines attempt to account for potential harms associated with population-based screening of women younger than age 50 and older than age 75 while maximizing the benefits of screening for women who are at average risk (Jolivet, 2010). However, several professional organizations have voiced their objections to the new recommendations. The American Cancer Society, the American College of Radiology, the American College of Obstetricians and Gynecologists, and several other expert groups recommend that clinicians and patients continue to receive yearly mammography beginning at age 40 and continuing as long as the woman is in good health. According to the American Geriatrics Society, mammography screening beyond the age of 85 should be reserved for those women most likely to benefit by virtue of excellent health and functional status, and for those who feel strongly that they will benefit from such screening, either in peace of mind or improved quality of life (Schonberg, 2010; Schonberg, Breslau, & McCarthy, 2013; Somerall, 2013).

Because mammography is considered a less useful screening and diagnostic tool in women younger than age 40, the health-care provider must determine the use of mammography in this patient population on an individual basis. When compared with film mammography, full-field digital mammography has been determined to be more accurate, especially for women younger than age 50, those with dense breast tissue, and those who are premenopausal or perimenopausal.

Optimizing Outcomes— Recognizing mammography barriers to enhance counseling and empower women

Women may be reluctant to obtain a mammogram for a number of reasons, including a fear of pain associated with the test and a fear of the test findings. Other barriers to breast cancer screening include older age, cultural patterns and health beliefs, lack of knowledge and information, lack of time, lack of motivation, expense, lack of availability of mammography services, lack of physician referral, lack of health-related social support, cancer fatalism, and the presence of disabilities (Barr, Giannotti, Van Hoof, Mongoven, & Curry, 2008; Farmer, Reddick, D'Agostino, & Jackson, 2007; Kang, Thomas, Kwon, Hyun, & Jun, 2008; Kim & Kim, 2008; Makuc, Breen, Meissner, Vernon, & Cohen, 2007; Wang, Mandelblatt, Liang, Ma, & Schwartz, 2009). Also, owing to fear of abnormal results, some women may delay following up on an incomplete or abnormal mammogram (Fang & Shu, 2009). Nurses can empower women by providing factual information and promoting shared decision making, by identifying local facilities that provide inexpensive or free mammograms, by addressing specific concerns, and by working with other professionals to help remove barriers to screening. Compliance with mammography guidelines may be improved by strategies such as reminder postcards or telephone calls and direct health-care provider referrals (Feldstein et al., 2011; Hale & deValpine,

2014; Kelleher, 2010). In addition, it has been shown that mobile mammography for underserved women may provide another opportunity for improved participation in breast cancer screening services (Buzek, 2010).

"What to say" — *Preparing for a mammogram*

Nurses can counsel women about strategies to enhance mammography results and minimize discomfort associated with the procedure. For example, the nurse can provide the following information:

- Choose a mammography facility that is accredited by the American College of Radiology; ensure that the mammogram is performed by a registered technologist and that the radiologist is trained specifically to interpret mammography.
- Remove powder, deodorant, and perfume prior to the mammogram (these substances may create shadows).
- Schedule the mammogram when the breasts are less tender (e.g., after the menstrual period).
- Ask for the use of a soft pad to cushion the breasts during mammography compression.
- Take acetaminophen, ibuprofen, or aspirin as needed for relief of discomfort.

BREAST TOMOSYNTHESIS: A NEW TOOL FOR BREAST CANCER SCREENING

Mammography, which produces a two-dimensional x-ray image of the breast, is the traditional first-choice modality for the early detection of breast cancer. However, mammography interpretation, especially in women with dense, fibroglandular breasts, has inherent limitations. With a standard mammogram, normal breast structures are superimposed on each other, creating an overlapping image that may mimic or mask a lesion and lead to false-positive or false-negative findings. Tomosynthesis, approved by the FDA in 2011, is a new advancement in breast imaging. This modality produces breast views in numerous thin slices, providing a three-dimensional image (and better visualization) of breast tissue. Similar to mammography, the breast is compressed with the tomosynthesis technique and the total radiation dose is comparable to the dose of a single-view mammogram. Complementary to standard mammography, tomosynthesis is performed along with a standard mammogram, at the same time and on the same scanner. The main benefits of this imaging modality are lower recall rates and a slight increase in cancer detection. With fewer recalls, tomosynthesis may reduce the number of women who experience anxiety associated with screening (ACOG, 2013; Freimanis & Yacobozzi, 2014; Yates, 2014).

---

⑤ Now Can You— Discuss methods of breast awareness and cancer screening?

1. Explain what is meant by the term breast awareness and identify the recommended guidelines for clinical breast examinations and screening mammography?
2. Teach a patient the proper procedure for breast self-examination?
3. Explain how to prepare for a mammogram?

Benign Breast Masses

It has been estimated that at some time during adulthood, 50% of women will experience a breast problem. Fortunately, most breast tumors are benign. Breast cysts are a common finding; they may be fluid-filled or solid. Fluid-filled cysts, also termed **fibrocystic changes**, are often tender and fluctuate in size with the menstrual cycle. These changes are the most common benign breast condition and occur most often during the childbearing years. During the clinical exam, palpation reveals lumpy or nodular tissue and patients often complain of pain (mastalgia) or tenderness. Patients may also report a change in breast size and density as the menstrual cycle progresses. Although the cause is unknown, an imbalance of estrogen and progesterone may play a role in the development of fluid-filled breast masses (Chase, Wells, & Eley, 2011).

Therapeutic interventions involve differentiating between fibrocystic changes and breast cancer. Screening methods include clinical breast examinations, mammography, and ultrasonography. The physician may choose to aspirate fluid-filled cysts for evaluation to determine if malignant cells are present. Patients should be advised that although aspiration may eliminate the cysts, they frequently re-form (Chase et al., 2011).

---

⑤ Optimizing Outcomes— Teaching about fibrocystic breast changes and mastalgia

When teaching women about breast health, nurses can include information about fibrocystic changes, palpable thickening in the breasts often associated with pain and tenderness that fluctuates with the menstrual cycle. Nurses can reassure them that fibrocystic changes are common and benign and tend to appear during the second and third decades of life and suggest strategies for coping with mastalgia: use of a well-fitting supportive bra, analgesics, NSAIDs (e.g., oral ibuprofen; topical diclofenac gel for localized breast pain), and consumption of dietary flaxseed (25 g/day) (Chase et al., 2011; Rosolowich, Saettler, & Szuck, 2006).

Fibroadenomas are solid cysts composed of stromal (connective) and glandular tissue. They are usually moveable and nontender. Fibroadenomas are the second most common benign breast condition (fibrocystic changes are the most common) and are usually located in the upper outer quadrant of the breast. This tumor occurs most often in women who are in their 20s and 30s. The use of oral contraceptives before age 20 has been linked to the risk of fibroadenomas (ACS, 2013; Pearlman & Griffin, 2010).

Lipomas are mobile, nontender fat tumors that are soft with discrete borders. Lipomas may develop anywhere in the body, including the breasts. **Intraductal papillomas** are small, wartlike growths in the lining of the milk ducts near the nipple. These rare, benign tumors usually produce a clear or bloody nipple discharge. They may be felt as a small lump behind or next to the nipple.

Mammary duct ectasia is an inflammation of the ducts located behind the nipple. Occurring most often in perimenopausal and postmenopausal women, this condition produces a thick, sticky nipple discharge that may be purple, brown, or white in color. Upon inspection, the nipple and adjacent breast tissue may be tender and red and the nipple may be pulled inward. Duct ectasia may resolve spontaneously, or it may require treatment with warm compresses and antibiotics. In some situations, surgical removal of the abnormal duct is necessary. This lesion does not increase the risk of breast cancer.

✳ Nursing Insight— *Nonproliferative and proliferative breast lesions*

The presence of cysts in the breasts does not necessarily increase a woman's risk for breast cancer. It has been estimated that approximately 70% of fibrocystic changes are nonproliferative lesions; 26% of changes are proliferative lesions without atypical or unusual growing cells (termed "atypia"), and proliferative lesions with atypical hyperplasia represent the remainder of fluid-filled breast lesions. Nonproliferative (multiplying) lesions do not affect breast cancer risk. Proliferative lesions without atypia may slightly increase cancer risk, and proliferative lesions with atypical hyperplasia raise the risk of cancer (ACS, 2013).

Mastitis is an infection of the breast that occurs when bacteria enter the mammary ducts through a nipple. Most often, bacteria (e.g., *Staphylococcus aureus*, *S. epidermidis*, *Streptococcal* species) are introduced during breastfeeding. Localized pockets of infection produce tender, warm lumps and the adjacent axillary lymph nodes are frequently enlarged and painful. Mastitis is usually treated with antibiotics and warm compresses. If there is no improvement in symptoms following antibiotic therapy, further screening is indicated to rule out inflammatory carcinoma, a rare form of breast cancer that may cause redness, warmth, swelling, and skin texture changes in the affected breast (Kosir et al., 2013).

Breast trauma or **injury** may produce an accumulation of blood at the site (hematoma) or destruction of the mammary fatty tissue ("fat necrosis"), which can appear as a lump. A biopsy may be performed to rule out malignancy. There is no evidence that breast injury causes cancer.

Evaluating Breast Abnormalities

Over the past decade, breast cancer screening methods, especially mammography, have become more precise, allowing for earlier diagnosis. Improved screening and increased public awareness have accounted for the dramatic increase in the detection of breast cancer. Earlier diagnosis has resulted in a decrease in mortality rates.

If an area of abnormal breast tissue is detected during the clinical breast examination, unless there is a high index of suspicion, the woman is usually asked to return for a second evaluation after her next menstrual period. In many situations, she is also referred for a mammography. A limitation of mammography is the inability of this modality to differentiate between solid and cystic masses. An ultrasound examination (ultrasonography; sonography) may be performed at the time of the mammography to determine whether the lump is solid or fluid-filled.

Further testing is indicated if the breast mass persists after the next menstrual period, or if any abnormality is identified on mammography or sonography. If the ultrasound examination reveals that the lump is solid, the suspicious tissue is biopsied for further analysis. If the mass is fluid-filled, a needle aspiration is performed, and the woman is monitored for the development of additional cysts. Ultrasound may be used to guide the needle aspiration. If a distinct, palpable lump persists despite normal findings on mammography, immediate follow-up and evaluation are indicated.

A biopsy of any suspicious area is needed to provide a tissue sample for analysis so that a definitive diagnosis can be made. Although mammography is considered the best detection method for early breast cancer, it is often unable to distinguish between benign and malignant tumors. The American Cancer Society estimates that four out of every five biopsy results are not cancer (ACS, 2013).

Breast MRI is used with increasing frequency to evaluate abnormal breast findings and to screen women at high risk for breast cancer. This screening modality is especially beneficial for breast masses that are not visualized mammographically, for lobular cancers, and for patients at risk for bilateral disease. MRI of the breast has shown an overall sensitivity to breast cancer of 95%. Recent evidence suggests that this diagnostic method can detect cancer in the contralateral breast that was missed by mammography in women with recently diagnosed breast cancer. Although MRI does not involve the use of radiation, effective cancer screening does require the use of a nonradioactive intravenous contrast agent. Hence, women with an allergy to the contrast agent, or poor renal function, or those who are pregnant are not candidates for this modality. Also, patients with certain devices (e.g., pacemakers) cannot undergo MRI, and highly claustrophobic patients may not tolerate the procedure (ACS, 2013; Freimanis & Yacobozzi, 2014).

The American Cancer Society recommends both MRI scans and mammograms once per year for women considered as high risk—those whose chance of developing breast cancer during their lifetime is greater than 20%—beginning at age 30. Younger women frequently develop more aggressive cancers and they tend to have denser breasts, a factor that makes it more difficult to detect cancerous changes via mammography alone (ACS, 2013).

Optimizing Outcomes— Algorithms to Enhance Evaluation of Breast Masses

Algorithms to facilitate the health-care provider's evaluation of breast masses are available on the Internet. The "Every Woman Counts" resource, which includes a downloadable booklet, can be accessed at https://qap.sdsu.edu/screening /breastcancer/bda/index.html. The CRICO breast care management algorithm, which has been continuously updated since 1995, is available at http://www.rmf.harvard.edu /Clinician-Resources/Guidelines-Algorithms/2010/Breast -Care-Management-Algorithm.

BIOPSY

Most often, the diagnosis and treatment of breast abnormalities form a two-step process: A biopsy is obtained and evaluated and then based on this information, decisions are made regarding the treatment. Palpation alone cannot determine whether or not a suspicious mass or lump is cancer. Likewise, neither the clinical breast examination nor available technology can provide definitive proof that a suspicious lesion is cancerous. All that can be concluded from these modalities is that "no evidence of cancer is found." Confirmation of cancer can be made only by examining the suspicious tissue. A number of different biopsy procedures may be used to obtain a sample of breast tissue or fluid within the breast tissue for evaluation. These include fine needle aspiration, core needle aspiration, and surgical or open biopsy.

Fine Needle Aspiration (FNA)

The FNA technique involves the use of a fine needle that is carefully guided into the suspicious area while the practitioner palpates the lump. It is usually conducted in the office setting. If the abnormality is too small to feel, ultrasound or a stereotactic biopsy can be used to help locate and ensure an adequate sampling of the suspicious tissue. In the latter technique, the biopsy is conducted with the aid of mammography. The needle is guided to the area by computer-assisted x-ray, which can help the examiner precisely control the needle placement. Then suction is applied to the needle. FNA is used to determine whether the lump is a fluid-filled cyst or a solid tumor (Fig. 3-6).

clinical alert

Indications for breast biopsy

A biopsy obtained by FNA with a stereotactic core needle or by surgical excision is usually recommended for any breast mass that does not resolve spontaneously within one or two menstrual cycles and for all postmenopausal women. It is important to note that negative results from mammography and ultrasonography are not always accurate enough to rule out cancer (Venes, 2013).

If fluid is aspirated, the FNA procedure may eliminate the lump altogether and provide a preliminary diagnosis. In some situations, it is necessary to perform further testing. Additional evaluation may be indicated if the fluid is dark in color, or if the fluid-filled cyst has recurred several

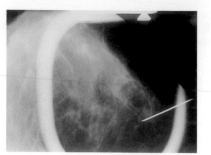

Figure 3-6 Fine needle breast biopsy.

times, or if the sample has been obtained from a post-menopausal woman, who would not be expected to have breast cysts because of low estrogen levels. Clear fluid is usually indicative of a benign cyst; cloudy or bloody fluid may be present in benign or malignant tumors.

If no fluid is aspirated or if a residual thickened area remains after aspiration of the fluid, a core needle biopsy is performed. The false-positive rate for needle aspiration is almost zero. False-negative results occur more frequently because the needle may have missed the abnormal tissue. If no abnormalities are found with aspiration, follow-up mammography or sonography is recommended in approximately 2 to 4 months to assess for recurrence of the cyst.

Core Needle Biopsy

In this technique, a large-bore needle is used to remove a small cylinder of tissue. The needle placement is often guided as with the fine needle aspiration procedure. Core needle biopsy may be performed with the use of a local anesthetic in the office setting. The procedure may be painful, but there is usually little or no scarring. The core needle biopsy is preferred over the FNA, as this method can identify invasive cancer and provide prognostic biomarkers to help direct the course of treatment (Kentley, 2011).

Optimizing Outcomes— With stereotactic biopsy

The Mammotome and the Advanced Breast Biopsy Instrument (ABBI) are stereotactic biopsy methods that remove more tissue than a core needle biopsy. The Mammotome is a type of vacuum-assisted biopsy that uses a hollow probe instrument to remove about twice as much tissue as would a core biopsy. Performed in the outpatient setting under local anesthesia, this procedure requires no stitches and leaves minimal scarring. The ABBI method uses a rotating circular knife equipped with a thin heated electrical wire to remove a large cylinder of abnormal tissue. This procedure requires sutures and is more likely to leave a minimal scar. In some centers, the biopsy is guided by an MRI, which locates the tumor, plots its coordinates, and precisely aims the stereotactic biopsy instrument into the tumor. Automated Tissue Excision and Collection (ATEC) is a biopsy technique that combines vacuum-assisted breast biopsy with MRI-assisted guidance. This method, which allows many samples to be taken through one small cut in the skin, requires only a local anesthetic. It is being studied in women who have had a personal or family history of breast cancer, in those who have had previous breast surgery, and in women with dense breast tissue who cannot be accurately screened with tests such as mammography or sonography (ACS, 2013).

Surgical or Open Biopsy

In many instances, removal of all or a portion of the tissue for microscopic analysis may be indicated. When this is the case, a number of decisions must be made concerning the amount of tissue needed, because the goal is to obtain surgical margins that are free of possible malignant tissue. If possible, the incision is made near the areola of the nipple to minimize scarring and disfigurement. The surgical or open biopsy is considered the most accurate biopsy technique for large masses or for large areas under suspicion and may involve removal of the entire tumor (excisional biopsy) or a small part of a large tumor (incisional biopsy) (ACS, 2013). Depending on the situation, the procedure may be performed using local anesthesia or regional anesthesia; if the tumor is deep inside the chest, general anesthesia may be required.

Skin ("Punch") Biopsy

A punch biopsy may be used to confirm a diagnosis of inflammatory breast cancer or Paget's disease (carcinoma of the mammary ducts) of the nipple.

Testing for Estrogen and Progesterone Receptors

Normal breast tissue contains hormone receptors that respond to the stimulatory effects of estrogen and progesterone. An estrogen receptor is a cellular protein that binds the female sex steroid hormones. When circulating estrogens attach to it, they stimulate the cells to transcribe DNA and manufacture proteins. This process typically leads to cellular growth and proliferation. Many types of breast cancers retain estrogen receptors, and for these particular tumors, estrogen enhances proliferation of the malignant cells. The same situation occurs with tumors having progesterone receptors.

An important component in the evaluation of a woman with early breast cancer is to test for the presence of hormone receptors. The estrogen and progesterone receptor proteins are present in the cell cytoplasm and may be located on the surface of some of the breast cancer cells. When present, the receptors bind to the estrogen or progesterone, and the binding promotes growth of the malignant cells. A malignant breast tumor may have estrogen receptors, progesterone receptors, or both types. Determining the patient's hormone receptor status through biological testing of the tumor type provides valuable information concerning the predicted response to hormone manipulation therapy. Tumors that lack hormone receptors will not respond to hormone therapy. In general, postmenopausal women tend to be estrogen receptor positive; premenopausal women tend to be estrogen receptor negative (Venes, 2013).

Evaluating Breast Symptoms

Breast symptoms may occur in benign and malignant conditions. For example, the woman may experience nipple discharge, skin changes, or breast pain. It is important that each symptom be evaluated to determine its significance and the need for further testing or treatment.

NIPPLE DISCHARGE

Any spontaneous nipple discharge should be promptly evaluated. In most cases, nipple discharge results from a physiological event (e.g., infection) or hormonal imbalance. However, a small percentage of women who experience this symptom are diagnosed with a serious pituitary disorder or malignancy.

Optimizing Outcomes— **Use of the ductogram to evaluate nipple discharge**

A ductogram is sometimes performed to determine the cause of nipple discharge. Also called a "galactogram," this test involves the placement of radiopaque dye (instilled via a tiny plastic tube) into the nipple. An x-ray is then taken to determine the presence of a ductal mass.

Galactorrhea (the continuation of milk secretion after breastfeeding has ceased) is characterized by a spontaneous bilateral, milky, sticky discharge. Galactorrhea normally occurs during pregnancy due to increased circulating levels of prolactin. Elevated prolactin levels may also be associated with a thyroid disorder, a pituitary tumor, chest wall surgery, or trauma. Some women develop galactorrhea during therapy with certain neuroleptic drugs or oral contraceptives. In addition to evaluation of serum prolactin levels, diagnostic testing may also include a ductogram, microscopic analysis of the nipple discharge, a thyroid profile, pregnancy testing, and mammography.

Serous or bloody nipple discharge may be caused by an intraductal papilloma, a rare, benign condition of unknown etiology that develops in the terminal nipple ducts. Purulent nipple discharge is typically associated with breast infection. Occasionally, breast cancer produces a spontaneous unilateral discharge that may be bloody, serous, or watery. The bloody discharge associated with breast cancer ranges from bright red to black and the serous discharge is thin, sticky, and yellow to light orange in color (ACS, 2013).

False discharge is a term that refers to fluid that appears on the nipple or areola but is not secreted by breast tissue. False discharge may be bloody, clear, colored, purulent, serous, or viscous. Various conditions such as eczema, dermatitis, nipple trauma, and Paget's disease may be associated with false nipple discharge.

Nursing Insight— *Recognizing symptoms that may point to Paget's disease*

Paget's disease is an inflammatory, malignant neoplasm that originates in the nipple. This rare tumor accounts for only 1% of all cases of breast cancer. It usually occurs with invasive ductal carcinoma and can cause scaling, bleeding, oozing, and crusting of the nipple. The woman may complain of burning or itching in the affected area. Nurses should remind women that an important component of breast awareness and self-examination involves visualization and inspection of the nipples and that any changes should be promptly reported.

SKIN CHANGES

Erythema, or reddening of the skin, may be related to benign or malignant conditions. Infection, the most common cause of breast erythema in young women, is usually accompanied by increased tenderness and localized warmth. Infection is treated with a course of antibiotic therapy. Reddening that occurs at the end of the nipple may be associated with Paget's disease, and a biopsy is required for diagnosis. Changes in the breast skin color and texture that resemble orange peel (*peau d'orange*) may result from inflammatory breast cancer and require immediate evaluation. Other skin changes associated with inflammatory breast cancer include the presence of pink, purplish, or bruised skin; a pitting or ridging of the skin; and a nipple newly turning inward. **Mondor disease** of the breast is a rare, self-limiting condition characterized by thrombophlebitis of the superficial veins. Symptoms include skin redness, edema, and pain in the affected area. The condition may occur after trauma or appear without apparent cause. Although Mondor disease is usually benign, it may be associated with breast cancer and hypercoagulability (Venes, 2013).

BREAST PAIN (MASTALGIA)

Evaluation of breast pain begins with a comprehensive health history. It is important to inquire about the type of pain and its relationship to menses, the duration, location, impact on activities of daily living, factors that aggravate and alleviate the pain, and other medical problems along with a list of the current medications and use of alternative therapies and/or herbal remedies. The most common type of breast pain occurs cyclically and is associated with the period of time that immediately precedes the onset of menses. It usually begins during the luteal phase of the menstrual cycle, when ovulation occurs and the estrogen-to-progesterone ratio is highest. While the exact etiology is unknown, cyclical breast pain has been linked to hormonal imbalances. The pain, often described as dull and aching, may be experienced in one or both breasts; it may also radiate into the axillary region and arm (Flynn & Tipton, 2011).

In the past, women with cyclical breast pain were counseled to avoid caffeine and other sources of methylxanthines such as coffee, black tea, chocolate, and theophylline and encouraged to use vitamin E and other supplements (e.g., isoflavones, evening primrose oil, ginseng, chasteberry), including diuretics, to minimize or reduce symptoms. Although these strategies may be of varying benefit to some women, to date, research has failed to provide clear evidence that they are effective. Instead, reassurance and support, along with broad lifestyle recommendations, can improve comfort and overall quality of life (ACOG, 2011; Chase et al., 2011; Flynn & Tipton, 2011; Institute for Clinical Systems Improvement [ICSI], 2012; Pearlman & Griffin, 2010; Rosolowich et al., 2006).

Noncyclical breast pain does not vary with menses and is less common than cyclic pain. Usually unilateral and more localized than cyclical pain, the discomfort, frequently described as a sharp, stabbing pain, is generally experienced by older women (40s or 50s) and extends into the postmenopausal years. Although the cause may be related to breast trauma, mastitis, or benign tumors, the cause may never be identified. Inflammatory breast cancer (see later discussion) may produce noncyclical pain (Chase et al., 2011; Flynn & Tipton, 2011).

Extra-mammary pain, the third type of breast pain, describes pain that originates in areas other than the breast, such as musculoskeletal pain, cardiac pain, gastrointestinal pain, and Tietze syndrome (a form of costochondritis of the upper front of the chest). Shingles may also produce pain, which is unilateral and accompanied by the characteristic zoster rash (Chase et al., 2011). Extra-mammary pain is typically treated by managing the underlying cause. In general, breast pain is not associated with breast cancer, although women with breast cancer may complain of a localized tightening or pulling sensation or a localized burning or itching.

Now Can You— Discuss breast abnormalities?

1. Describe the following types of breast masses: fibrocystic changes, fibroadenomas, intraductal papillomas, mammary duct ectasia?
2. Identify and describe four methods for evaluating breast abnormalities?
3. Explain the significance of testing for estrogen and progesterone receptors?

Breast Cancer

RISK FACTORS

Risk factors for breast cancer may be related to demographics, personal health history, lifestyle choices, and defects in certain genes. As is the case with many other diseases, the greater the number of risk factors that are present, the greater the likelihood of developing breast cancer. A listing of specific risk factors is presented in Box 3-1. It is important to note, however, that approximately 70% to 80% of women who develop breast cancer have none of the known risk factors (ACS, 2013). Nurses may assist women in assessing their personal risk for breast cancer with the Breast Cancer Risk Assessment Tool.

Optimizing Outcomes— The Breast Cancer Risk Assessment Tool

The National Cancer Institute (NCI) and the National Surgical Adjuvant Breast and Bowel Project (NSABP) have developed an interactive computer tool to estimate a woman's risk of developing invasive breast cancer. The tool, designed for use by health professionals, has recently been updated for African American women. The tool predicts a woman's risk of breast cancer in 5 years and over the lifetime (to age 90 years). Various risk factors, including present age, number of first-degree relatives affected, age at menarche, age at first live birth, the number of breast biopsies, and a history of abnormal hyperplasia in breast biopsy specimens, are assessed. The tool is available at the Web site http://www.cancer.gov/bcrisktool/ (NCI, 2011).

Demographics and Personal Health History

Advancing age constitutes the single most important risk factor for breast cancer. A woman's risk increases as her age increases. According to the American Cancer Society, approximately one out of eight invasive breast cancer diagnoses are made among women younger than age 45; approximately two out of three women with invasive breast cancer are aged 55 or older when they are diagnosed. Breast cancer is more prevalent in women than in men. In males, breast cancer accounts for only 0.7% of all breast cancer diagnoses (ACS, 2013).

Caucasian women are more likely to develop breast cancer than are African American women. Statistically, however, African American women are more likely to die from their disease than are Caucasian women, and they are also more likely to be diagnosed with higher-grade tumors associated with a poorer prognosis. Reasons for this finding may include an inability to obtain health care or screening mammography, not following up after receiving abnormal test results, distrust of the health-care system, and the belief that mammograms are not needed (USDHHS, 2010). Also, higher-grade tumors may occur more frequently in African American women, even those who receive regular screening. Asian, Hispanic, and Native American women have an overall lower risk of developing and dying from breast cancer (ACS, 2013; CDC, 2012; Silva, 2012).

Cultural Diversity: Chinese American Immigrant Women and Breast Cancer

Through focus group discussions, Lee-Lin, Menon, Nail, and Lutz (2012) explored beliefs of Chinese American immigrant women related to breast cancer and mammography. They found that although the women share beliefs with other minority women in the United States, some culturally related barriers (e.g., alienation owing to cultural reasons for not sharing the diagnosis with others, beliefs about the efficacy of Eastern versus Western medicine) might affect adherence to screening and treatment. It is important that nurses and other primary health-care providers take into account various culturally driven motivations and barriers to mammography adherence among Chinese American immigrant women, and focus interactions to

---

Box 3-1 Risk Factors Associated With Breast Cancer

- Defects in breast cancer gene 1 *(BRCA1)* or breast cancer gene 2 *(BRCA2)*
- Gender: 100 times more likely to occur in females than in males
- Age: Increasing age—two out of three invasive breast cancers occur in women aged 55 and older
- Personal history of breast cancer in at least one breast
- Family history of breast cancer
- Exposure to chest radiation
- Excess weight
- Exposure to estrogen: early onset of menarche, late menopause, or use of hormonal therapy
- Race: Caucasians more likely to develop breast cancer than Hispanics or African Americans
- Smoking
- Exposure to carcinogens
- Excessive use of alcohol
- Diagnosis of precancerous breast changes
- Increased breast density revealed on mammography*
- Exposure to diethylstilbestrol (DES)—mothers and female offspring

Source: American Cancer Society (2013).
* According to a recent study (Gierach et al., 2012), women with high mammographic breast density do not appear at increased risk of dying from breast cancer.

include discussion about breast cancer risks and screening harms and benefits.

Women who currently have or have been previously diagnosed with cancer in one breast have three to four times the risk of developing new cancer in the same or other breast than do their counterparts who have never had breast cancer (ACS, 2013). A history of a family member, especially a mother or sister, who received a diagnosis of breast cancer also increases the risk, especially if the cancer occurred prior to menopause. Interestingly, however, approximately 70% to 80% of women who develop breast cancer do not have a family history of this disease.

Lifestyle-Related Factors

Women who have had no children or who had their first child after age 30 have a slightly increased risk of breast cancer, owing to increased exposure to estrogen. Also, women who use oral contraceptives (OC) have a slightly greater risk of breast cancer than women who never used them. However, after discontinuation of OC use, the risk decreases; approximately 10 years after discontinuing the OC, there is no increased risk of breast cancer. Postmenopausal combined hormone therapy (i.e., estrogen + progestin) is associated with an increased risk of breast cancer; the use of estrogen alone for less than 10 years does not appear to increase the risk. Breastfeeding, especially for 1 to 2 years, appears to slightly reduce the risk for breast cancer (ACS, 2013).

Being overweight or obese increases breast cancer risk, especially for postmenopausal women, and especially if the extra weight has been gained in adulthood and is accumulated at the waist. Following menopause, adipose tissue becomes the primary source of estrogen. Postmenopausal weight loss lowers circulating estrogen levels, and because estrogens are directly related to the risk of breast cancer, it is believed that weight loss may decrease the risk. Regular exercise also appears to reduce breast cancer risk; the American Cancer Society recommends 45 to 60 minutes of intentional physical activity 5 or more days a week (ACS, 2013; Guimond, 2014).

Recent research suggests an inverse relationship between vitamin D deficiency and breast cancer. Vitamin D comprises a group of fat-soluble compounds naturally found in fish-liver oils, fatty fish, mushrooms, egg yolks, and liver. The two physiologically relevant forms of vitamin D are D_2 (ergocalciferol) and D_3 (cholecalciferol). Vitamin D_3 is photosynthesized in the skin by ultraviolet B (UVB) radiation; vitamin D_2 is produced by the UV irradiation of ergosterol (a sterol found in fungi). Active vitamin D, which functions as a hormone, maintains serum calcium and phosphorus concentrations within a normal range by enhancing the efficiency of the small intestine to absorb these minerals from the diet (Bergren & Heuberger, 2010).

Crew and colleagues (2009) examined the association between levels of 25-hydroxyvitamin D (the specific vitamin D metabolite measured in serum) and the incidence of breast cancer. Women with 25-hydroxyvitamin D levels above 40 ng/mL (optimal range is 32.0–100.0 ng/mL) were less likely to develop breast cancer than women with a vitamin D deficiency (25-hydroxyvitamin D levels less than 20 ng/mL). Investigations by other researchers (John, Schwartz, Dreon, & Koo, 1999; McCullough et al., 2005;

Nunez, Carbajal, Belmonte, Moreiras, & Varela, 1996; Shinn et al., 2002) have also provided evidence of an inverse relationship between active vitamin D levels and a risk of breast cancer. Moreover, findings from a meta-analysis conducted by Mohr, Gorham, Kim, Hofflich, and Garland (2014) suggest that breast cancer patients with high serum levels of vitamin D are more likely to survive the disease than patients with low levels. Nurses can educate women about simple strategies to boost vitamin D intake: Consume fatty fish and fortified foods; obtain 15 to 20 minutes of direct sun exposure (without sunscreen) to the face and arms three times a week; and take vitamin D_3 supplements (Bergren & Heuberger, 2010; BreastCancer.org, 2012; Hoffman, 2010).

Family Teaching Guidelines . . .

TOPIC: Tips for Reducing Breast Cancer Risk

Nurses can teach families about simple at-home strategies that may reduce breast cancer risk:

Diet and exercise: Reducing calories and engaging in regular exercise may slow tumor growth and lower the amount of circulating leptin, a fat-released protein that has been linked to breast cancer.

Extra-virgin olive oil: This oil contains polyphenol compounds that suppress a breast cancer-promoting gene.

Apples: Phenols found in apples may combat malignant tumors.

Vitamin D: This vitamin prevents the division of cancer cells and activates a tumor-suppressing protein.

Folate: Consuming foods that contain the B-vitamin folate (e.g., leafy green vegetables, beans, and fortified cereals) may help to mitigate the increased breast cancer risk associated with drinking alcohol.

Soy supplements: Soy contains isoflavones, substances that act like estrogen and may stimulate the growth of certain types of breast cancers. Supplements that contain concentrated amounts of isoflavones should be avoided. However, healthy soy foods such as edamame, soy milk, and tofu are not considered harmful.

Alcohol use increases breast cancer risk, especially for women who drink more than one alcoholic beverage per day. Women who consume two to five alcoholic drinks daily have about one and a half times the risk of women who consume no alcohol. According to the American Cancer Society (2013), women should limit their alcohol consumption to no more than one drink a day. Smoking or secondhand exposure to tobacco smoke as a risk factor for breast cancer is controversial; all women should be counseled to stop smoking and avoid secondhand smoke as a health-promoting strategy (ACS, 2013).

Nursing Insight— *Controversial breast cancer risk factors*

It has been suggested that various factors, including dietary fat, antiperspirants, bras, breast implants, environmental chemicals, abortions, and night work, increase the risk for breast cancer. It is important for nurses to know about these claims so that they can address their patients' concerns and provide appropriate counseling. The dietary intake of fat has not been clearly linked with an increased risk for breast cancer. However, high-fat diets can lead to obesity, which is a breast cancer risk factor. Although one postulate is that the absorption of chemicals in underarm antiperspirants may lead to cancer, there is no evidence to support this theory. Bras, purported to obstruct lymph flow, have also been implicated in the development of breast cancer. However, there is no scientific evidence to support this claim. Although breast implants do not increase breast cancer risk, scar tissue associated with the silicone implants may make mammography interpretation more difficult. According to a recent (2013) systematic review conducted by Lavigne and colleagues, cosmetic breast augmentation adversely affects survival of women who are subsequently given a diagnosis of breast cancer. Presently, there are no data supporting a definite link between breast cancer and environmental chemicals (e.g., DDE [a pesticide]; polychlorinated biphenyls [PCBs]). Neither induced nor spontaneous abortions are related to an increased risk for breast cancer. Some researchers have proposed that, owing to a disruption in the hormone melatonin, there is a link between working at night and breast cancer; this theory is currently undergoing investigation (ACS, 2013; Kaunitz, 2013; Lavigne et al., 2013).

Gene Defects

Approximately 5% to 10% of breast cancer cases are hereditary, resulting from gene defects, or mutations, passed on from a parent. The identification of the BRCA1 and BRCA2 genes was a pivotal discovery that clearly demonstrated the role of heredity and genetic mutations in the development of breast and ovarian cancer. It is estimated that approximately 10% of ovarian cancer cases and 3% to 5% of breast cancer cases are due to genetic mutations in BRCA1 and BRCA2. Hereditary breast and ovarian cancer syndrome is an inherited cancer-susceptibility syndrome (ACOG, 2009; ACS, 2013; Griffin & Pearlman, 2010).

clinical alert

Recognizing hallmarks of hereditary breast and ovarian cancer syndrome

Women of childbearing age who are BRCA-positive are not only at increased risk for hereditary breast and ovarian cancer syndrome; they also have a 50% chance of passing the mutation on to their offspring. When taking the patient history, nurses must be aware of the following indicators of hereditary breast and ovarian cancer syndrome: multiple family members with breast cancer or ovarian cancer or both; the presence of both breast cancer and ovarian cancer in a single individual; and early age of breast cancer onset. Women with these risk factors can be referred for clinical genetic testing for gene mutations. Information gained from the testing allows for the identification of individuals who are at substantial risk of breast cancer and ovarian cancer and the timely institution of screening and prevention strategies to reduce the woman's personal risk (ACOG, 2009; Bingham, 2012; Guimond, 2014).

Approximately 1 in 300 to 1 in 800 individuals in the general population are estimated to carry a mutation in BRCA1 or BRCA2. Normally, BRCA1, located on chromosome 17,

and BRCA2, located on chromosome 13, help to prevent cancer by manufacturing proteins that halt the abnormal growth of cells. However, individuals who inherited a mutated copy of either gene from a parent have an increased risk of developing breast and/or ovarian cancer. For a woman with a BRCA1 mutation, the risk of ovarian cancer is 39% to 46%. For a woman with a BRCA2 mutation, the risk of ovarian cancer is 12% to 20%. The estimated lifetime risk of breast cancer with a BRCA1 or BRCA2 mutation is 65% to 74%. For women with breast cancer, the 10-year actuarial risk of developing subsequent ovarian cancer is 12.7% for BRCA1 mutation carriers and 6.8% for BRCA2 mutation carriers. In the United States, BRCA mutations occur most often in Jewish women of Ashkenazi (Eastern European) origin. In fact, an estimated 1 in 40 Ashkenazi Jews carries a specific "founder mutation" in BRCA1 or BRCA2. Other rare gene mutations, such as ATM, p53, CHEK2, PTEN, and CDH1, are less common causes of inherited breast cancer. Genetic testing to identify mutations in the BRCA and other genes is available; women who seek this testing should be offered counseling to help them make an informed decision (ACOG, 2009; ACS, 2013).

Across Care Settings: Preparing patients for genetic testing

In the United States, genetic testing is available for consenting adults at age 18. Prior to the testing, it is essential that patients be prepared for the various medical, psychological, and social implications that accompany it. For example, patients should understand that a positive test result would most likely prompt recommendations for more frequent and invasive strategies to prevent cancer or to detect it early. The patient and her family should be prepared for long-term psychological implications that can accompany the test results. Concern about genetic discrimination is not unusual, and women should be informed about the federal Genetic Information Nondiscrimination Act of 2008 that protects against health and employment discrimination based on genetic information. However, patients should be aware that life insurance, disability insurance, and long-term care may fall outside the protection of existing laws (Hudson, Holohan, & Collins, 2008; Lebensohn, Kingham, Chun, & Kurian, 2011).

TUMOR TYPES

There are several types of breast cancers. The majority of breast cancers represent a type of adenocarcinoma, which arises from the glandular tissue (i.e., ducts and lobules of the breast). Four subtypes account for most breast cancers. Occasionally, a single breast tumor can have a combination of these types or a mixture of invasive and in situ cancer. The term in situ indicates that the cancer cells remain confined to the ducts (ductal carcinoma in situ) or lobules (lobular carcinoma in situ); they have not penetrated into deeper breast tissues or spread to other organs in the body. Invasive carcinomas have grown beyond the layer of cells where the cancer originated. Most breast cancers are invasive carcinomas—either invasive ductal carcinoma or invasive lobular carcinoma (ACS, 2013).

Ductal Carcinoma In Situ (DCIS) and Lobular Carcinoma In Situ (LCIS)

The most common type of noninvasive breast cancer, ductal carcinoma in situ, is confined within the ducts and has not spread into the surrounding breast tissue. Ductal carcinoma in situ (DCIS) accounts for approximately one in five new breast cancer cases. It is most often detected by mammography and has an excellent cure rate (ACS, 2013). In 2013, a team of scientists convened by the National Cancer Institute proposed a change in the classification of some cancers, and recommended reserving the word *cancer* for lesions with a reasonable likelihood of lethal progression if left untreated. Under the proposed classification, DCIS, which has a low potential for malignancy, would no longer be labeled as a cancer or neoplasia, and the word *cancer* would be removed from the name (National Cancer Institute, 2014).

Lobular carcinoma in situ (LCIS) (sometimes termed "lobular neoplasia") begins in the milk-producing glands and does not penetrate the wall of the lobules. LCIS is not considered a true cancer, although this neoplasm is sometimes classified as a type of noninvasive breast cancer. LCIS is rarely an invasive cancer, but women with this type have a higher risk of developing an invasive breast cancer in the same breast or in the opposite breast (ACS, 2013).

Invasive (Infiltrating) Ductal Carcinoma (IDC)

The most common type of breast cancer, invasive (infiltrating) ductal carcinoma (IDC), originates in a mammary duct, penetrates through the ductal wall, and grows into the fatty tissue of the breast (Fig. 3-7). Metastasis (spread) to other parts of the body may occur through the lymphatic system and bloodstream. Approximately 8 out of 10 invasive breast cancers are infiltrating ductal carcinomas. Women with this type of tumor usually present with a discrete, solitary breast mass (ACS, 2013).

Invasive (Infiltrating) Lobular Carcinoma (ILC)

Invasive (infiltrating) lobular carcinoma (ILC) originates in the lobules (milk-producing glands). Like invasive ductal carcinoma, this neoplasm has spread into the fatty tissue and can metastasize to other parts of the body. Approximately 1 out of 10 invasive breast cancers is an ILC, and women with this type are more likely than those with other cancers to have bilateral disease. ILC may be harder to detect by mammography; breast MRI is often helpful in the diagnosis (ACS, 2013).

Inflammatory Breast Cancer (IBC)

Inflammatory breast cancer (IBC) is a rare neoplasm that tends to grow more quickly and aggressively than the more common types of breast cancers. There is usually no lump or tumor, and the skin often exhibits changes similar to an infectious process such as mastitis. The affected breast may

appear inflamed: red, thickened, tender, itchy, or larger than the unaffected breast. *Peau d'orange*, another characteristic physical finding, is an edematous thickening and pitting of the skin that develops from edema surrounding the hair follicle. Because metastasis has usually occurred by the time of diagnosis, the cure rate is lower with IBC than it is with other types of breast cancers (Nelson, Patel, & Mancuso, 2011).

 Optimizing Outcomes— Teaching about inflammatory breast cancer

Although inflammatory breast cancer is rare, nurses should educate women about the signs and symptoms (ACS, 2013):

* Breast swelling, which is usually sudden with one breast much larger than the other
* Itching
* A pink, red, or dark-colored area, sometimes with a texture like the skin of an orange (*peau d'orange*)
* Ridges and thickened areas of the skin
* Sensation of heat in the breast
* Heaviness or fullness in the breast
* Nipple retraction
* Breast pain, burning, or aching

In the early stages, IBC may be mistaken for infection, resulting in a delay in diagnosis. Also, because there is no defined lump, this neoplasm may not be detected by mammography. Breast ultrasonography may reveal axillary lymphadenopathy and tumors. MRI, which allows for precise measurement of the associated skin changes, is the most sensitive imaging test for IBC. Positron emission tomography (PET) scanning combined with computed tomography (CT) may be used to detect areas of metastasis (lymph nodes and organs) (ACS, 2013). However, skin and tissue biopsies taken from the affected areas of the breast constitute the gold standard for IBC diagnosis (Nelson et al., 2011).

Cultural Diversity: African American Women and Inflammatory Breast Cancer

Inflammatory breast cancer accounts for approximately 1% to 3% of all breast cancers diagnosed in the United States. Symptoms (e.g., redness, increased warmth, changes in the skin texture) that occur with this rare type of breast cancer are related to interference with lymph drainage by the malignant cells. Inflammatory breast cancer tends to occur at a younger age (age 52 versus age 57 for noninflammatory breast cancer), and it is more common among women who are overweight or obese. Also, African American women appear to be at a higher risk than white women (ACS, 2013).

INDICATORS OF DISEASE PROGNOSIS

A number of variables, such as the cancer stage, type, and tumor size; the presence of lymph node involvement (Fig. 3-8); and the presence of hormone receptor levels and HER2/neu (human epidermal growth factor receptor 2) in the tumor tissue, are associated with the likelihood of breast cancer recurrence.

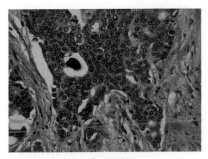

Figure 3-7 Invasive ductal carcinoma.

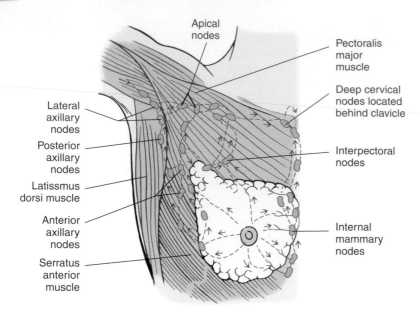

Apical
nodes

Pectoralis
major
muscle

Deep cervical
nodes located
behind clavicle

Lateral
axillary
nodes

Posterior
axillary
nodes

Latissmus
dorsi muscle

Interpectoral
nodes

Anterior
axillary
nodes

Internal
mammary
nodes

Serratus
anterior
muscle

Figure 3-8 Breast cancer: possible paths of lymphatic spread.

Nursing Insight— *Understanding about human epidermal growth factor receptor 2 (HER2/neu)*

Human epidermal growth factor receptor 2 (HER2/neu), a protein involved in normal cell growth, is found on some types of cancer cells, including breast and ovarian. Approximately 20% of breast cancers have an amplification (or overexpression) of the *HER2/neu* gene. Overexpression of this receptor in breast cancer is associated with increased disease recurrence and a worse prognosis. All newly diagnosed breast cancers should be tested for HER2/neu because HER2-positive cancers are more likely to benefit from treatment with medications that specifically target the HER2/neu protein, such as trastuzumab (Herceptin), pertuzumab (Perjeta), and lapatinib (Tykerb) (ACS, 2013; NCI, 2013).

Identification of these factors allows for development of an individualized plan of treatment. The majority of women with negative lymph nodes (approximately 60% of women diagnosed with breast cancer today) will be cured by surgery alone. Approximately 30% of women with breast cancer will develop recurrent disease within 10 years of the initial treatment. In addition to identifying hormone receptor status and the histological tumor type, information concerning the status of the axillary lymph nodes and the overall tumor size is useful in determining the disease prognosis (ACS, 2013).

Axillary Nodes

It has long been recognized that tumor involvement of the axillary nodes is an important indicator for breast cancer prognosis. Clinical assessment of the axillary nodes is associated with a 30% false-positive and false-negative rate. Thus, pathological staging of the patient's lymph nodes is an essential step in the development of the treatment plan. Seventy percent of women with negative nodes survive 10 years following their breast cancer treatment. The disease prognosis worsens as the number of positive lymph nodes increases. Recurrence of breast cancer occurs in approximately 75% of women who have multiple positive nodes (ACS, 2013).

Sentinel node mapping and biopsy target selected lymph nodes to remove for an excisional biopsy. A radioactive tracer (dye) injected into the region of the tumor travels through the lymphatic system to a lymph node. This node, termed the "sentinel node," is the first node that receives lymphatic drainage from the tumor. If no cancer is detected in this node, the patient is able to avoid more extensive lymph node surgery with its accompanying side effects, such as lymphedema (an accumulation of fluid and protein in the extravascular space from trauma to the lymphatic system or supporting structures; results in swelling of the arm) (ACS, 2013).

Tumor Size

There is a direct relationship between the size of the tumor and the risk of recurrence. Prior to the widespread use of mammography, fewer than 8% of women with node-negative breast cancer had tumors that were less than 1 cm in diameter. Tumors of this size are associated with a relative 5-year survival that approaches 99%. Women with tumors that measure 1–3 cm have a relative 5-year survival rate of approximately 91%, and those with tumors that measure greater than 3 cm have a 5-year survival of approximately 85%. Women whose tumors are greater than 3 cm have a breast cancer recurrence rate that exceeds 50% (ACS, 2013).

Cancer Staging System

The stage of cancer is based on the size of the tumor, the number of lymph nodes involved, and whether the cancer has spread. The American Joint Committee on Cancer TNM system is the most commonly used system to describe the stages of breast cancer. The *clinical stage* is based on findings from the physical examination, biopsy, and imaging tests; the *pathological* stage combines these three diagnostic modalities with the results of surgery. Pathological staging, which includes detailed information about the breast mass and adjacent lymph nodes, provides a more accurate description of the tumor.

⑤ Optimizing Outcomes— Staging cancer to guide development of a treatment plan

The TNM staging system classifies cancers based on their T, N, and M stages:

T = Tumor: size and spread within the breast and to nearby organs

N = Nodes: spread to the lymph nodes

M = Metastasis: spread to distant organs

Additional letters or numbers are added after the T, N, and M to provide further details about the tumor, lymph nodes, and metastasis to distant organs, such as the bones, lungs, brain, and liver. Breast cancer stage grouping is a process that combines the T, N, M information to allow for the identification of cancers with similar stages, which are usually treated in a similar way. Stage is delineated in Roman numerals and progresses from Stage I (least advanced) to Stage IV (most advanced); Stage 0 identifies non-invasive cancer (ACS, 2013) (Box 3-2).

Box 3-2 The Breast Cancer Staging System

Stage 0: Ductal carcinoma in situ (DCIS), the earliest form of breast cancer. (Note: Under a new classification system proposed by the National Cancer Institute, DCIS would no longer be labeled as "cancer" or "neoplasia.")

Stage I: The tumor measures 2 cm in diameter or less and there is no involvement of the lymph nodes and no distant metastasis.

Stage II: The tumor measures 2.0 cm in diameter (or less) to 5.0 cm. Depending on the specific findings, the cancer may have spread to the axillary or internal mammary lymph nodes but has not spread to distant sites.

Stage IIIA: One of the following applies:

1. The tumor is not more than 5 cm across and has spread to four to nine axillary lymph nodes, or it has enlarged the internal mammary lymph nodes; no distant metastasis.
2. The tumor is larger than 5 cm across and does not grow into the chest wall or skin. It has spread to one to nine axillary nodes or to internal mammary nodes; no distant metastasis.

Stage IIIB: The tumor has grown into the chest wall or skin and one of the following applies:

1. No spread to the lymph nodes; no distant metastasis.
2. Spread to one to three axillary lymph nodes and/or small amounts of cancer are found in the internal mammary lymph nodes (per sentinel lymph node biopsy); no distant metastasis.
3. Spread to four to nine axillary lymph nodes, or enlargement of the internal mammary lymph nodes; no distant metastasis.

Stage IIIC: The tumor is any size, and one of the following applies:

1. Cancer has spread to 10 or more axillary lymph nodes; no distant metastasis.
2. Cancer has spread to the lymph nodes beneath the clavicle; no distant metastasis.
3. Cancer has spread to the lymph nodes above the clavicle; no distant metastasis.
4. Cancer involves the axillary lymph nodes and there is enlargement of the internal mammary lymph nodes; no distant metastasis.
5. Cancer has spread to four or more axillary lymph nodes, small amounts of cancer are present in the internal mammary lymph nodes (per sentinel lymph node biopsy); no distant metastasis.

Stage IV: The cancer can be any size (any "T"), may or may not have spread to nearby lymph nodes (any "N"). It has metastasized ("M") to distant organs or to distant lymph nodes.

Sources: ACS (2013); National Cancer Institute (2014).

---

⑤ Now Can You— Discuss aspects of breast cancer diagnosis and staging?

1. Identify and describe at least 12 risk factors associated with breast cancer?
2. Describe at least six signs and symptoms associated with inflammatory breast cancer?
3. Explain why the hormone receptor status, tumor type and size, and presence of positive axillary lymph nodes are important indicators for the overall breast cancer prognosis?
4. Explain what is meant by the TNM cancer staging system and why this information is useful?

BREAST CANCER TREATMENT

Medical management of breast cancer is complicated and may require a multitreatment approach, including surgery and adjunctive treatment, such as radiation, chemotherapy, and hormone therapy. The simplest surgical treatment option is a lumpectomy, also referred to as breast conservation therapy (BCT): The lump and an area of surrounding normal tissue are removed. Factors that indicate BCT instead of mastectomy (surgical removal of the breast) include the tumor size, location, number, and patient preference. The lumpectomy is usually followed by radiation treatment to remove any remaining cancerous cells. A partial or segmental mastectomy involves removal of the tumor, the surrounding breast tissue, a portion of the lining of the chest wall, and some of the axillary lymph nodes. This procedure is usually followed with radiation therapy as well. A simple mastectomy involves the removal of all the breast tissue along with the area surrounding the nipple and areola. Radiation, chemotherapy, or hormone therapy may follow this surgical procedure. In a modified radical mastectomy, the entire breast and several axillary lymph nodes are removed, leaving the chest wall intact. Although this procedure makes breast reconstruction easier for the patient, complications including lymphadenopathy and paresthesia are more likely to occur (ACS, 2013; Kentley, 2011).

⑤ Optimizing Outcomes— Counseling women about potential health issues associated with breast cancer treatment

Breast cancer treatment is associated with a myriad of potential gynecological health issues such as fertility (may be compromised from medication and/or surgery; pregnancy after breast cancer is not thought to increase breast cancer recurrence), contraceptive management (options include barrier methods, the copper intrauterine device, and sterilization; all hormonal methods are contraindicated), menopause (hormone-blocking medications may produce menopausal changes such as vasomotor symptoms and urogenital atrophy in premenopausal women), sexual function (patients who undergo chemotherapy are at higher risk of sexual dysfunction), and osteoporosis (in postmenopausal women, treatment with aromatase inhibitors is associated with decreased bone mineral density) (ACOG, 2012a; Chism, 2012; Kim, 2011; Knobf & Visinski, 2012; Minkin, 2012; Trolice, 2012).

When counseling patients about expected side effects from chemotherapy, nurses can reassure them that there are medications available now that are highly effective in reducing nausea and vomiting, the major symptoms traditionally associated with chemotherapy. Other side effects include a change in appetite, loss of hair, mouth or vaginal sores, cognitive disturbances, suppression of the immune system that leads to an increased chance of infection, anemia, fatigue, menstrual cycle changes, and infertility. With the exception of infertility, most of the side effects are temporary.

Many women choose to undergo breast reconstruction after a mastectomy. This surgical option, performed by a plastic surgeon, is a personal decision that requires considerable individualized counseling and education. Because the reconstruction can be performed at the same time as the mastectomy, it is important to consider the options early. Breast reconstruction methods include use of a synthetic breast implant or reconstruction using one's own tissue. Synthetic implants typically are composed of a silicone shell filled with a saline solution. A tissue expander may be needed to cover the implant. To accomplish tissue expansion, an empty implant shell is placed under the skin and muscles and is gradually filled with the saline solution over several months. Once the skin is stretched sufficiently, the expander is removed and replaced with a permanent implant. Recovery usually takes several weeks.

Women who choose to undergo breast reconstruction using their own tissue may have a transverse rectus abdominis myocutaneous (TRAM) flap procedure. The breast is reconstructed using fat and muscle tissue taken from the abdomen, back, and buttocks. Recovery following the procedure usually takes 6 to 8 weeks, and there is an increased risk of infection and tissue necrosis. Deep inferior epigastric perforator (DIEP) reconstruction is a slightly less complicated surgical procedure. This method is similar to the TRAM flap procedure, but the abdominal muscles are left intact. The DIEP procedure is associated with fewer complications and less postoperative pain. Following reconstruction of the breast tissue, the surgeon can reconstruct the nipple and areola using tissue from other areas of the body. A small mound is constructed to resemble a nipple, and tattooing may be used to create an areola. In this situation, the surgeon applies a skin graft to the areolar region, slightly raises the skin, and then tattoos the skin graft.

Adjuvant therapies may include radiation therapy, chemotherapy, or hormone-blocking therapy. Radiation is usually begun 3 to 4 weeks after surgery, and treatments are given 5 days per week for 5 to 6 weeks. Chemotherapy that includes a combination of two or more drugs may also be prescribed. Chemotherapeutics may be administered orally or intravenously and usually require four to eight treatments over 3 to 6 months. Hormone-blocking therapy is most commonly used to treat advanced metastatic cancer or as an adjuvant treatment to prevent recurrence of cancer. Normally, estrogen and progesterone bind to receptor sites in the breast tissue and encourage growth of cancerous cells. Prescribed hormone medications bind to the sites instead and prevent estrogen from reaching them. Medications used in hormone-blocking treatment include tamoxifen (Nolvadex), a selective estrogen receptor modulator (SERM), and aromatase inhibitors, which block the conversion of androgens into estrogen.

Nursing Insight— *Anti-angiogenesis therapy for cancer treatment*

Angiogenesis, which comes from the Greek words *angio* ("making new blood vessels") and *genesis* ("beginning"), is the process of making new blood vessels. Anti-angiogenesis is a targeted therapy that uses drugs or other substances to halt the tumor's production of new blood vessels. New anti-angiogenesis drugs that may prove useful in the treatment of breast cancer are currently under development and investigation (ACS, 2013).

Optimizing Outcomes— **Using genomics to guide breast cancer care**

Genomic medicine encompasses the disciplines of gene mapping and sequencing and the study of the functions and interactions of all genes in the genome (a complete copy of the genetic material in an organism). Genomics focuses on developing tests that are both prognostic (i.e., based on factors such as tumor size, lymph node involvement, hormone receptor status) and predictive. *Prognostic* testing identifies the likelihood of cancer recurrence; *predictive* testing identifies the relative resistance of a cancer to specific treatments. Breast cancer specialists use information from genomics-driven specialized tests (e.g., Mammoprint; Oncotype DX; HOXB13/IL17BR) to develop an individualized treatment approach based on recurrence risk and predicted benefits of specific therapies.

NURSING CARE FOR WOMEN DEALING WITH BREAST CANCER

Nurses must be sensitive to the fact that once a woman has received a diagnosis of breast cancer, her life is forever changed. Compassionate care during this difficult time includes providing emotional support; empowering the patient and her family with current, evidence-based information; assisting them with immediate needs; and directing them to available resources. Personal and professional resources are essential as the woman works her way through the diagnostic process, the necessary decision making concerning treatment and possible breast reconstruction, the surgery and adjuvant therapies, and the future with its uncertainties. Women who are confronted with breast cancer frequently discover an inner strength that they did not know existed. Examples of appropriate nursing diagnoses for women who have received a diagnosis of breast cancer are listed in Box 3-3.

Nursing Insight— *Breast cancer in women desirous of childbearing*

Both alkylating chemotherapeutic agents and selective estrogen receptor modulating agents are routinely used in treatment for premenopausal women with invasive breast cancer. Unfortunately, these medications can exert profound effects on ovarian hormonal function and fertility. Nurses should ensure that women who desire future childbearing receive detailed information about the impact of breast cancer treatment on fertility and fully understand options for fertility preservation prior to initiating treatment (Howard-Anderson, Ganz, Bower, & Stanton, 2012; Pearlman & Miller, 2013; Trolice, 2012).

Nurses can be a tremendous source of support and advocacy for women who are diagnosed with breast cancer. It is important to encourage patients to carefully consider all options and seek other opinions or other providers if they do not feel comfortable with recommendations. Nurses can direct women to the wealth of reliable information about breast cancer treatment and recovery available in books and on Internet sites and to the opportunities for personal sharing through local and national support groups.

Collaboration in Caring— *Resources for women with cancer*

An important nursing role in the care of women with cancer centers on sharing information about the various resources that are available to them. These include:

- National Breast and Cervical Cancer Early Detection Program, NCCDPHP, CDC
- National Cancer Institute, NIH, HHS
- Office of Minority Health, OPHS, OS, HHS
- American Cancer Society
- Cancer.net
- BreastCancerTrials.org
- Celebrating Life Foundation
- Sisters Network Inc.
- Susan G. Komen
- LiveStrong Cancer Survivorship Center
- NCI Community Cancer Centers Program
- National Coalition for Cancer Survivorship
- Living Beyond Breast Cancer

In 2013, Living Beyond Breast Cancer (LBBC) and the Metastatic Breast Cancer Network (MBCN) released a free publication, *The Metastatic Breast Cancer Series: Guide for the Newly Diagnosed*, to address the needs of women in the first few months after receiving a diagnosis of metastatic (Stage IV) breast cancer. The publication is designed to help women make the best and most informed decisions for themselves and their families when facing a breast cancer diagnosis and when considering various options for treatment. Additional information is available at

http://www.lbbc.org/Understanding-Breast-Cancer/Guides-to-Understanding-Breast-Cancer/Metastatic-Breast-Cancer-Series-Guide-for-the-Newly-Diagnosed.

For many, holistic medicine offers an additional healing approach to assist the body, mind, and spirit through the rigors of cancer diagnosis and treatment and to foster healing throughout the recovery process. The woman's immune system can be supported and enhanced naturally through dietary and safe herbal remedies, along with practices that reduce stress and help restore physical and emotional harmony and balance. For example, patients may benefit from imagery, aromatherapy, meditation, music therapy, dance therapy, journal writing, humor, art therapy, and hypnosis. Other modalities such as acupuncture, Ayurveda, Qigong, yoga, and tai chi may provide relief from unpleasant symptoms and be instrumental in lifting the body and spirit during the journey to recovery.

Complementary Care: *CAM for cancer patients*

Many women find that various complementary and alternative medicine (CAM) therapies help to relieve cancer side effects and discomforts and enhance and enrich their lives during treatment and into recovery. Nurses can empower women with specific information and direct them to available resources. The American Cancer Society provides an up-to-date Internet source for complementary and alternative therapies. It is available at http://www.cancer.org/cancer/breastcancer/detailedguide/breast-cancer-treating-c-a-m.

An increasing number of studies have demonstrated the value of exercise in enhancing certain outcome variables (e.g., cardiovascular fitness, fatigue, nausea, malnutrition, preservation of lean body mass, immune system functioning) and quality of life among cancer survivors (Mohr & Whyte, 2013). *Strength & Courage: Exercises for Breast Cancer Survivors*, available as a traditional DVD or as a digital download (can be viewed on tablets and smartphones), is a home-based exercise program specially designed to help breast cancer survivors regain strength and mobility during and following breast cancer treatment. At the same time, the program strives to enhance a woman's ability to lead an active life after breast cancer surgery. The exercises, which can be started as soon as 1 day after surgery, focus on increasing muscle strength and flexibility and range of motion, which can help reduce fatigue during and after treatment. Information about the program and DVD/digital download is available at http://www.strengthandcourage.net/.

Today, there are an estimated 13.7 million cancer survivors living in the United States, and that number will grow to almost 18 million by 2022. Nurses who care for women across the life span are likely to see patients who are dealing with the psychosocial and physical effects of cancer treatments, which may occur for months or years after the treatment has ended. Development of a cancer survivorship care plan can help to ensure coordination of care and appropriate follow-up and empower the woman to understand and participate in her continuing care. Cancer survivorship care plans have been recommended by a variety of groups, including the Institute of Medicine (IOM), which, along with the National Research Council, produced a major report on cancer survivorship in 2006 (ACS and the National Cancer Data Base, 2012).

Optimizing Outcomes— With a cancer survivorship care plan

First introduced for survivors of childhood cancers, cancer survivorship care plans have recently been recommended for adult survivors. Components of the survivorship plan, which should be provided to the patient's primary care physician, include a summary of treatment, the possible short- and long-term effects of treatment, late toxicity monitoring, monitoring for primary cancer recurrence or a second cancer, identification of the provider responsible for survivor care, psychological and vocational needs, community support resources, and recommendations for preventive care and practices. For women, additional information should include genetic issues, the effects of treatment on future pregnancy and fertility, and menopausal issues.

Nurses are perfectly situated to provide cancer survivor care. With a holistic and family-centered approach that emphasizes patient education, health promotion, and preventive care practices, nursing can fully embrace the cancer survivorship movement to empower women and their providers with a comprehensive, holistic plan for continuing care in the aftermath of cancer. Owing to the dynamic nature of the survivorship plan, evolving scientific evidence about the specific cancer type, management of short- and long-term treatment sequelae, and the need for screening for recurrence and other cancers can be readily incorporated into the plan. This information can help to inform the woman's decision making and allow her and her care provider to be proactive in both the planning and management of her health after cancer (Knobf & Visinski, 2012; Ruhl, 2009; Zalewski, Beikman, Ferrari, Slavish, & Rosenzweig, 2010).

? Global Health Case Study Eduedima T.

Breast Cancer

Eduedima T. is a 56-year-old postmenopausal Nigerian woman who received a diagnosis of early-stage breast cancer approximately 6 months ago. Eduedima's treatment, which included a lumpectomy followed by radiation therapy, was uncomplicated and her physician has told her that her chance for a cure is "excellent."

Today, during an interview at the woman's health clinic, Eduedima confides in the nurse that she is concerned about herself because she feels "down and out." She admits that physically, she feels just fine and is very relieved to have the treatment behind her. Lately, however, she has been concerned about "the way my body looks." As a result of the surgery and radiation therapy, Eduedima has experienced a decrease in breast size in the affected breast. Although she acknowledges that "in the grand scheme of things, this change is a minor thing," the alteration in breast appearance is concerning to her.

critical thinking questions

1. What is a priority nursing intervention for Eduedima?

2. What information should the nurse provide to Eduedima?

3. What other actions should the nurse take?

◆ See suggested answers to case studies on DavisPlus.

Now Can You— Discuss aspects of breast cancer treatment?

1. Identify four treatment modalities for breast cancer?
2. Describe the nurse's role in breast cancer treatment care?
3. Identify the components of a cancer survivorship care plan and explain why this information is useful?

Summary Points

◆ Maintaining breast health is an essential strategy for maintaining optimal physical and psychological health.

◆ Nurses are in an ideal position to educate women about breast health and strategies for the identification of benign and malignant breast disease.

◆ Breast cancer is the most common cancer in women in the United States, except for skin cancer, and it is the second leading cause of cancer deaths in women.

◆ Dietary, socioeconomic, and environmental factors most likely contribute to the development of breast cancer.

◆ A number of screening and diagnostic methods, including mammography, ultrasonography, magnetic resonance imaging, and biopsy, may be used in the clinical evaluation of the breasts.

◆ Risk factors for breast cancer may be related to demographics, personal health history, lifestyle choices, and defects in certain genes.

◆ The cancer staging system, based on the size of the tumor, the number of lymph nodes involved, and the presence of metastasis, is used to guide the development of a treatment plan for breast cancer.

◆ Breast cancer treatment may include surgery, radiation, chemotherapy, hormone therapy, and complementary and alternative therapies.

◆ The nursing role in caring for women with breast cancer includes providing emotional support, empowering the patient and her family with current information, assisting them with immediate needs, and directing them to available resources.

Review Questions

Multiple Choice

1. When teaching women how to perform proper breast self-examination (BSE), the nurse advises:
   A. Avoid the axillary area
   B. Refrain from squeezing the nipples
   C. Place the arm adjacent to the breast being examined in a relaxed position alongside the thigh
   D. Use the finger pads to apply light, medium, and firm pressure

2. Breast magnetic resonance imaging (MRI) is useful in screening:
   A. Women with recently diagnosed breast cancer
   B. Postmenopausal women
   C. All women
   D. Women whose screening mammograms are satisfactory

3. Ultrasound can reveal whether a breast mass is:
A. Malignant
B. Benign
C. Fluid-filled or solid
D. Potentially malignant

4. Known risk factors for breast cancer include:
A. Slender body type
B. Pregnancy before the age of 20
C. Age greater than 50
D. Menopause before the age of 50

5. Treatment for breast cancer may include:
A. Estrogen therapy
B. Anti-angiogenesis drugs
C. Lactation suppressants
D. Oral contraceptives

REFERENCES

Aliotta, H.M., & Schaeffer, N.J. (2011). Breast conditions. In K.D. Schuiling & F.E. Likis, (Eds.), *Women's gynecologic health* (2nd ed., pp. 377–403). Sudbury, MA: Jones & Bartlett Learning.

Allen, T.L., Van Groningen, B.J., Barksdale, D.J., & McCarthy, R. (2010). The breast self-examination controversy: What providers and patients should know. *The Journal for Nurse Practitioners—JNP, 6*(6), 444–451.

American Cancer Society (ACS). (2013). *Breast cancer overview.* Retrieved from http://www.cancer.org/cancer/breastcancer/overviewguide/breast-cancer-overview-key-statistics

American Cancer Society and the National Cancer Data Base. (2012). *Cancer treatment and survivorship facts & figures 2012–2013.* Retrieved from http://www.cancer.org/research/cancerfactsfigures/cancertreatment survivorshipfactsfigures/index

American College of Obstetricians and Gynecologists (ACOG). (2009). Hereditary breast and ovarian cancer syndrome. Practice Bulletin No. 103. *Obstetrics and Gynecology, 113*(4), 957–966.

American College of Obstetricians and Gynecologists (ACOG). (2011). Breast cancer screening. (Practice Bulletin No. 122). *Obstetrics and Gynecology, 118*(8), 372–382.

American College of Obstetricians and Gynecologists (ACOG). (2012a). Management of gynecologic issues in women with breast cancer. Practice Bulletin No. 126. *Obstetrics & Gynecology, 119*(3), 666–682.

American College of Obstetricians and Gynecologists (ACOG). (2012b). Well woman visit. Committee Opinion No. 534. *Obstetrics & Gynecology, 120*(8), 421–424.

American College of Obstetricians and Gynecologists (ACOG). (2013). Digital breast tomosynthesis. (Technology Assessment No. 9). *Obstetrics and Gynecology, 121*(6), 1415–1417.

American College of Obstetricians and Gynecologists (ACOG). (2014). Management of women with dense breasts diagnosed by mammography. Committee Opinion No. 593. *Obstetrics & Gynecology, 123*(4), 910–911.

Are You Dense Advocacy. (2014). About D.E.N.S.E. Retrieved from http://Areyoudenseadvocacy.org/

Association of Women's Health, Obstetric & Neonatal Nursing (AWHONN). (2010). Position Statement: Breast cancer screening. *Journal of Obstetric, Gynecologic & Neonatal Nursing, 39*(5), 608–610. doi:10.1111/j.1552-6909.2010.01177.x

Barr, J.K., Giannotti, T.E., Van Hoof, T.J., Mongoven, J., & Curry, M. (2008). Understanding barriers to participation in mammography by women with disabilities. *American Journal of Health Promotion, 22*(6), 381–385.

Bergren, T., & Heuberger, R. (2010). Vitamin D and breast cancer prevention. *Nursing for Women's Health, 14*(5), 368–375. doi:10.1111/j.1751-486X.2010.01575.x

Bingham, R. (2012). Hereditary breast and ovarian cancer. *Nursing for Women's Health, 16*(4), 319–324. doi:10.1111/j.1751-486X.2012.01750.x

Bleyer, A., & Welch, H.G. (2012). Effect of three decades of screening mammography on breast-cancer incidence. *New England Journal of Medicine, 367*(21), 1998–2005. doi:1056/NEJMoa1206809

BreastCancer.org. (2012). *U.S. breast cancer statistics.* Retrieved from http://www.breastcancer.org/symptoms/understand_bc/statistics

Buzek, N. (2010). Mobile mammography for underserved women. *Advance for Nurse Practitioners, 18*(5), 29–32.

Centers for Disease Control and Prevention (CDC). (2012). *Breast cancer rates by race and ethnicity.* Retrieved from http://www.cdc.gov/cancer/breast/statistics/race.htm

Centers for Disease Control and Prevention (CDC), Office of Minority Health & Health Disparities. (2010). *Native Hawaiian & Other Pacific Islander Populations (NHOPI).* Retrieved from http://www.cdc.gov/omhd/Populations/NHOPI/NHOPI.htm

Champion, V.L., & Scott, C.R. (1997). Reliability and validity of breast cancer screening belief scales in African American women. *Nursing Research, 40*(4), 331–337.

Chase, C., Wells, J., & Eley, S. (2011). Caffeine and breast pain: Revisiting the connection. *Nursing for Women's Health, 15*(4), 286–294. doi:10.1111/j.1751-486X.2011.01649.x

Chism, L. (2012). Breast cancer and menopause. *Advance for NPs & PAs, 3*(10), 21–25.

Cibulka, N. (2011). Update on breast cancer screening. *The Journal for Nurse Practitioners—JNP, 7*(1), 67–68. doi:10.1016/j.nurpra.2010.10.001

Crew, K.D., Gammon, M.D., Steck, S.E., Hershman, D.L., Cremers, S., & Dworakowski, E., et al. (2009). Association between plasma 25-hydroxyvitamin D and breast cancer risk. *Cancer Prevention Research, 2*(6), 598–604.

Fang, S., & Shu, B. (2009). Adherence characteristics after abnormal screening results between mammogram and Papanicolaou test groups. *Cancer Nursing, 32*(6), 437–444.

Farmer, D., Reddick, B., D'Agostino, R., Jr., & Jackson, S.A. (2007). Correlates of mammography screening in older African American women. *Oncology Nursing Forum, 34*(1), 117–123.

Feldstein, A.C., Perrin, N., Rosales, A.G., Schneider, J., Rixx, M., & Glasgow, R. (2011). Patient barriers to mammography identified during a reminder program. *Journal of Women's Health, 20*(3), 421–428. doi:10.1089/jwh2010.2195

Flynn, G.B., & Tipton, C. (2011). An algorithm for managing breast pain. *The Clinical Advisor, 14*(10), 47–54.

Freimanis, R.I., & Yacobozzi, M. (2014). Breast cancer screening. *North Carolina Medical Journal, 75*(2), 117–120.

Gierach, G., Ichikawa, L., Kerlikowske, K., Brinton, L., Farhat, G., Vacek, P., . . . Sherman, M. (2012). Relationship between mammographic density and breast cancer death in the Breast Cancer Surveillance Consortium. *Journal of the National Cancer Institute, 104*(16), 1218–1227.

Griffin, J.L., & Pearlman, M.D. (2010). Breast cancer screening in women at average risk and high risk. *Obstetrics & Gynecology, 116*(6), 1410–1421.

Guimond, M.E. (2014). Confronting confirmation bias about breast cancer screening with the Four C's. *Nursing for Women's Health, 18*(1), 29–37. doi:10.1111/1751-486X.12091

Gulian, H.J. (2012). Pairing up: Shared decision making in cancer screening. *Advance for NPs & PAs, 3*(1), 19–23.

Hale, P.J., & deValpine, M.G. (2014). Screening mammography: Revisiting assumptions about early detection. *The Journal for Nurse Practitioners, 10*(3), 183–188. doi:dx.doi.org/10.1016/j.nurpra.2013.11.001

Ho, R., Muraoka, M., Cuaresma, C., Guerrero, R., & Agbayani, A. (2010). Addressing the excess breast cancer mortality in Filipino women in Hawai'i through AANCART, an NIC community network program. *Hawaii Medical Journal, 69*(7), 164–166.

Hoffman, R.L. (2010). What lies behind the vitamin D revolution? *The Clinical Advisor, 13*(3), 31–37.

Howard-Anderson, J., Ganz, P., Bower, J., & Stanton, A. (2012). Quality of life, fertility concerns, and behavioral health outcomes in younger breast cancer survivors: A systematic review. *Journal of the National Cancer Institute, 104*(5), 1386–1405.

Hudson, K.L., Holohan, M.K., & Collins, F.S. (2008). Keeping pace with the times—the Genetic Information Nondiscrimination Act of 2008. *New England Journal of Medicine, 358*(25), 2661–2663.

Institute for Clinical Systems Improvement. (2012). *Health care guideline: Diagnosis of breast disease* (14th ed., pp. 1–45). Retrieved from https://www.icsi.org/_asset/v9l91q/DxBrDis-Interactive0112.pdf

John, E.M., Schwartz, G.G., Dreon, D.M., & Koo, J. (1999). Vitamin D and breast cancer risk: The NHANES I epidemiologic follow up study, 1971–1975 to 1992. National Health and Nutrition Examination Survey. *Cancer Epidemiology Biomarkers and Prevention, 8*(5), 399–406.

Jolivet, R.R. (2010). Current resources for evidence based practice, March/April 2010. *Journal of Obstetric, Gynecologic & Neonatal Nursing, 39*(2), 199–200. doi:10.1111/j.1552-6909.2010.01107.x

Kang, H.S., Thomas, E., Kwon, B.E., Hyun, M.S., & Jun, E.M. (2008). Stages of change: Korean women's attitudes and barriers toward mammography screening. *Health Care for Women International*, 29(2), 151–164.

Kaunitz, A.M. (2013). Do cosmetic breast implants hinder the detection of malignancy and reduce breast cancer-specific survival? *OBG Management*, 25(7), 64–65.

Kelleher, K. (2010). Pink ribbons and beyond. *Nursing for Women's Health*, 14(5), 409–412.

Kentley, D. (2011). Early-stage breast cancer treatment. *The Clinical Advisor*, 14(4), 80–88.

Kim, J.H., & Kim, O. (2008). Predictors of perceived barriers to mammography in Korean women. *Asian Nursing Research*, 2(2), 74–81.

Kim, S.S. (2011). Preserving fertility in patients who have cancer. *Contemporary OB/GYN*, 56(5), 48–60.

Knobf, M.T., & Visinski, S. (2012). Managing bone health in breast cancer survivors. *The American Journal for Nurse Practitioners*, 16(7/8), 6–11.

Kosir, M.A., Chism, L., Bland, K., Choi, L., Gorski, D., & Simon, M.S. (2013). Common breast symptoms: When to refer to a breast surgeon. *Advance for NPs & PAs*, 4(10), 12–16.

Lavigne, Holowaty, E.J., Pan, S.Y., Villeneuve, P.J., Johnson, K.C., Fergusson, D.A., . . . Brisson, J. (2013). Breast cancer detection and survival among women with cosmetic breast implants: Systematic review and meta-analysis of observational studies. *British Medical Journal*, 346:f2399. doi:10.1136/bmj.f2399

Lebensohn, A., Kingham, K.E., Chun, N.M., & Kurian, A.W. (2011). Hereditary cancer: Counseling women at risk. *Contemporary OB-GYN*, 56(4), 30–40.

Lee-Lin, F., Menon, U., Nail, L., & Lutz, K.F. (2012). Findings from focus groups indicating what Chinese American immigrant women think about breast cancer and breast cancer screening. *Journal of Obstetric, Gynecologic, & Neonatal Nursing*, 41(5), 627–637. doi:10.1111/j.1552-6909.2012.01348.x

Lowe, N.K. (2010). What's a woman to do about the new breast and cervical cancer screening recommendations? *Journal of Obstetric, Gynecologic & Neonatal Nursing*, 39(2), 133–134. doi:10.1111/j.1552-6909.2010.01099.x

Makuc, D.M., Breen, N., Meissner, H.I., Vernon, S.W., & Cohen, A. (2007). Financial barriers to mammography: Who pays out-of-pocket? *Journal of Women's Health*, 16(3), 349–360.

Mark, K., Temkin, S., & Terplan, M. (2014). Breast self-awareness: The evidence behind the euphemism. *Obstetrics & Gynecology*, 123(4), 734–746. doi:10.1097/AOG.0000000000000139

McCullough, M.L., Rodriguez, C., Diver, W.R., Feigelson, H.S., Stevens, V.L., & Thun, M.J. (2005). Dairy, calcium, and vitamin D intake and postmenopausal breast cancer risk in the Cancer Prevention Study II Nutrition Cohort. *Cancer Epidemiology, Biomarkers and Prevention*, 14(12), 2898–2904.

Minkin, M.J. (2012). Quality of life for breast cancer survivors. *The Female Patient*, 37(4), 37–42.

Mohr, C.R., & Whyte, J. (2013). The role of exercise for patients with cancer. *Consultant*, 53(5), 363–366.

Mohr, S., Gorham, E., Kim, J., Hofflich, H., & Garland, C. (2014). Meta-analysis of vitamin D sufficiency for improving survival of patients with breast cancer. *Anticancer Research*, 34(3), 1163–1166.

Moorhead, S., Johnson, M., Maas, M. L., & Swanson, E. (2013). *Nursing outcomes classification (NOC)* (5th ed.). St. Louis, MO: Elsevier Mosby.

Mounga, V., & Maughan, E. (2012). Breast cancer in Pacific Islander women. *Nursing for Women's Health*, 16(1), 24–35. doi:10.1111/j.1751-486X.2012.01697.x

National Cancer Institute. (2011). *Breast Cancer Risk Assessment Tool*. Retrieved from http://www.cancer.gov/bcrisktool/

National Cancer Institute. (2014). Ductal carcinoma in situ. Retrieved from http://www.cancer.gov/cancertopics/pdq/treatment/breast/health professional/page4

National Cancer Institute. (2012). *Mammograms*. Retrieved from http://m.cancer.gov/topics/factsheets/mammograms

National Cancer Institute. (2013). *Targeted therapies for breast cancer tutorial*. Retrieved from http://www.cancer.gov/cancertopics/understandingcancer/targetedtherapies/breastcancer_htmlcourse/page2

National Comprehensive Cancer Network. (2013). *Breast screening*. Retrieved from http://www.nccn.org/professionals/physician_gls/f_guidelines.asp

Nelson, H.D., Tyne, K., Naik, A., Bougatsos, C., Chan, B., Nygren, P., & Humphrey, L. (2009). *Screening for breast cancer: Systematic evidence review update for the U.S. Preventive Services Task Force* (Evidence Syntheses, No. 74). Rockville, MD: Agency for Healthcare Research and Quality.

Nelson, J.A., Patel, D., & Mancuso, P. (2011). Inflammatory breast cancer. *Advance for NPs & PAs*, 2(10), 25–28.

Nunez, C., Carbajal, A., Belmonte, S., Moreiras, O., & Varela, G. (1996). A case control study of the relationship between diet and breast cancer in a sample from 3 Spanish hospital populations. Effects of food, energy and nutrient intake. *Revista Clinica Espanola*, 196(2), 75–81.

Pearlman, M.D. (2014). Separating the baby from the bath water: Breast self-awareness and breast self-examination. *Obstetrics & Gynecology*, 123(4), 731–732.

Pearlman, M.D., & Griffin, J.L. (2010). Benign breast disease. *Obstetrics & Gynecology*, 116(3), 747–758.

Pearlman, M.D., & Griffin, J.L. (2013). Breast health. *OBG Management*, 25(3), 35–41.

Phillips, J., & Cohen, M.Z. (2011). The meaning of breast cancer risk for African American women. *Journal of Nursing Scholarship*, 43(3), 239–247.

Registe, M., & Porterfield, S.P. (2012). Health beliefs of African American women on breast self-exam. *The Journal for Nurse Practitioners—JNP*, 8(6), 446–451. doi:http://dx.doi.org/10.1016/j.nurpra.2011.09/025

Rosolowich, V., Saettler, E., & Szuck, B. (2006). *SOGC clinical guideline: Mastalgia*. Ottawa, Ontario, Canada: Society of Obstetricians and Gynaecologists of Canada. Retrieved from http://www.sogc.org/guidelines/public/170E-CPG-January2006.pdf

Ruhl, C. (2009). Cancer survivor care planning: A dynamic approach to cancer survivors' futures. *Nursing for Women's Health*, 13(5), 427–431.

Schonberg, M. (2010). Breast cancer screening: At what age to stop? *Consultant*, 50(5), 196–205.

Schonberg, M., Breslau, E., & McCarthy, E. (2013). Targeting of mammography screening according to life expectancy in women aged 75 and older. *Journal of the American Geriatrics Society*, 51(3), 388–395. doi:10.1111/jgs.12123

Shinn, M.H., Holmes, M.D., Hankinson, S.E., Wu, K., Colditz, G.A., & Willett, W.C. (2002). Intake of dairy products, calcium, and vitamin D and risk of breast cancer. *Journal of the National Cancer Institute*, 94(17), 1301–1311.

Silva, A. (2012, October 28). *Minority women and higher-grade breast cancer tumors*. Paper presented at the fifth AACR Conference on the Science of Cancer Health Disparities in Racial/Ethnic Minorities and the Medically Underserved, San Diego, CA.

Somerall, D.W. (2013). Screening for breast and cervical cancer: Understanding the different recommendations. *Nursing for Women's Health*, 17(4), 331–335. doi:10.1111/1751-486X.12052

Susan G. Komen for the Cure. (2012). *Racial & ethnic differences: Breast cancer differences*. Retrieved from http://ww5.komen.org/uploaded-Files/Content_Binaries/806-373a.pdf

Susan G. Komen for the Cure. (2013). *Clinical breast exam*. Retrieved from http://ww5.komen.org/BreastCancer/ClinicalBreastExam.html

Trolice, M.P. (2012). Preservation of fertility in patients receiving radiation and chemotherapy. *The Female Patient*, 37(9), 32–36.

U.S. Department of Health & Human Services (USDHHS). (2010). *Minority women's health: Breast cancer*. Retrieved from http://womenshealth.gov/minority-health/african-americans/breast-cancer.cfm

U.S. Department of Health and Human Services (USDHHS). (2011). *Healthy People 2020*. Retrieved from http://www.healthypeople.gov/2020/topicsobjectives2020/default.aspx

U.S. Food and Drug Administration. (2012). *FDA approves first breast ultrasound imaging system for dense breast tissue*. Retrieved from http://www.fda.gov/NewsEvents/Newsroom/PressAnnouncements/ucm319867.htm

U.S. Preventive Services Task Force (USPSTF). (2009a). *Screening for breast cancer. Guide to preventive services, 2009, Section 2. Recommendations for adults*. Retrieved from http://www.uspreventiveservicestaskforce.org/uspstf/uspsbrca.htm

U.S. Preventive Services Task Force (USPSTF). (2009b). Screening for breast cancer: U.S. Preventive Services Task Force recommendation statement. *Annals of Internal Medicine*, 151(10), 716–726.

Venes, D. (Ed.). (2013). *Taber's cyclopedic medical dictionary* (22nd ed.). Philadelphia, PA: F.A. Davis.

Wang, J.H., Mandelblatt, J.S., Liang, W., Yi, B., Ma, I-Jung, & Schwartz, M.D. (2009). Knowledge, cultural, and attitudinal barriers to mammography screening among nonadherent immigrant Chinese women. *Cancer*, 15(20), 4828–4838.

Wu, T., & Bancroft, J. (2006). Filipino American women's perceptions and experiences with breast cancer screening. *Oncology Nursing Forum*, 33(4),71–78. doi:10.1188/06.ONF.E71-E78

Yankaskas, B.B., Haneuse, S., Kapp, J., Kerlikowske, K., Geller, B., & Buist, D. (2010). Performance of first mammography examination in women younger than 40 years. *Journal of the National Cancer Institute, 102*(10), 692–701. doi:10.1093/jnci/djq090

Yates, J. (2014). Does screening mammography save lives? *OBG Management, 26*(4), 62–72.

Zalewski, M.A., Beikman, S., Ferrari, S., Slavish, K., & Rosenzweig, M. (2010). Breast cancer follow-up: Strategies for successful collaboration between cancer care specialists and primary care providers. *The Journal for Nurse Practitioners—JNP, 6*(6), 452–463.

 DavisPlus | For more information, go to **http://www.davisplus.fadavis.com/.**

CONCEPT MAP

Cysts:
- Fibrocystic: fluid-filled
- Fibroadenoma: solid
- Lipoma
- Intraductal papilloma: wart-like growth

Mammary duct ectasia:
- Inflammation of ducts behind nipple

Mastitis:
- Infection of the breast

Breast trauma → results in hematoma formation or fat necrosis

Benign Breast Masses

Promoting Breast Health

Breast Cancer

Risk Factors:
- Advanced age
- Being Caucasian
- Previous or current cancer in one breast
- Family history; especially mother or sister
- No children; first child after age 30
- Use of oral contraceptives
- Postmenopausal combined hormone therapy
- Obesity
- Having more than one alcoholic drink per day
- Genetic defects/mutation in BRCA1 and BRCA2

Types of Breast Cancer:
("In situ"= confined to ducts or lobules; no spread)
- Ductal carcinoma in situ
- Lobular carcinoma in situ
- Invasive ductal carcinoma
- Invasive lobular carcinoma
Inflammatory breast cancer
  - Rare; grows quickly and aggressively
  - No lump or tumor
  - Mimics an infection
- **Invasive carcinoma**

Multitreatment Approach:
- Surgery
- Radiation
- Chemotherapy
- Hormone therapy
- Reconstructive surgery

Clinical Alert:
- Breast biopsy is recommended for masses that do not spontaneously resolve either in menstruating women in one or two cycles or in all postmenopausal women
- Recognize hallmarks of hereditary breast and ovarian syndrome

Evaluating Breast Abnormalities:
- Biopsy
  - Fine needle aspiration
  - Core needle
  - Surgical/open
  - Skin "punch"
- Breast MRI
- Testing breast cancer cells for the presence of hormone receptors

Evaluating Breast Symptoms:
- Nipple discharge
- Skin changes
- Breast pain (mastalgia)

Breast Cancer Screening:
- BSE: breast self-exam/breast awareness
- CBE: clinical breast exam: performed by a trained health care professional
- Mammography following current guidelines
- MRI: select populations
- Breast tomosynthesis: newer tool; three-dimensional image

Cultural Diversity:
- Breast cancer screening practices differ in women from different ethnic backgrounds
- African American women are at higher risk for IBC
- Culture-related barriers may affect adherence to screening and treatment in Chinese immigrant women

Nursing Care → Patient with Breast Cancer Includes:
- Providing emotional support
- Using evidence-based information to empower patients as they consider treatment options
- Providing care to meet actual needs during treatment
- Directing the patient to appropriate/ available resources
- Providing information about additional healing approaches such as holistic medicine

What To Say:
When teaching patients about breast health:
- With age, breast tissue sags; breasts drop; skin covering the breasts becomes thinner
- Nipples can vary in size and location; a third nipple is not uncommon; pregnancy darkens nipple color; hair surrounding nipples not uncommon
- Fluctuating hormone levels during monthly cycle cause changes in breast tissue
- Schedule CBE to be performed 1 week after menstruation
- Breast implants still pose health risks
- Bacteria can grow between the breasts due to oil and sweat accumulation
- Regular exercise of pectoral muscles can reduce sagging
- The left breast is usually larger than the right; breasts do not reach their full size until age 20
- Strategies to decrease discomfort during mammography

Optimizing Outcomes:
- A holistic approach to breast care includes prevention/health promotion strategies that empower women and meet an important goal of Healthy People 2020
- For early cancer detection: breast self-awareness, monthly BSE, annual CBE, and routine mammography
- Collaboration with other health-care professionals is necessary to address and remove barriers to breast cancer screening
- Teaching about breast health includes information about fibrocystic changes, mastalgia, and symptom relief
- NCI has a tool to estimate a woman's risk for invasive breast cancer
- Teach women about inflammatory breast cancer signs and symptoms
- Reassure patients that new medications are highly effective against chemotherapy-associated nausea and vomiting
- Help patients develop a Cancer Survivorship Plan
- Tools on Internet to evaluate breast masses

Where Research And Practice Meet:
- There is a link between absence of breast symptoms and the belief that no exam is needed in Korean women
- SEER data → mammography increases the detection of early stage breast cancer; screening has minimal effect of death rates

Nursing Insight:
- Breast cancer is the most commonly diagnosed cancer in US women
- Current recommendations → teach women both benefits and harms of BSE
- Screening and diagnostic mammography differ
- Type of fibrocystic breast changes determines cancer risk
- Be aware of nipple changes that may indicate Paget's disease
- No scientific evidence that certain factors increase risk for breast cancer (e.g., diet, bras, abortions, antiperspirants, night work)
- Overexpression of HER2/neureceptor is associated with increased reoccurrence of and worse prognosis for breast cancer
- Anti-angiogenesis → new targeted therapy for certain breast tumors
- Teach women who wish to bear children the impact of cancer treatment on fertility

Now Can You:
- Discuss breast health promotion?
- Discuss the term "breast awareness"?
- Identify common breast abnormalities?
- Identify risk factors for breast cancer?
- Develop a holistic plan of care for the woman being treated for breast cancer?

Promoting Reproductive Health Through an Understanding of Various Gynecological Disorders

Both within the family and without,
our sisters hold up our mirrors,
our images of who we are and of
who we can dare to become.

—Elizabeth Fishel

LEARNING TARGETS *At the completion of this chapter, the student will be able to:*

◆ Describe various gynecological disorders and discuss implications for patient counseling and teaching.

◆ Develop a nursing plan of care for a patient with a diagnosis of endometriosis.

◆ Develop a nursing plan of care for a patient with a diagnosis of polycystic ovary syndrome.

◆ Identify signs and symptoms that may be associated with vaginal, ovarian, endometrial, and vulvar carcinoma.

◆ Describe a strategy for increasing women's awareness of potential ovarian cancer symptoms.

◆ Teach a woman how to perform vulvar self-examination.

PICO(T) Questions

The intent of Evidence-Based Practice (EBP) is to provide nursing care that integrates the best available evidence. An initial step in EBP is to write a PICO(T) question that effectively guides the research. A PICO(T) question is an acronym that stands for population (P), intervention or issue (I), comparison of interest (C), outcome (O), and time frame (T). Depending on the question, all or some of the question components are used in the research process.

Use these PICO(T) questions to spark your thinking as you read the chapter.

1. What (I) complementary or alternative practices (O) are beneficial for (P) women with symptoms of dysmenorrhea?

2. Does (I) routine screening for symptoms that could indicate ovarian cancer lead to (O) earlier detection of the disease in (P) women over age 60 (C) compared with women under age 60?

Evidence-Based Practice

Billhult, A., & Stener-Victorin, E. (2012). Acupuncture with manual and low frequency electrical stimulation as experienced by women with polycystic ovary syndrome: A qualitative study. *BMC Complementary and Alternative Medicine, 12*(32), 1–6.

The purpose of this study was to describe the experience of acupuncture for women diagnosed with polycystic ovary syndrome (PCOS). Approximately 5% to 10% of women of reproductive age are affected with PCOS. Associated complications include obesity and insulin resistance, conditions that increase the risk for type 2 diabetes and cardiovascular disease. Additional issues associated with PCOS include a reduced quality of life, anxiety, and depression. Although frequently effective, pharmacological treatments for PCOS are associated with numerous side effects and there is no "gold standard" for long-term treatment. Women's use of acupuncture as a PCOS treatment modality is reported to be as high as 22% in U.S. fertility clinics; PCOS patients in Australia and the United Kingdom also report use of this therapy. Acupuncture treatments with a combination of electrical and manual stimulation of the needles, both in uncontrolled trials and in randomized controlled trials, have been shown to improve menstrual bleeding patterns, ovulation, and hyperandrogenism. Qualitative studies have reported on the extent of physical, social, and emotional challenges faced by women experiencing PCOS.

Participants in this study included eight women recruited from a previous randomized controlled trial on the use of acupuncture as a treatment modality for PCOS. All eight participants demonstrated symptoms of hyperandrogenism and oligoamenorrhea, and none had been medicated for the 3 months prior to the beginning of the study. The mean age of the participants was 31.9 years; ages ranged from 23 to 38 years. The participants' occupations varied and included students as well as professional, clerical, and blue-collar workers. The mean period of time between the last acupuncture treatment and the time of the study interview was 6.75 months. None of the women received acupuncture or other treatments for PCOS between the time of the intervention and the interview. The intervention consisted of acupuncture with manual and electrical (low frequency) needle stimulation twice weekly for 2 weeks, once weekly for 6 weeks, and once every other week for 8 weeks (14 treatments total) administered by a physical therapist trained in Western medical acupuncture. Each treatment lasted 30 minutes. Data were gathered during an interview conducted after completion of the treatment intervention. The interviewer used open-ended questions and encouraged participants to elaborate about the procedure and how they felt. On average, the interviews lasted approximately 30 minutes, and each was recorded and transcribed verbatim.

Data were analyzed using qualitative research methodology. Interviews were categorized and organized into the following themes: (1) the experience of hope, (2) acupuncture triggered things, (3) feelings of responsibility, (4) skepticism and proof of effect, and (5) feeling normal. The participants described living with problems associated with PCOS and voiced concern over the fact that they might never find a solution and treatment or bear children. Before entering the study, the women held on to the idea that their PCOS was untreatable. Acupuncture gave the participants a "sense of hope" not previously experienced. In regard to "triggered things about their body," more than half of the participants noted a change in their health states related to symptoms of PCOS. Specifically, the acupuncture treatments were associated with a decrease in body hair growth and acne, improved mood, and improved menstrual regularity. One participant reported becoming pregnant.

The acupuncture intervention gave the participants "insight into change and a feeling of responsibility," (p. 3) which inspired a desire to change habits in their lives that could possibly prolong the positive effects of the treatment. Participants reported feelings of responsibility to take charge and attempt to influence their condition; these feelings were perceived as inspirational and empowering.

Participants who had no expectations for improvement or who were skeptical regarding the treatment's effectiveness expressed surprise when change and improvements occurred.

Many participants found that their bodies had the possibility of normal functions, such as regaining a regular menstrual period. Rather than feeling tired, bloated, and having a craving for sweets, some expressed a feeling of wellness strongly connected to bodily functions. Several of the participants expressed feeling more positive about their ability to become pregnant, especially as their visible symptoms (i.e., excess hair growth, acne) decreased.

The researchers concluded that, based on their findings, acupuncture is a promising treatment for the symptoms associated with PCOS. Acupuncture provides a possibility for patients to gain hope as they experience positive results. Furthermore, acupuncture empowers women to take responsibility for their future well-being, even when they may have been initially skeptical to try the modality.

1. How is this information useful to clinical nursing practice?

2. Based on these findings, what are implications for further research?

See Suggested Responses for Evidence-Based Practice on Davis*Plus*.

Introduction

This chapter explores several gynecological disorders in women. To deliver safe, effective care, nurses who care for women should be familiar with the special aspects of various gynecological conditions. It is important to remember that the human body functions as a whole system. Although a gynecological problem may initially appear to be confined to the pelvis, it could actually result from a host of other influences, activities, and imbalances. For example, amenorrhea, or absence of menses, may be related to excessive exercise, eating disorders, obesity, weight loss, stress, chronic illness, or endocrine disorders that adversely affect the normal functioning of the menstrual cycle.

Mutual trust and respect in the nurse–patient relationship help to facilitate appropriate discussion of questions and concerns about various health issues. Women's emotional responses to certain gynecological disorders may profoundly affect their quality of life and ability to function. The nurse must always remain sensitive to women's unique problems related to the functioning of their reproductive systems and offer holistic, individualized care that empowers them to seek and embrace strategies to restore balance and control over their lives.

Menstrual Disorders

Menstrual disorders, specifically amenorrhea, irregular bleeding, and dysmenorrhea, constitute some of the most common reproductive problems in women. Premenstrual syndrome, another problem frequently encountered in the clinical setting, is discussed in Chapter 2. Potential nursing diagnoses for women with various menstrual disorders are presented in Box 4-1.

AMENORRHEA

Under normal circumstances, the menstrual cycle is dependent on the integrated functioning of the hypothalamus, pituitary gland, ovaries, uterus, cervix, and vagina. Amenorrhea, or a lack of menstruation, may result from abnormalities of the structure or function of any of these organs.

The term *amenorrhea* is rooted in the Greek "a" = no + "men" = month + "rhoia" = flow = "no monthly flow." Amenorrhea may be classified as "primary" or "secondary." With primary amenorrhea, menstruation never takes place. With secondary amenorrhea, menstruation starts but then stops. The nurse should refer the patient for an evaluation for amenorrhea when the following circumstances are present:

Primary

- Lack of secondary sex characteristics by age 14 to 15
- Lack of menarche (the initial menstrual period) by age 15
- Lack of menses within 3 years after breast development (thelarche) or the appearance of pubic or axillary hair (pubarche or adrenarche) (American College of Obstetricians and Gynecologists [ACOG], 2006a)

Primary amenorrhea may be caused by a number of conditions, including pregnancy, lactation, missed abortion, eating disorders (e.g., anorexia nervosa, bulimia), obesity,

---

Box 4-1 Potential Nursing Diagnoses for Women With Menstrual Disorders

- Ineffective Coping related to emotional and physical effects that stem from the disorder
- Knowledge Deficit related to the cause, treatment, and self-care strategies of the disorder
- Disturbed Body Image related to sexual dysfunction associated with the disorder
- Situational Low Self-Esteem related to an inability to conceive
- Acute Pain related to the menstrual disorder

---

hyperthyroidism, hypoglycemia, cystic fibrosis, Crohn's disease, genetic abnormalities, congenital absence of the cervix and/or vagina, and polycystic ovary syndrome.

Secondary

Secondary amenorrhea is defined as an absence of menses for at least 3 months in a woman who has previously had regular monthly menses, or a lack of menses for at least 6 to 12 months in a woman who normally experiences irregular menses. The term *delayed menses* is used in situations wherein the amenorrhea occurs for a shorter period of time. Pregnancy, lactation, premature ovarian failure (menopause before age 40), weight loss, eating disorders, and obesity are conditions that may cause secondary amenorrhea. Other causes include hormonal contraceptive effects and post–oral contraceptive pill amenorrhea, pituitary gland dysfunction (e.g., hyperprolactinemia), polycystic ovary syndrome, emotional or physical stress, frequent strenuous exercise, chronic illness (e.g., colitis, kidney failure, cystic fibrosis), cancer chemotherapy, ovarian cysts or tumors, and certain endocrine disorders such as Cushing's syndrome and thyroid dysfunction (ACOG, 2006a; Nelson & Baldwin, 2011).

When evaluating a patient for amenorrhea, the first step is to test for pregnancy. Once pregnancy has been ruled out, the patient undergoes a thorough physical examination and, depending on the findings, additional testing that may include laboratory and diagnostic testing (e.g., ultrasonography). In many situations, a careful review of the woman's health history can provide clues as to the cause(s) of the amenorrhea (Nelson & Baldwin, 2011).

 ***Nursing Insight*—** *Perspectives on amenorrhea*

Amenorrhea is a symptom, not a condition. In the United States, approximately 2% to 5% of all women of childbearing age are affected by amenorrhea. Although the cause is generally not a life-threatening condition, amenorrhea can be associated with significant potential morbidity. In most situations, amenorrhea is reversible with treatment for the underlying condition (Nelson & Baldwin, 2011).

ABNORMAL GENITAL BLEEDING

Any bleeding other than what is expected in a normal ovulatory cycle is considered abnormal genital bleeding. This condition constitutes one of the most frequent reasons for patient visits to the clinic or private office and accounts for approximately 19% of all gynecological complaints. The source of the bleeding may be the rectum, urinary tract, vulva, vagina, cervix, or uterus. Conditions that may cause abnormal bleeding include pregnancy and pregnancy-related complications, trauma, infection, endocrine abnormalities, lesions, or tumors (ACOG, 2006a, 2012a; Nelson & Baldwin, 2011).

***Nursing Insight*—** *Understanding correct terminology for abnormal genital bleeding*

Nurses who care for women should be familiar with terminology for abnormal genital bleeding, which is classified by the timing of the bleeding and the duration of the flow. The use of accurate terminology helps to promote effective communication and justifies appropriate work-ups and therapies. Patient-recorded menstrual calendars and pictorial bleeding assessment calendars are beneficial in facilitating the accurate documentation of bleeding patterns.

Menorrhagia* is excess bleeding (80 mL or more, or bleeding that lasts longer than 7 days) during the expected time of menstrual flow.

Metrorrhagia† is bleeding that occurs at abnormal times during an ovulatory cycle—that is, the woman experiences bleeding more frequently than every 21 days.

Menometrorrhagia is a combination of the above two bleeding abnormalities—the woman experiences excessive bleeding and frequent bleeding at abnormal times during the cycle.

Polymenorrhea is bleeding that occurs at short intervals (less than 21 days).

Intermenstrual bleeding is bleeding of variable amounts that occurs between regular menses.

Oligomenorrhea is bleeding that occurs less frequently than every 35 days.

Postcoital bleeding is bleeding that occurs after sexual intercourse.

---

*The definition for menorrhagia is used for research purposes and, in practice, excessive blood loss should be used based on the patient's perception (ACOG, 2012a, 2013a, 2013b; Nelson & Baldwin, 2011).

†According to the new classification system, the descriptive terms *heavy menstrual bleeding* and *intermenstrual bleeding* now replace the terms *menorrhagia* and *metrorrhagia*.

Several possible diagnoses are associated with bleeding disorders. Although many factors influence a woman's menstrual patterns, one of the first considerations is the patient's age. In an adolescent female, approximately 20 hormonal cycles occur before ovulation takes place on a regular basis. Bleeding that is irregular in both timing and amount tends to be the rule rather than the exception during early adolescence. Similarly, perimenopausal women commonly experience an increased variation in their menstrual intervals and in the quantity of flow during the 5 years that precede menopause. The cause of abnormal genital bleeding can range from simple to complex. Evaluation requires a careful and thorough history and work-up, including a physical examination, laboratory tests, and appropriate diagnostic tests such as ultrasonography (ACOG, 2012a, 2013a, 2013b; Jacobs, 2012; Nelson & Baldwin, 2011; Rydz & Jamieson, 2013).

Optimizing Outcomes— Using patient age to guide the work-up for abnormal genital bleeding

The patient's age is an important consideration in the evaluation of abnormal genital bleeding. For example, during adolescence, a common cause is persistent anovulation, or failure to ovulate, which may be related to contraception, pregnancy, polycystic ovary syndrome, or coagulopathies.

During *midlife* (30s–40s), women most often develop abnormal genital bleeding from pregnancy, structural lesions (e.g., leiomyomata [fibroid tumors], polyps), and anovulation, including that caused by polycystic ovary syndrome, hormone therapy, and endometrial hyperplasia.

During *menopause*, bleeding most often results from hormone therapy, endometrial atrophy, leiomyomata, endometrial hyperplasia, and malignancy (ACOG, 2012a, 2013a, 2013b; Nelson & Baldwin, 2011).

DYSMENORRHEA

Dysmenorrhea, defined as painful menstruation, is one of the most common gynecological problems occurring in women of all ages. For most, the pain develops during or shortly before the onset of menstruation and is most intense in the suprapubic region or in the lower abdomen. Symptoms including nausea, vomiting, diarrhea, headaches, and light-headedness may accompany the pain. Dysmenorrhea can cause significant disruption with daily activities each month, resulting in absence from school and missed time from work. Dysmenorrhea may be classified as primary (intrinsic and usually early onset) or secondary (results from some other physical cause and usually has a later onset) (Nelson & Baldwin, 2011).

Primary dysmenorrhea usually begins within 1 to 3 years following menarche and results from physiological causes—no pathology is present. In general, women with primary dysmenorrhea are ovulatory and thus produce progesterone in the luteal phase. Progesterone stimulates the production of prostaglandins in the base of the endometrium. Found in various tissues throughout the body, prostaglandins are substances that control local functions such as vasodilation and vasoconstriction. Women with primary dysmenorrhea produce excessive amounts of prostaglandin F2-alpha, which increases the force of the uterine contractions. Uterine contractions reduce blood flow to the uterus, causing ischemia and pain. The pain usually begins at the onset of menstrual flow and persists for 8 to 48 hours. During menstruation, the highest levels of prostaglandins are released during the first 48 hours. When the prostaglandins are introduced into the general circulation by uterine contractions, they can produce symptoms of headache, nausea, vomiting, and diarrhea (Nelson & Baldwin, 2011).

Secondary dysmenorrhea is due to some other physical cause and usually is of a later onset. Women with secondary dysmenorrhea also complain of painful uterine cramping with menstruation but frequently have other accompanying complaints, such as dyspareunia or nonmenstrual pelvic pain. By definition, pain that occurs with secondary dysmenorrhea is related to uterine or pelvic pathology. The treatment for secondary dysmenorrhea should be targeted to the underlying cause and should be reflective of the patient's desire for fertility. When surgical intervention is not required, the treatments helpful for primary dysmenorrhea are often successful in reducing the symptoms of secondary dysmenorrhea (Nelson & Baldwin, 2011).

The most common causes of secondary dysmenorrhea are adenomyosis, endometriosis, pelvic adhesions, and neoplasia. Adenomyosis is a condition characterized by the presence of endometrial glands and stoma that are embedded in the myometrium (the deep muscle layer of the uterus). Adenomyosis most commonly occurs in parous women. Each month, normal ovarian hormonal changes cause stimulation of the ectopic (abnormally located) endometrial tissue and produce sloughing within the myometrium. In addition to dysmenorrhea, women with adenomyosis may also experience heavy menses and perimenstrual pain. The uterus is enlarged, boggy, and tender immediately before and during menses (Nelson & Baldwin, 2011).

Endometriosis is a condition characterized by implantation of endometrial tissue outside the uterus. Women with endometriosis experience painful menses due to the cyclical shedding of the ectopic endometriotic implants and the local inflammatory response triggered by the shedding. The pain associated with endometriosis often occurs just prior to the onset of menses. (See later discussion of endometriosis.) Pelvic adhesions may also cause secondary dysmenorrhea. Pelvic adhesions are fibrous bands that may result from previous pelvic inflammatory disease, appendicitis, and pelvic or abdominal surgery. *Neoplasia* is a term that refers to the abnormal proliferation of benign or malignant cells (Nelson & Baldwin, 2011). (See later discussion about various neoplastic processes.)

Health-care teaching for women experiencing dysmenorrhea should be holistic in nature and include relaxation and breathing techniques, the use of heat to reduce uterine contractions and increase blood flow to the uterine tissues, exercise or rest, and the use of NSAIDs to inhibit the synthesis of prostaglandin. These drugs not only improve the cramping pain but also reduce backache, headaches, and gastrointestinal symptoms. When taken at the onset of menses, NSAIDs reduce the release of prostaglandins and considerably decrease menstrual blood loss. Other therapeutic interventions for dysmenorrhea include hormonal contraceptives (e.g., combined oral contraceptive pills, depot medroxyprogesterone acetate [Depo-Provera], and the levonorgestrel-releasing intrauterine systems [LNG-IUS]), which reduce menstrual blood loss and decrease the production of prostaglandins (Nelson & Baldwin, 2011; Perriera & Greenfield, 2011). Findings from research (Lasco, Catalano, & Benvenga, 2012) suggest that vitamin D, which decreases prostaglandin synthesis and increases prostaglandin inactivation, may be useful in decreasing dysmenorrheal cramps; further studies are indicated (Rutecki, 2012).

🌸 Complementary Care: *Measures for relief from dysmenorrhea*

Throughout the ages, women have resorted to the use of various herbal remedies such as cramp bark, wild yam, black haw, ginger, and raspberry leaf to ease the pain of menstrual cramps. The nurse should counsel patients that because herbal preparations may be toxic and also interact with other medications, only preparations obtained from reputable companies should be used. Other strategies for relief from menstrual pain include the application of heat or cold, massage, meditation, acupuncture, and progressive relaxation. Exercise is beneficial for some women. Physical activity enhances blood flow to the pelvis and reduces pelvic congestion. Dietary strategies include the use of natural diuretics such as peaches, parsley, and cranberry juice to reduce edema and limiting the intake of meat (Robinson & Wiczyk, 2011; Sego, 2012; Woo & McEneaney, 2010).

🌀 Now Can You— **Discuss abnormal genital bleeding and dysmenorrhea?**

1. Define the terms *heavy menstrual bleeding* and *intermenstrual bleeding*?
2. Differentiate primary dysmenorrhea from secondary dysmenorrhea and identify three possible causes of secondary dysmenorrhea?
3. Develop a holistic teaching plan for women who experience dysmenorrhea?

Common Vaginal Infections

Under normal circumstances, the vaginal environment functions as an ecosystem that maintains a steady state as it interacts with the environment outside the vagina. Many organisms, including certain bacteria and yeast, normally reside in the vagina. In fact, at any given time, from 5 to 10 different types of microorganisms are normally present in the vaginal flora. *Lactobacillus* is the dominant bacterial genus. It plays an essential role in helping to maintain the vaginal balance by producing by-products such as lactic acid and hydrogen peroxide. These by-products allow the vagina to maintain a healthy acidic pH of less than 4.5, which prevents the overgrowth of less desirable vaginal microorganisms. If the delicate balance of microorganisms is upset, the potentially pathogenic minor bacteria can proliferate to a concentration that causes symptoms (ACOG, 2006b; Gura & Baresic, 2011; Marazzo & Cates, 2011).

🌸 Nursing Insight— *Understanding vaginal infections*

During the reproductive years, the normal vaginal pH range is between 3.8 and 4.2, which falls within the acidic spectrum of the pH scale. Anaerobic bacteria are unable to colonize and thrive in the normally acidic vaginal environment, and lactobacilli become the predominant bacteria. When anaerobic bacteria are able to colonize, they eradicate the lactobacilli, creating an alkaline environment that allows continued colonization. Vaginal infections primarily occur in two ways: An imbalance and overgrowth of organisms that normally inhabit the vagina proliferate and cause symptoms, or organisms are introduced into the vagina, usually from intimate sexual contact. Factors that may cause an alteration in the normal vaginal environment include stress, douching, feminine hygiene products, harsh soaps, dietary changes (e.g., an increase in sugar, caffeine), sexual intercourse, barrier contraceptive methods (e.g., condoms, diaphragms), spermicides, synthetic underwear or tight-fitting pants, illness, chronic metabolic conditions (e.g., diabetes), immunosuppression, certain medications, and pregnancy (ACOG, 2006b; Gura & Baresic, 2011; Schwartz & Gabelnick, 2011).

🌀 Optimizing Outcomes— **Teaching women strategies for promoting vaginal health**

Nurses can be instrumental in promoting vaginal health by teaching women about the normal functioning of their bodies. Women can be taught that leukorrhea is a normal vaginal discharge that undergoes hormonally mediated changes throughout the menstrual cycle. In the early (proliferative) phase, estrogen promotes a clear, thin, stretchy vaginal discharge. Later, the discharge becomes thick and tacky in response to the effects of progesterone, the dominant hormone during the second half of the cycle. The normal vaginal discharge varies in quantity from woman to woman, and often from cycle to cycle. Nurses can help patients explore ways to promote a balanced vaginal environment through alterations in lifestyle and choice of birth control method. Women should be taught that douching is discouraged, as it has a drying effect on the vagina and disrupts the normal vaginal flora. Douching can also cause an increase in the amount of vaginal discharge normally present and has been shown to contribute to serious infection of the upper reproductive tract (ACOG, 2012c; Marazzo & Cates, 2011).

A number of infections and conditions that involve the vaginal environment are commonly seen in women with gynecological disorders. These include candidiasis, sexually transmitted diseases (STDs), cervicitis, and pelvic inflammatory disease (PID). Cervicitis may be accompanied by a purulent discharge, which may be a symptom of infection with gonorrhea or Chlamydia. Less commonly encountered conditions include vaginal carcinoma (primary, which is rare, or secondary, which results from the spread of cancer to the vagina from another site), cancer associated with in utero exposure to diethylstilbestrol (DES), and toxic shock syndrome (TSS). STDs and PID are discussed in a separate chapter.

BACTERIAL VAGINOSIS

Bacterial vaginosis (BV) was previously called nonspecific vaginitis, *Haemophilus vaginitis,* or *Gardnerella.* BV is the most common vaginal infection in women, and although it is a sexually associated condition, it is not usually considered to be a specific STD. This vaginal infection is related to a lack of hydrogen peroxide–producing lactobacilli (microorganisms that normally maintain a low vaginal pH) and a dramatic overgrowth of the vaginal resident bacterium *Gardnerella vaginalis* and anaerobic bacteria (e.g., *Mycoplasma hominis, Mobiluncus, Bacteroides, Prevotella, Peptostreptococcus, Eubacterium, Escherichia coli*, and group B streptococci). Anaerobic bacteria thrive in a low-oxygen environment (Marazzo & Cates, 2011; Waldman, 2012).

🌸 *Cultural Diversity: Prevalence of Bacterial Vaginosis*

Bacterial vaginosis affects approximately 30% of reproductive-age women. In the United States, black women are infected with BV at three times the rate of white women. The prevalence rate of BV is highest in black women without Hispanic heritage (50.3%) and Mexican American women (28.8%) when compared with non-Hispanic white women (22.4%) (Coughlin & Secor, 2010; Johns Hopkins University, 2011).

Women with BV may be asymptomatic. When present, symptoms include a thin white or gray adherent vaginal discharge with a "fishy" amine odor, and women often report that the odor is worse after intercourse and following menses. The diagnosis is made on the basis of a positive finding on the "whiff" test—the characteristic amine odor is produced when a sample of the discharge is combined with a 10% solution of potassium hydroxide (KOH). Microscopic examination of the vaginal fluid (i.e., a wet mount) reveals the presence of clue cells, which are sloughed vaginal epithelial cells coated with bacteria that cling to the edges of the cells. Clue cells have a granular appearance with indistinct, blurry borders (Fig. 4-1).

🌸 *Nursing Insight*— *The vaginal wet mount*

A wet mount, also known as a "wet-prep" or "wet smear," is frequently used in the clinical setting to diagnose three of the

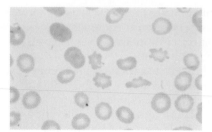

Figure 4-1 Clue cell. (Venes, D. [Ed.]. [2009]. *Taber's cyclopedic medical dictionary* [21st ed., p. 397]. Philadelphia, PA: F.A. Davis.)

most common vaginal infections: bacterial vaginosis, trichomoniasis, and yeast (candidiasis). To perform this test, the clinician inserts a speculum and uses a moist cotton swab to take a sample of the discharge from the posterior vaginal fornix. The discharge is then placed on a glass slide and viewed under a microscope. Alternately, a dry swab may be used: The sample is placed in 1 mL of saline, mixed, and placed on a slide, or a drop of saline is placed on a slide and the sample is added to it. A cover slip is then applied and the slide is promptly viewed.

Typically, when BV is present, the vaginal pH is above the normal value of 4.5. Because BV may occur concurrently with other STDs (e.g., chlamydia, gonorrhea, genital herpes), it is important to screen for STDs as well (Marazzo & Cates, 2011).

🌸 *Across Care Settings:* **Vaginal swab testing kits for home and clinical use**

Self-diagnosis of vaginal infections based on symptoms alone is inaccurate approximately 50% of the time. Over-the-counter vaginal pH screening tests can help distinguish vaginal symptoms that require attention from a health-care provider. One such product, the Vagisil Screening Kit, contains plastic wands with attached pH paper; the woman touches the wand to the vaginal wall to moisten the pH paper and withdraws the device. The vaginal pH level is then compared with the color on the pH guide. A pH value of 4.5 suggests that the vaginal symptoms are due to candidiasis (yeast); a pH reading of 5.0 or higher indicates that the vaginal symptoms are likely due to BV, trichomoniasis, or a mixed infection, and office follow-up is necessary.

The VS-SENSE PRO is a swab-based test to detect vaginitis in the clinical setting. The VS-SENSE indicates by color change the elevated vaginal acidity levels associated with bacterial vaginosis and trichomoniasis. The screening test offers immediate results and assists in detecting BV and trichomoniasis even when *Candida* (yeast) symptoms mask the more serious infections. Other kits (e.g., NuSwab VG, APTIMA) allow for clinician or patient collection of vaginal swab specimens to test for multiple vaginitis-causing microorganisms such as *Chlamydia trachomatis, Neisseria gonorrhoeae*, vulvovaginal candidiasis, and *Trichomonas vaginalis* (Waldman, 2012).

Findings from an investigation by Xu and colleagues (2011) suggested that in sexually transmitted disease (STD) and family planning clinics, the use of home-based, self-obtained vaginal swabs resulted in significant increases in STD rescreening rates, compared with rescreening in the clinic. The investigators concluded that home-based vaginal specimen collection could be an alternative to clinic-based rescreening for Chlamydia infection in women.

When BV is detected in an asymptomatic woman, it is usually not treated unless the patient will be undergoing an invasive surgical procedure, such as abortion, hysterectomy, or insertion of an intrauterine device. These procedures increase the risk of pelvic infection in the presence of BV. Bacterial vaginosis has also been shown to be associated with various pregnancy complications, such as spontaneous abortion, preterm birth, and infection following cesarean birth (Coughlin & Secor, 2010; Marazzo & Cates, 2011).

Symptomatic women are typically treated with metronidazole (Flagyl), which is given either orally (500 mg twice a day for 7 days) or vaginally (metronidazole gel, 0.75% [Metro-Gel], 5 grams intravaginally for 5 days). Flagyl should not be used in women with a history of seizures. No alcohol should be ingested 24 hours before or after taking this medication, because the combination of metronidazole and alcohol causes abdominal discomfort, nausea, vomiting, and headache. Because nausea is the most common side effect, nurses should advise women to always take the medication with food. Metronidazole readily crosses the placenta and should not be taken during the first trimester of pregnancy; it is also contraindicated in breastfeeding women. Clindamycin (Cleocin) given orally (300 mg twice a day for 7 days) or in a 2% vaginal cream (5 grams intravaginally for 7 days) or in a vaginal ovule (100 mg at bedtime for 3 days) is also used to treat bacterial vaginosis. This medication is especially useful in individuals with an allergy or intolerance to metronidazole. Tinidazole (Tindamax), an oral medication, may also be used to treat BV in nonpregnant, adult women. The recommended dose is 2 grams once daily for 2 days, or 1 gram once daily for 5 days, and this medication should be taken with food. The half-life of this medication is twice as long as that of metronidazole, and it has fewer side effects. Alcohol should be avoided during the 3 days after taking tinidazole because of its longer half-life. Because treatment of male sexual partners has no effect on the recurrence rate in female partners, male treatment is not indicated (Centers for Disease Control and Prevention [CDC] 2011a; Coughlin & Secor, 2010; Marazzo & Cates, 2011). Health professionals should consult the CDC Web site (http://www.cdc.gov/std/treatment/2010/vaginal-discharge.htm#a1) for the most current guidelines on BV treatment.

CANDIDIASIS

Commonly known as a yeast infection, candidiasis is generally caused by *Candida albicans* (Fig. 4-2). Other related yeast species (e.g., *C. tropicalis, C. glabrata, C. parapsilosis, C. krusei, C. lusitaniae*), however, can also be causative agents as well. Infection with candidiasis is usually characterized by intense vulvar pruritus (itching) and irritation and a thick, white, cottage cheese–like vaginal discharge that may have a sour odor. The discharge may be observed on the vaginal walls, cervix, and labia, and the vulva and labial folds are red and edematous. The patient may complain of dyspareunia and dysuria, although symptoms are subtler in some women. The diagnosis of candidiasis is made on the basis of microscopic examination of the vaginal discharge. A saline and KOH wet smear reveals budding

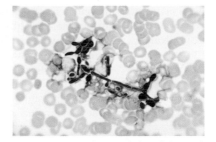

Figure 4-2 Gram's stain of *Candida albicans* (purple) in blood (x 640). (Venes, D. [Ed.]. [2009]. *Taber's cyclopedic medical dictionary* [21st ed., p. 354]. Philadelphia, PA: F.A. Davis.)

yeast or pseudohyphae. The vaginal pH is usually unaltered, although it may be slightly more acidic than normal. During the examination, it is important to rule out STDs.

Optimizing Outcomes— Recognizing factors that are associated with vulvovaginal candidiasis

Certain factors are associated with vulvovaginal candidiasis, such as the use of broad-spectrum antibiotics and systemic corticosteroids, which can cause a reduction in the normal protective vaginal flora; high-dose oral contraceptives; and uncontrolled diabetes and allergies, especially allergic rhinitis. Spermicidal creams have also been associated with vaginal yeast infections. Nurses can advise women who use these medications or products about strategies to enhance the normal vaginal environment and reduce the likelihood of vulvovaginal candidiasis (Marazzo & Cates, 2011).

Candidiasis is treated with antifungal medications, and many over-the-counter agents such as miconazole (Monistat) and clotrimazole (Gyne-Lotrimin) are available. Most of the commercial products are fungistats that inhibit the organisms from reproducing, so the woman's immune system can suppress the yeast. Patients can apply a topical antifungal cream to the vulva as well as the intravaginal cream or suppositories. It is important to remind women that creams and vaginal suppositories are oil based and may weaken latex condoms or diaphragms. Although these medications are available without prescription, the nurse should advise patients to avoid self-treatment without first undergoing a clinical evaluation to confirm the diagnosis of vulvovaginal candidiasis. Treatment of asymptomatic sexual partners is not generally necessary (CDC, 2011a; Marazzo & Cates, 2011).

Complementary Care: *Measures for vaginal candidiasis*

Nurses can educate women about strategies to relieve symptoms of candidiasis and help prevent recurrent yeast infections. For example, women can be advised to take sitz baths for comfort and add Aveeno powder to the bath. Boric acid, 600 mg in size 0 gelatin capsules inserted in the vagina each night for 14 days, has been reported to be effective against resistant infections. Vaginal suppositories containing acidophilic bacteria, as well as long-term (6 months) daily ingestion of dairy products or powders, capsules, or tablets that contain *Lactobacillus acidophilus*, are other strategies that anecdotally have been associated with prevention and relief of symptoms, although the evidence supporting this intervention is conflicting (Nyirjesy et al., 2011). Nurses can also teach women to wear cotton underwear to enhance ventilation of the genital area, avoid wearing tight-fitting pants or wet clothing (e.g., bathing suits) for prolonged periods of time, and avoid potential irritants such as perfumed soaps; bubble baths; hot tubs; and the application of perfumes, sprays, or powder near the vaginal area.

Stronger antifungal prescription medications are available in creams or suppositories, along with oral preparations, including fluconazole (Diflucan), itraconazole (Sporanox), and ketoconazole (Nizoral). Although the oral medications are associated with various side effects (e.g., nausea, vomiting, diarrhea, abdominal pain, headache), they tend to be well tolerated by most women. Ketoconazole is associated with hepatotoxicity, and baseline and ongoing liver function monitoring is recommended. Oral antifungals and boric acid suppositories should not be used during pregnancy. Topical antifungals have limited systemic absorption and are considered safe for maternal use. Women who have recurrent yeast infections should be evaluated for diabetes and infection with HIV (CDC, 2011a; Marazzo & Cates, 2011).

Now Can You— Discuss various aspects of vaginitis?

1. Develop an educational tool for teaching women about promoting a healthy vaginal environment?
2. Compare and contrast bacterial vaginosis and vaginal candidiasis?
3. Describe strategies intended to relieve symptoms and help prevent recurrence of vaginal candidiasis?

Vaginal Carcinoma

Vaginal carcinoma is any type of cancer that forms in the tissues of the vagina. Vaginal carcinomas can be primary or secondary or related to in utero diethylstilbestrol (DES) exposure. Vaginal cancer is extremely rare, occurs primarily in women over age 50, and accounts for only 1% to 2% of gynecological malignancies. It is frequently asymptomatic and first detected during a routine gynecological examination. Abnormal vaginal bleeding constitutes the most common symptom of this type of cancer, and the bleeding may be postcoital, intermenstrual, prepubertal, or postmenopausal. Other symptoms include foul-smelling vaginal discharge, dysuria, dyspareunia, and pelvic pain.

There are two primary types of vaginal cancer: squamous cell carcinoma and adenocarcinoma. Most lesions (85% of cases) are squamous cell carcinomas that arise from the thin, flat squamous cells that line the vagina. These kinds of cancers develop over a period of many years and are usually found in women between the ages of 60 and 80. Vaginal squamous cell carcinoma occurs most often in women with a history of infection with human papillomavirus (HPV) (genital warts) or cervical or vulvar cancer. The time from HPV infection to the development of invasive cancer is believed to be from 5 to 10 years. In most cases, the cancer initially spreads superficially within the vaginal wall and later invades the paravaginal tissues and the parametria (the connective tissue and fat adjacent to the uterus). Distant metastases occur most commonly in the lungs and liver (National Cancer Institute [NCI], 2013).

Vaginal adenocarcinoma (occurring in approximately 5% to 10% of cases) arises from the glandular or secretory cells that line the vagina and produce some vaginal fluids. Adenocarcinoma is more likely than squamous cell cancer to spread to the lungs and lymph nodes. The most common type of vaginal adenocarcinoma usually develops in women over the age of 50. Clear cell adenocarcinoma is another type of vaginal cancer that usually occurs in women who were exposed to diethylstilbestrol (DES) in utero.

Nursing Insight— Understanding diethylstilbestrol (DES)

Diethylstilbestrol (DES) is a nonsteroidal, synthetic estrogen that is several times more potent than natural estrogens. In the United States, DES was prescribed to approximately 5 to 10 million mothers during the late 1930s until the early 1970s as a preventive treatment to reduce the likelihood of spontaneous abortion or preterm birth (Smith, 1948). It was taken off the market when study results revealed that DES was linked to abnormalities in both male and female offspring of women who received this drug during pregnancy. Structural alterations, changes in the tissue of the vagina and cervix, and infertility have been linked to in utero DES exposure. The incidence of DES-related clear cell adenocarcinoma is highest for those women who were exposed during the first 3 months of their mother's pregnancy. The highest incidence of occurrence is between ages 17 and 21. The incidence of vaginal clear cell adenocarcinoma peaked in the early 1970s and is now rare, because DES use during pregnancy diminished during the early 1960s and was banned in the early 1970s (NCI, 2011).

Other less common forms of vaginal cancer include germ cell tumors (e.g., teratoma, endodermal sinus tumors), which are rare and found most often in infants and children; malignant melanoma; and sarcoma botryoides, a rhabdomyosarcoma that is also found most often in infants and children. Screening for malignancies of the vagina is similar to screening for cervical cancer. In addition to a history and physical examination, diagnostic testing for vaginal carcinoma includes a pelvic exam, Pap test, biopsy, and colposcopy (an examination of the cervix, using a lighted instrument that magnifies the tissues). Other diagnostic modalities may include laboratory testing and imaging studies (NCI, 2013).

The prognosis for vaginal carcinoma depends primarily on the type and stage of the condition at the time of diagnosis, but survival is reduced in women who are older than 60 years of age, are symptomatic at the time of diagnosis, have lesions of the middle and lower third of the vagina, or have poorly differentiated tumors. Treatment modalities depend on the stage of the condition; surgery or radiation therapy is highly effective in the early stages, while radiation therapy is the primary treatment for the more advanced stages. Chemotherapy has not been shown to be curative for advanced vaginal cancer (NCI, 2013).

Toxic Shock Syndrome

Toxic shock syndrome (TSS) is a rare, sometimes fatal condition that affects many body systems. Although this disorder is not well understood, TSS is believed to be associated with tampon use during menses. However, TSS can also occur in children, men, and nonmenstruating women. Nonmenstrual TSS risk is increased for women who use vaginal barrier contraceptives. The incidence of TSS peaked during the late 1970s and 1980s, most likely because of the widespread availability of superabsorbent tampons. A few specific tampon designs and high-absorbency tampon materials were found to have some association with an increased risk of TSS; these products are no longer sold in the United States. Today, the overall rate of TSS is one to three cases per 100,000 people per year, and only 55% of current cases are associated with menstruation (Eckert & Lentz, 2012).

legal alert— Teach about toxic shock syndrome

Women who use a diaphragm, cervical cap, or contraceptive sponge should be aware of the possible association between these devices and toxic shock syndrome. Common signs of TSS include fever of sudden onset greater than 102.2°F (38.9°C), diffuse, macular (flat) erythematous rash, vomiting, diarrhea, malaise, muscle aches, disorientation, platelets less than 100,000/mm³, and hypotension with a systolic blood pressure less than 90 mm Hg. Patients who experience these symptoms should seek medical care immediately; left untreated, TSS can be fatal within hours (Eckert & Lentz, 2012).

Toxic shock syndrome is caused almost exclusively by toxins produced by some strains of the colonized bacterium *Staphylococcus aureus*. Toxins produced from the bacterium *Streptococcus pyogenes* may also cause TSS (sometimes referred to as toxic shock–like syndrome [TSLS] or streptococcal toxic shock syndrome [STSS]). Although the exact mechanism of cause is unknown, several conditions are believed to contribute to the development of menstrual TSS. These include alterations in the normal vaginal flora, a neutral vaginal pH, mechanical blockage of menstrual flow, contamination of tampons by the bacterium *S. aureus*, absorption of bacteria-resistant cervical fluids, the superabsorbent or synthetic materials found in some tampons, and damaged cervical or vaginal tissue. The toxin implicated in menstrual TSS is capable of entering the bloodstream by crossing the vaginal wall in the absence of ulcerations (Eckert & Lentz, 2012; Venes, 2013).

Optimizing Outcomes— Strategies to reduce risk for menstrual TSS

Nurses can teach women about strategies to minimize the risk of contracting menstrual TSS. For example, menstruating women may use sanitary pads or choose a tampon with the minimum absorbency needed to manage the menstrual flow and use the tampons only during active menstruation. Women can be taught to change tampons frequently (at least every 6 hours) and alternate sanitary pads with tampons, especially during the night. Nurses should emphasize that if symptoms suggestive of TSS occur, the tampon should be removed and medical attention sought immediately.

The diagnosis of TSS is made on the basis of physical examination findings and symptoms, along with results of a complete blood count, which often shows an elevated white blood cell count indicative of an acute infectious process. Treatment of this potentially life-threatening condition involves immediate hospitalization with fluid replacement and aggressive antibiotic therapy. Antibiotics should cover both *S. aureus* and *S. pyogenes* and may include a combination of cephalosporins, penicillins, and vancomycin, along with clindamycin or gentamicin. With appropriate care and prompt treatment, patients usually recover within 2 to 3 weeks (Eckert & Lentz, 2012; Venes, 2013).

Nursing Insight— Formulating appropriate nursing diagnoses for patients with TSS

Nursing diagnoses for patients with TSS may focus on Hyperthermia (related to the inflammatory process/hypermetabolic state and dehydration), Deficient Fluid Volume (related to increased gastric losses, fever, and decreased intake), Acute Pain (related to the inflammatory process, effects of circulating toxins, and skin disruptions), and Impaired Skin/Tissue Integrity (related to the effects of circulating toxins and dehydration).

Urinary Tract Infections

Because of the widespread prevalence of urinary tract infections in women, a brief description of the problem is included in this discussion of gynecological disorders. Urinary tract infection (UTI) is defined as significant bacteriuria in the presence of symptoms. UTIs occur more frequently in women than in men because of the shorter route from the external environment to the bladder in women, along with the close proximity of the urethra to the vaginal and anal areas. UTIs account for a significant number (>6 million) of physician/health clinic visits each year, and it is estimated that 20% of women will be affected by a UTI at some time during their lifetime (ACOG, 2008d).

Under normal circumstances, the flow of urine keeps bacteria flushed from the urinary tract, and the entire urinary system remains sterile. The bladder wall possesses antibacterial properties, and the urine is usually acidic, which inhibits growth of bacteria.

A & P review   The Female Urinary Tract and Bacterial Exposure

The female and male urinary tracts are relatively the same except for the length of the urethra. Owing to this difference, women are 30 times more likely to develop UTIs than are men. The female urethra is approximately 1.5 inches long; the male urethra is approximately 8 inches long. In women, bacteria from fecal matter can be easily transferred to the vagina or the urethra (Figs. 4-3 and 4-4). Most UTIs arise from one type of bacteria, *Escherichia coli*, which normally lives in the colon. Other common culprits include *Enterococcus faecalis*, *Staphylococcus saprophyticus*, *Klebsiella pneumoniae*, and *Proteus mirabilis*. Chlamydia and mycoplasma may also cause UTIs in both women and men, but these infections tend to remain limited to the urethra and reproductive system. Unlike *E. coli*, chlamydia and mycoplasma may be sexually transmitted (Minkin, 2011). ◆

Risk factors for UTIs include extremes of age, altered immunity, diabetes, urinary tract obstructions, pregnancy,

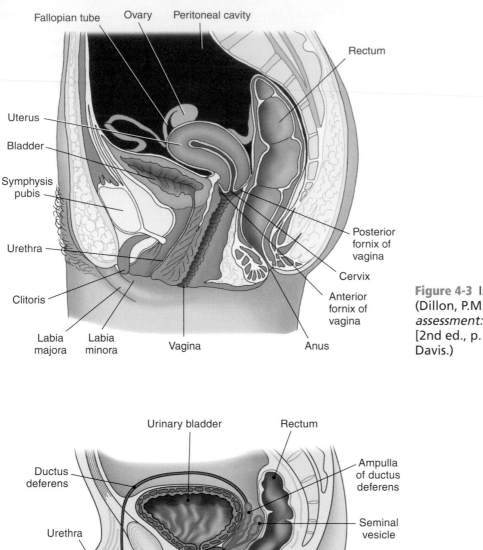

Figure 4-3 Internal female genitalia. (Dillon, P.M. [2007]. *Nursing health assessment: A critical thinking approach* [2nd ed., p. 612]. Philadelphia, PA: F.A. Davis.)

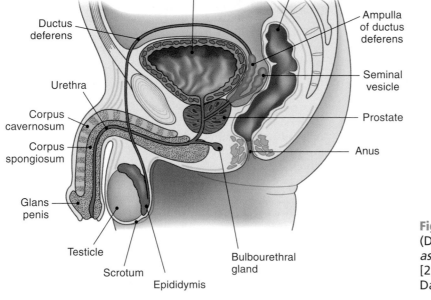

Figure 4-4 Male genitourinary system. (Dillon, P.M. [2007]. *Nursing health assessment: A critical thinking approach* [2nd ed., p. 651]. Philadelphia, PA: F.A. Davis.)

sexual activity, and diaphragm use. Irritation of the urethra during sexual activity can cause bacteria to migrate upward into the urinary tract. Spermicides may alter the vaginal pH and decrease levels of normal protective bacteria, allowing harmful bacteria to grow in the vagina, which can then migrate to the bladder. Allergy to certain ingredients in soaps, vaginal creams, bubble baths, or other chemicals used in the genital area may cause tissue injury that can allow for the introduction of bacteria.

Nursing Insight— *Recognizing signs and symptoms of a UTI*

Nurses should be alert to certain patient symptoms that may be indicative of a UTI. Dysuria (pain with urination), urinary frequency, urgency, a sensation of bladder fullness, suprapubic tenderness, and cloudy, foul-smelling urine are classic symptoms associated with a UTI. If the infection has ascended to the kidneys, the woman may experience pain in the lower back region where the vertebrae and ribs meet (costovertebral angle tenderness), and fever may be present.

Diagnosis for a UTI varies according to the location and extent of the infection. *Cystitis* is the term used for infection of the lower genitourinary tract; *pyelonephritis* is the term used for infection of the upper tract. Symptoms associated with cystitis include dysuria and increased urinary frequency and urgency; symptoms associated with pyelonephritis include fever (temperature greater than 38°C [100.4°F]), chills, flank pain, and nausea and vomiting. For uncomplicated infection of the lower urinary tract, the diagnosis is made on the basis of symptoms and urinalysis, including the microscopic examination of a clean-catch (midstream) urine sample (Procedure 4-1) for the presence of white or red blood cells and bacteria. Complicated cases require a urine culture and sensitivity. In some practice settings, a leukocyte esterase (an enzyme present in white blood cells) or nitrite urine dipstick screening test to detect bacteriuria in women with suspected uncomplicated urinary tract infections is used (ACOG, 2008d, Nostl, Arnold, & Iglesia, 2013; Rubin, 2013).

Teach the patient to recognize common signs of a UTI:

* Dysuria—pain (burning sensation) on urination
* Urinary urgency and frequency associated with small amounts of urine
* Hematuria—blood or red blood cells in the urine

❝What to say❞ — *If the woman is unable to obtain a urine specimen*

If the patient has no beverage with her, offer her a beverage such as bottled water. Ask her to drink the beverage in its entirety and then remain nearby until she is able to obtain a urine specimen.

Treatment for uncomplicated lower urinary tract infections may be initiated in nonpregnant women with antibiotic therapy given over a 3-day course. Medications commonly used include trimethoprim/sulfamethoxazole (e.g., Bactrim, Septra TMP/SMX), nitrofurantoin monohydrate macrocrystals (e.g., Macrodantin), and amoxicillin/clavulanate (e.g., Augmentin). If the woman complains of intense dysuria, a

---

⚙ Procedure 4-1 Obtaining a Midstream Urine Sample

Purpose

To assist the woman in providing a suitable urine specimen for laboratory testing

Preparation

1. Complete the information requested on the container label. Include the patient's full name and the date and time of collection of the specimen. If a requisition is needed, note the date and time on the requisition.

2. Explain the procedure to the woman to ensure she understands why a urine sample is requested, the purpose of any tests to be performed, and directions on how to obtain a midstream urine sample.

Equipment

Approved empty sterile container for collection
Towelette for cleaning in between the labia
Tissue

Procedural Steps

Instruct the patient to do the following:

1. Wash and dry your hands thoroughly or use an alcohol-based hand rub.

   RATIONALE: *To reduce the risk of specimen contamination. Alcohol-based hand rubs are fast acting, reduce the number of microorganisms on the skin, and may cause less skin irritation or dryness.*

2. Remove the container cap and set it on a clean, even surface with the inner surface pointing up. Do not touch the inner surface of the lid or the container.

   RATIONALE: *To reduce the risk of specimen contamination.*

3. Sit on the toilet seat and separate the labia (vaginal lips) using your nondominant hand. Clean the urogenital area from the front to back with the towelette provided. Wipe for only one stroke and then discard the towelette.

   RATIONALE: *To reduce the risk of specimen contamination and to reduce the number of microorganisms on the skin. Cleansing from front to back prevents bringing rectal contamination forward.*

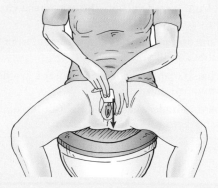

4. Holding the labia apart, begin to pass urine. Allow the beginning urine go directly into the toilet.

   RATIONALE: *The initial stream of urine washes urethral microorganisms and other debris away from the urethral meatus. The midstream collection ensures that a sterile specimen is obtained.*

5. Continue to urinate and hold the container under the urine stream. Avoid touching the inside of the container. Remove the container when it is approximately half full.

(Continued)

Procedure 4-1 Obtaining a Midstream Urine Sample—cont'd

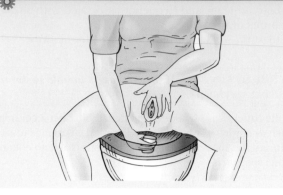

6. Carefully replace the cap and secure tightly.

RATIONALE: *Placing the cap on the container prevents inadvertent spilling and possible contamination of the urine specimen.*

7. Wash your hands again after the specimen collection.

Clinical Alert Pregnant women are at an increased risk for developing urinary tract infections, especially if they are diabetic or have gestational diabetes. Urinary tract infections may also predispose the woman to the onset of preterm labor.

bladder analgesic such as phenazopyridine (Pyridium), given for 1 to 2 days, is beneficial in alleviating the bladder discomfort (ACOG, 2008d; Vallerand & Sanoski, 2013).

"What to say" — *Teaching women about strategies to promote bladder health and decrease the incidence of UTI*

Nurses can teach women about strategies to promote bladder health and decrease the likelihood of developing a UTI. For example, the nurse may advise the patient to:

- Void frequently (every 2–4 hours); avoid postponing urination (allowing urine to remain in the bladder allows bacteria to multiply).

- Empty the bladder before and after intercourse; drink liquids before and after intercourse.

- Remain hydrated to keep bacteria flushed out of the urinary tract system.

- Drink fruit juices to acidify the urine; take vitamin C regularly to inhibit bacterial growth.

- Wipe the urethral meatus and perineum from front to back after voiding.

- Avoid harsh soaps, powders, and sprays; avoid bubble baths and bath oils.

- Wear cotton underwear; avoid tight-fitting underwear and pants.

? Global Health Case Study Inger P.

Urinary Tract Infection

Inger P. is a 20-year-old foreign exchange student from Norway. She visits the campus student health center complaining of mild dysuria and urinary frequency and urgency for the past 3 days. Inger explains to the nurse that her symptoms were "mild" at first, but have grown progressively worse and this morning she noticed blood in her urine. She denies fever, chills, flank pain, or other symptoms and states that she has never experienced any similar symptoms. Inger is sexually active and uses oral contraceptives for birth control. Her menstrual history is normal and she uses tampons. She has no known allergies.

critical thinking questions

1. What testing/evaluation does the nurse anticipate?

2. What will most likely happen next?

Inger's physical examination is unremarkable, she appears to be in no acute distress, and her vital signs, including temperature, pulse, respirations, and blood pressure, are within normal limits. She does complain of suprapubic tenderness on palpation. A laboratory dipstick test is performed on the urine sample and is positive for blood and leukocyte esterase.

3. Based on results of the physical examination and laboratory testing, what is the diagnosis?

4. What can the nurse teach Inger about her medication?

5. What other information should the nurse provide?

Now Can You— Discuss various aspects of vaginal carcinoma, toxic shock syndrome, and urinary tract infections?

1. Identify risk factors for vaginal carcinoma?
2. Develop an educational program to teach women about toxic shock syndrome?
3. Discuss urinary tract infections and describe five strategies to reduce risk for a UTI?

Endometriosis

First described by Dr. John Sampson in the 1920s, endometriosis is defined as the growth, adhesion, and progression of endometrial glands and tissue outside of the uterine cavity with cellular activity evident in lesions, nodules, and cysts. Women aged 30 to 40 years are most likely to develop endometriosis, and the condition is found in 20% to 50% of infertile women and in up to 87% of women with chronic pelvic pain. Endometrial lesions have been discovered on the ovaries, fallopian tubes, lining of the inside of the pelvic cavity, cervix, bladder, bowel, brain, nostrils, liver, and lungs (Fig. 4-5) (ACOG, 2010; Sampson, 1940).

Each month, the misplaced endometrial tissue responds to cyclical hormonal stimulation during the secretory and proliferative stages of the menstrual cycle, growing and

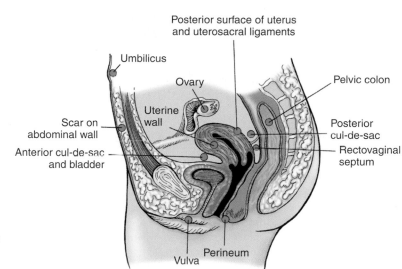

Figure 4-5 Possible sites of occurrence of endometriosis. (Venes, D. [Ed.]. [2013]. *Taber's cyclopedic medical dictionary* [22nd ed., p. 809]. Philadelphia, PA: F.A. Davis.)

thickening in a similar fashion to the endometrial tissue normally lining the uterus. During the ischemic and menstrual phases of the cycle, however, the misplaced endometrial tissue breaks down and bleeds into the surrounding tissue, causing inflammation. The released blood becomes trapped in the surrounding tissues, causing the development of blood-containing cysts. The recurrence of inflammation in the areas outside of the uterus eventually results in scarring, fibrosis, and the development of adhesions, scar tissue that binds the organs together, causing increased abdominal pain and a risk of infertility (ACOG, 2010; Speroff & Fritz, 2011).

> ✿ *Nursing Insight— Understanding terms associated with endometriosis*
>
> Endometriosis is the presence of endometrial glands and tissue outside the uterus. An *endometrioma* is a solitary, nonneoplastic mass that contains endometrial tissue. An *endometrioma* is also referred to as an *endometrioid* cyst. Endometrioid cysts, often filled with dark, reddish-brown blood, may range in size from 0.75 to 8 inches (19.05 mm–20.32 cm). An endometrioid cyst is sometimes called a *chocolate cyst* because it is filled with old blood.

ETIOLOGY, PATHOGENESIS, AND RISK FACTORS

The exact cause and pathogenesis of endometriosis is not known. One of the most widely accepted theories is Sampson's theory, or "retrograde menstruation." This theory postulates that during menstruation, endometrial tissue is transported through the fallopian tubes into the peritoneal cavity, where it implants on the ovaries and other structures. Although retrograde menstruation occurs in most women, it is not clear why some develop endometriosis and others do not. The level of functioning of the immune system is thought to be a factor in the development of endometriosis, although the exact mechanism is unknown. Interestingly, women with endometriosis tend to develop additional symptoms such as allergies, fibromyalgia, asthma, eczema, autoimmune inflammatory disease, chronic fatigue syndrome, and hypothyroidism. Also, there is a higher risk of breast cancer

in women diagnosed with endometriosis after age 40 because of their prolonged exposure to elevated endogenous estrogen (ACOG, 2010).

Risk factors for developing endometriosis include early age at menarche (onset of menstruation before age 11 years), short menstrual cycles (less than 27 days), low birth weight, nulliparity, and heavy, prolonged menstrual periods. Endometriosis also has a strong familial component: first-degree relatives of individuals with endometriosis are 7 to 10 times more likely to develop the disease. Higher parity and increased duration of lactation are associated with a decreased risk of endometriosis among parous women. Also, regular exercise (more than 4 hours per week) is associated with a reduced risk of developing endometriosis (ACOG, 2010; Falcone & Lebovic, 2011).

SIGNS AND SYMPTOMS

The signs and symptoms of endometriosis vary from woman to woman, and the severity of symptoms may increase over time. However, the most common symptom is pelvic pain. The pain, which usually begins 1 or 2 days before the expected menses, may be unilateral or bilateral and frequently lasts until the end of menstruation. Some patients experience a constant, debilitating pain that interferes with their normal daily activities. Bowel symptoms such as diarrhea, pain with defecation, constipation, and rectal bleeding with significant bowel involvement may also occur. Other symptoms include dyspareunia, dysuria, various gastrointestinal symptoms, low back pain, infertility, and menstrual dysfunction. Interestingly, the severity of pain does not correlate well with the extent of the condition. Thus, severe disease may go undetected (ACOG, 2010).

DIAGNOSIS

The diagnosis of endometriosis can be difficult to confirm owing to the wide variation in symptoms. Diagnostic laparoscopy to allow for visualization and biopsy of the lesions remains the gold standard for diagnosis, after other causes of pelvic pain (e.g., upper genital tract infection, pelvic inflammatory disease) have been ruled out. A vaginal ultrasound may also be performed to provide imaging of the displaced endometrial tissue or cyst(s), although it may be difficult to differentiate between other pathological entities such as tubal cysts, abscesses, and ectopic pregnancy (ACOG, 2010).

ⓢ Optimizing Outcomes— Endometriosis staging to guide care

The American Society for Reproductive Medicine (ASRM) has developed classification and staging guidelines to assist with endometriosis diagnosis, prognosis, treatment, and progress and communication among health professionals. Staging is based on the extent of the spread of the lesions, the density of pelvic adhesions, involvement of pelvic organs, and the degree of fallopian tube occlusion. In the standardized schema, endometriosis is classified into four stages: Stage 1—minimal, Stage 2—mild, Stage 3—moderate, and Stage 4—severe. Interestingly, women with minimal or mild endometriosis have been shown to have high degrees of pain and infertility, whereas women with Stage 4 disease have been asymptomatic and diagnosed during laparoscopy for various procedures such as tubal ligation (ASRM, 2012).

TREATMENT OPTIONS

Because endometriosis can persist during a woman's entire reproductive life, her treatment plan should be individualized and holistic. When determining the best approach for therapy, many factors must be taken into account, such as the woman's desire for future pregnancy, the size of her current family, and general lifestyle patterns. Although there are no ideal treatments for endometriosis, the planned course of therapy is based on the severity of symptoms and the woman's or couple's goals. Treatment plans generally begin with the least invasive approach and progress to more invasive therapies. Regardless of the treatment, however, approximately 10% to 20% of women with endometriosis experience a recurrence of the condition.

Medical Therapy

The goal of medical treatment is to reduce the amount of estrogen in the body so that menstruation and the subsequent growth of endometrial tissue are suppressed. To accomplish the suppression of endogenous estrogen, two main classes of drugs are used: GnRH-agonists and gonadotropin inhibitors. GnRH-agonists such as leuprolide (Lupron), goserelin (Zoladex), and nafarelin (Synarel) suppress the secretion of pituitary gonadotropins. This action causes anovulation and amenorrhea, which result in shrinkage of the endometrial tissue. The patient experiences significant pain relief and an interruption in the further development of endometrial lesions. Unfortunately, recurrence rates are high after the medication is discontinued. Common side effects are similar to those associated with natural menopause and include hot flashes; vaginal dryness; loss of libido; emotional lability; and mild, reversible bone loss. Treatment is limited to 5 months because of the decrease in bone mineral density associated with these medications (ACOG, 2010; Vallerand & Sanoski, 2013).

Danazol (Cyclomen) is a synthetic androgen that acts as a pituitary gonadotropin inhibitor. This medication causes anovulation by suppressing the secretion of follicle-stimulating hormone (FSH) and luteinizing hormone (LH). Pain relief results from the hypoestrogenic environment, endometrial

atrophy, and regression of the endometrial lesions. Because this medication is an androgenic synthetic steroid, masculinizing side effects such as acne, hirsutism, deepening of the voice, weight gain, decreased breast size, and oily skin are common. Other side effects include headaches, flushing, sweating, atrophic vaginitis, and edema. The duration of treatment is approximately 6 months because of the multitude of adverse side effects (ACOG, 2010; Falcone & Lebovic, 2011; Vallerand & Sanoski, 2013).

Contraceptive medications are also used to treat endometriosis. Combination oral contraceptives contain progestins and estrogen—hormones that suppress gonadotropins, prevent ovulation, and cause endometrial atrophy. Pain relief, related to a thinning of the endometrial lining and regression of the endometriotic implants, is achieved in approximately 75% of patients. Side effects include irregular bleeding, weight gain, headache, thrombophlebitis, benign liver tumors, and gallbladder disease. Medroxyprogesterone (Depo-Provera) is an injectable progesterone that also suppresses gonadotropins and thins endometrial tissue. Potential adverse side effects associated with this medication include weight gain, headache, abdominal discomfort, and irregular bleeding. Treatment outcomes are similar to those achieved with oral contraceptives (ACOG, 2010; ASRM, 2013; Vallerand & Sanoski, 2013).

Anastrozole (Arimidex) and letrozole (Femara) are aromatase inhibitors that decrease levels of circulating estrogen by inhibiting the peripheral conversion of androgens. Potential adverse effects include headache, nausea, diarrhea, hot flashes, and an increased risk of osteoporosis with long-term use. Treatment is limited to 6 months because of the decrease in bone mineral density. Up to 90% of patients experience alleviation of symptoms during and up to 15 months post-treatment (ACOG, 2010; Vallerand & Sanoski, 2013).

Surgical Treatment

Laparoscopy with biopsy of the lesions is the only accurate method to diagnose and determine the severity of endometriosis. During the laparoscopy, surgical removal of the lesions, adhesions, and cysts may be conducted via excision, electrocautery, or laser vaporization. The recurrence rate of endometriotic lesions after 5 years is 19% with laparoscopic removal of the lesions and 10% with hysterectomy (removal of the uterus) and bilateral oophorectomy (removal of the ovaries). Women who undergo a bilateral oophorectomy are usually treated with hormone therapy, as the benefits outweigh the risk of endometriosis recurrence (ACOG, 2010; ASRM, 2012; Falcone & Lebovic, 2011).

IMPLICATIONS FOR NURSES

Counseling and support constitute the cornerstone of nursing care for women diagnosed with endometriosis. It is incumbent upon nurses who care for women with this chronic condition to remain knowledgeable about endometriosis so that they can provide factual information about treatment options, including the risks and benefits of each. Therapeutic listening reflects respect and encourages patients to share intimate details about sensitive issues, such as dyspareunia. Teaching patients about endometriosis empowers them to participate in their treatment plan and explore approaches such as alternative methods of pain control and lifestyle and diet modifications (e.g., regular exercise and balanced nutrition) that may enhance well-being and improve functionality (Altman & Wolcyzk, 2010; Kaatz, Solari-Twadell, Cameron, & Schultz, 2010). Potential nursing diagnoses for women with endometriosis are presented in Box 4-2.

Complementary Care: *Therapies for endometriosis*

In addition to the traditional medical/surgical therapies for endometriosis, women may wish to engage in the following complementary therapies (Kaatz et al., 2010):

Yoga—to enhance stress reduction and relaxation, and to strengthen the abdominal and back muscles compromised by surgical trauma

Acupuncture—to provide pain control and fertility enhancement through increased pelvic blood flow

Stress reduction techniques—to diminish stress and enhance overall feelings of well-being

Massage—to enhance relaxation and promote release of endorphins

Physical therapy—to diminish symptoms of chronic pelvic pain and dyspareunia

Chinese herbal medicine—to provide symptomatic relief comparable to that achieved with hormonal agents, with fewer side effects (Flower et al., 2012)

Collaboration in Caring— *Assisting women with endometriosis*

Women with endometriosis can benefit from a multidisciplinary approach to treatment. The health-care team, composed of professionals with skills to address the many difficulties associated with this chronic condition, may include dietitians, physiotherapists, psychologists, and chronic pain specialists. Kaatz and colleagues (2010) described the role of the parish nurse in a community faith-based setting in providing physical, emotional, and spiritual care for women diagnosed with endometriosis. Also, nurses may suggest referral to local support groups and national organizations such as Resolve (http://www.resolve.org), an organization for infertile couples, or the Endometriosis Association (http://www.endometriosisassn.org). Nurses can remain up-to-date on evidence-based guidelines for the treatment of endometriosis through the European Society for Human Reproduction & Embryology (SHRE) Web site (http://www.guidelines.endometriosis.org) or the National Guideline Clearinghouse Web site (http://www.guideline.gov).

Box 4-2 Potential Nursing Diagnoses for Women With Endometriosis

- Knowledge Deficit related to endometriosis diagnostic work-up and treatment
- Acute Pain related to menstruation secondary to endometriosis
- Situational Low Self Esteem related to infertility secondary to endometriosis
- Anxiety related to possible invasive surgical interventions secondary to endometriosis
- Risk for Tissue Injury related to progression of endometriosis

---

Now Can You— Discuss various aspects of endometriosis?

1. Describe the chronic condition of endometriosis, and define the term *endometrioma*?
2. Discuss the modalities and goals of medical and surgical treatment for endometriosis?
3. Develop a nursing plan of care for a patient with endometriosis?

Leiomyomas (Fibroids)

Uterine leiomyomas (also called *fibroids*) are the most common solid pelvic tumors in women and the leading indication for hysterectomy. Fibroids arise from a singular neoplastic smooth muscle cell in the uterus and grow slowly. Although the exact cause is unknown, the growth of leiomyomas is dependent on estrogen; both estrogen and progesterone play a key role in the pathogenesis of leiomyomas. They are almost always benign (ACOG, 2008a; Falcone & Parker, 2013).

Nursing Insight— *Understanding terminology for uterine fibroid tumors*

A leiomyoma, or fibroid, is a benign tumor composed of nonstriated muscular tissue. The plural form of *leiomyoma* is either *leiomyomas* or *leiomyomata*.

Leiomyomas may be located in various places in and around the uterus. The most common fibroids form within the uterine wall. They can vary greatly in size and may protrude into the uterine cavity, bulge outward through the uterine wall and into the pelvic cavity, or grow on a stalk called a *pedicle* that can become twisted and cause pain. Leiomyomas are more common in African American women, and some studies report the presence of fibroids in 70% of white women and more than 80% of black women by age 50 years. Stimulated by estrogen and progesterone, the tumors occur more frequently with increasing age and regress after menopause. Other factors, such as nulliparity, cigarette smoking, and a prolonged menstrual cycle, are associated with an increased incidence (ACOG, 2008a; Garza-Cavazos & Loret de mola, 2012; Laughlin & Stewart, 2011).

SIGNS, SYMPTOMS, AND DIAGNOSIS

The two most common symptoms of uterine leiomyomas for which women seek medical treatment are abnormal uterine bleeding and pelvic pressure. Frequently, however, fibroids cause no symptoms and are first discovered during a routine bimanual pelvic examination. When abnormal bleeding is present, it is usually reported as heavy or prolonged menstrual bleeding, which may result in iron-deficiency anemia. In some situations, the bleeding significantly disrupts the woman's normal daily activities. The pelvic and abdominal discomfort is often described as "pressure." Depending on the location of the leiomyoma, pressure may be experienced in the bladder or rectal regions, leading to difficulty with urination or defecation or dyspareunia. Also, depending on their size and location, leiomyomas can interfere with fertility (ACOG, 2008a; Comerford & Hurst, 2012).

On examination, the uterus is nontender and may feel enlarged, irregularly shaped, or both. Pregnancy must always be ruled out. An ultrasound examination can confirm the presence of the leiomyoma and provide baseline measurements. Sometimes a hysteroscopy, an office procedure that uses an instrument to view the uterine cavity, or a laparoscopy, an outpatient hospital procedure that uses an instrument to view the uterus and surrounding structures, is performed to aid the diagnosis (ACOG, 2008a, 2011a).

✿❁ Diagnostic Tools Sonohysterography

Sonohysterography is the evaluation of the endometrial cavity using the transcervical injection of sterile fluid (e.g., normal saline solution) under real-time ultrasound imaging. The primary goal of this office-based diagnostic procedure is to visualize the endometrial cavity in more detail than is possible with routine transvaginal ultrasonography; it may also be used to assess tubal patency and is less painful than hysterosalpingography (dye test to evaluate tubal patency). Sonohysterography should be scheduled during the follicular phase of the menstrual cycle, after the menstrual flow has ceased, but before ovulation (i.e., by the 10th day of the menstrual cycle). Indications for use include evaluation of the following: abnormal uterine bleeding; congenital uterine anomalies; infertility; abnormalities detected on transvaginal ultrasonography; the presence of abnormalities in the uterine cavity (e.g., leiomyomas, polyps); and recurrent pregnancy loss. The procedure should not be performed in pregnant patients or in women with existing pelvic infections or unexplained pelvic tenderness (ACOG, 2011a, 2012b).

TREATMENT

In general, patients with leiomyomas are seen in the office every 3 to 6 months as long as they are experiencing mild symptoms. If heavy and prolonged bleeding or severe pain occurs, however, referral to a specialist for further evaluation is indicated. Interventions may include drug therapy; uterine artery embolization; myomectomy; hysterectomy; and laser surgery, electrocauterization, or magnetic resonance imaging (MRI)–guided focused ultrasound surgery.

Drug Therapy

Contraceptive steroids (estrogen and progestin combination and progestin alone) may be prescribed to control heavy periods and dysmenorrhea. The levonorgestrel intrauterine system (LNG-IUS) has been shown to be an effective means to decrease menorrhagia and improve quality of life. Gonadotropin-releasing hormone (GnRH) agonists, including leuprolide acetate (Lupron, Synarel), suppress the production of estrogen and progesterone and shrink the tumors, although the effects of these agents is temporary, with gradual recurrent growth of leiomyomas within several months following the cessation of treatment. Also, the significant menopausal symptoms such as vaginal dryness, hot flashes, and mood changes along with decreased bone mineral density limit use of these medications to no more than 6 months. Antiprogesterone agents such as mifepristone (Mifeprex) may also be useful in controlling leiomyoma symptoms. Recurrence of tumor growth following cessation of treatment tends to be slower than with other medications; however, further study is needed. Potential side effects include endometrial hyperplasia and alterations in liver functioning (ACOG, 2008a; Comerford & Hurst, 2012).

Uterine Artery Embolization (UAE)

Performed by interventional radiologists, this treatment involves the injection of polyvinyl alcohol pellets into selected blood vessels to block the blood supply to the fibroid and cause shrinkage and resolution of symptoms. UAE is performed under local anesthesia and conscious sedation. An incision is made into the groin, a catheter is threaded from the femoral artery into the uterine artery, and an arteriogram identifies the major blood vessels that supply the leiomyoma. Most tumors shrink in size by 50% within 3 months following treatment. Women who wish to undergo this procedure should be advised that data are lacking about the long-term effects on fertility and future pregnancies (ACOG, 2008a; Comerford & Hurst, 2012). Women who undergo UAE for the treatment of symptomatic uterine fibroids are just as satisfied with the outcome as women treated with myomectomy or hysterectomy (discussed below), according to a 2012 review from the *Cochrane Database* (Gupta, Sinha, Lumsden, & Hickey, 2012).

Myomectomy and Hysterectomy

For women who desire uterine preservation (e.g., those who desire future fertility), myomectomy (removal of the leiomyoma) may be an option. Depending on the size and number of tumors, this surgical procedure may be accomplished during a laparotomy, a laparoscopy, or a hysteroscopy. Myomectomy can be performed through a laparoscopic (conventional or robot-assisted) approach, an abdominal incision approach, or a vaginal (hysteroscopic) approach. The uterus (and therefore childbearing potential) is preserved, although most myomectomy patients will require a cesarean birth. Myomectomy is associated with significant improvements in symptoms and health-related quality of life. Hysterectomy (removal of the uterus) may be the treatment of choice if heavy, persistent bleeding cannot be controlled by any other means (ACOG, 2008a, 2011a; Comerford & Hurst, 2012; Falcone & Parker, 2013; Flyckt & Falcone, 2011; Wortman, 2012).

Laser Surgery, Electrocauterization, and MRI-Guided Focused Ultrasound Surgery

Laser surgery and electrocauterization may be used to destroy small leiomyomas with a vaginal (hysteroscopic) or abdominal (laparoscopic) approach. Laser coagulation vaporizes the fibroids and produces necrosis. However, although the uterus remains intact, endometrial scarring may diminish future fertility (ACOG, 2008a).

Magnetic resonance-guided focused ultrasound surgery (MRgFUS) is a noninvasive approach that uses magnetic resonance imaging (MRI) to deliver high-intensity ultrasound waves into the leiomyoma. The ultrasound energy penetrates soft tissue and causes necrosis. Adverse effects include heavy menses and persistent pain; further studies regarding the long-term efficacy of this treatment modality are indicated (ACOG, 2008a; Comerford & Hurst, 2012; Tulandi & Salamah, 2010).

⑤ Optimizing Outcomes— Following surgical intervention for leiomyomas

Nurses can educate women undergoing surgical interventions for leiomyomas about strategies to enhance comfort and promote healing. Nurses can teach women to:

- Take all prescribed medications.
- Contact the physician for symptoms including bleeding, cramping, fever of 39°C (102.2°F) or greater, gastrointestinal

changes, signs of wound infection (redness, swelling, heat, or pain at the incision site), urinary retention, abnormal vaginal discharge.
- Consume foods high in protein, iron, and vitamin C to facilitate tissue healing; drink plenty of fluids.
- Avoid straining during bowel movements.
- Follow the physician's recommendations regarding physical activity and driving.
- Follow the physician's orders regarding tub baths and the resumption of intercourse.

Abnormal Uterine Bleeding

Abnormal uterine bleeding, a common problem for women, may be associated with major disruptions in daily functioning. In the past, various inconsistent definitions were used to describe abnormal uterine bleeding, which was categorized as either *structural* or *dysfunctional;* the diagnosis of dysfunctional uterine bleeding was made only after all pathological causes of bleeding, such as leiomyomata, polyps, endometrial hyperplasia, and cancer, had been excluded. In 2011, the Federation of Gynecology and Obstetrics (FIGO) endeavored to create a universally accepted system of nomenclature to describe uterine bleeding abnormalities in reproductive-aged women. Adoption of the classification system (polyp, adenomyosis, leiomyoma, malignancy and hyperplasia, coagulopathy, ovulatory dysfunction, endometrial, iatrogenic, and not yet classified), known by the acronym PALM-COEIN, has been supported by ACOG (2012a) as a nomenclature system for standardizing the terminology used to describe abnormal uterine bleeding. The term *dysfunctional uterine bleeding* is not part of the new classification system, and its use is no longer recommended (Garcia, 2013; Munro, Critchley, Broder, & Fraser, 2011).

Prior to treatment, an accurate diagnosis for the cause of the bleeding should be established. Based on age alone, endometrial assessment to exclude cancer should be performed on any woman older than 35 years. In addition to a physical examination, diagnostic/laboratory tests used to evaluate women with abnormal uterine bleeding may include a pregnancy test to rule out ectopic pregnancy, Pap test, testing for the presence of *Chlamydia trachomatis,* complete blood count, evaluation for endocrine dysfunction (e.g., thyroid-stimulating hormone, prolactin), endometrial biopsy, transvaginal ultrasound, hysteroscopy, and dilation and curettage (D & C) (ACOG, 2011a, 2012a; Halloran, 2011). Owing to issues such as fatigue; anxiety; social embarrassment; and restrictions on social, leisure, and physical activities, heavy menstrual bleeding may significantly diminish women's quality of life; the diagnosis, evaluation, and treatment of heavy menstrual bleeding should be based on the "patient experience"—the woman's personal assessment of her blood loss and its effect on her life (Matteson et al., 2013; Moore, 2013).

"What to say" — *Asking about menstrual blood loss*

When interviewing patients about menstrual blood loss, the nurse may ask the following questions (Dominguez, 2012):
- How many days does your menstrual period usually last?
- Would you describe your monthly flow as "unusually heavy"?
- Do you ever pass large blood clots?
- What size/kind/brand of protection do you use—and on your heaviest days, do you need to use extra protection such as a tampon plus a napkin?
- Do you ever leak and stain your underclothes, outer clothes, or bed sheets?
- Do you ever miss school/work because of a heavy menstrual flow?
- Do you ever have to limit any activities because of a heavy menstrual flow?
- Does a heavy menstrual flow affect your relationships/sex life/quality of life?

ABNORMAL BLEEDING RELATED TO PALM: STRUCTURAL CAUSES

Structural causes of uterine bleeding include Polyps, Adenomyosis (a condition in which endometrial tissue grows into the myometrium), Leiomyomata, and Malignancy and hyperplasia. Uterine fibroid tumors are often asymptomatic and first detected during a bimanual pelvic examination. Precancerous or cancerous conditions of the uterus or cervix can also cause abnormal bleeding (ACOG, 2012a).

ABNORMAL BLEEDING RELATED TO COEIN: NONSTRUCTURAL CAUSES

Nonstructural causes of uterine bleeding, which include Coagulopathy, Ovulatory dysfunction, Endometrial, Iatrogenic, and Not yet classified (entities that are poorly defined or not well examined), produce noncyclical menstrual blood flow that is derived from the endometrium. The bleeding may range from spotty to excessive and may be prolonged. It is most commonly caused by hormonal imbalances, which account for approximately 75% of cases of irregular bleeding. Heavy bleeding is a common problem for women during the perimenopausal period between the ages of 40 and 50. As ovulation becomes more erratic, levels of progesterone decrease. An important function of progesterone is to stabilize the uterine endometrial lining. In the absence of progesterone, the bleeding may become unpredictable, excessive, or prolonged. Abnormal uterine bleeding may also occur during adolescence, before a pattern of regular ovulatory cycles has been established. Other conditions that may cause abnormal bleeding include thyroid or adrenal gland disorders, polycystic ovary syndrome, clotting disorders, liver or kidney disease, and leukemia. Taking herbal preparations, such as ginseng, or medications, such as anticoagulants, may also cause abnormal bleeding (ACOG, 2012a, 2013b; Speroff & Fritz, 2011).

> **Nursing Insight**— *Clotting disorders may cause abnormal uterine bleeding*
>
> Nurses should be aware that abnormal uterine bleeding may be related to an undiagnosed coagulopathy such as defects in primary hemostasis, platelet deficiency (e.g., leukemia, idiopathic thrombocytopenia), platelet dysfunction (e.g., von Willebrand disease), and abnormalities of secondary homeostasis (congenital factor deficiencies). Von Willebrand disease is a genetic bleeding

disorder caused by a defect or deficiency of a blood-clotting factor (von Willebrand factor). This condition occurs in approximately 1% of all women and is the most common inherited bleeding disorder among American women (ACOG, 2012a, 2013c).

TREATMENT

Depending on the cause, treatment for abnormal uterine bleeding may include drug therapy and/or surgery. Medical management is the preferred method of therapy for anovulatory uterine bleeding. The goals of medical treatment are to alleviate the acute bleeding, prevent future episodes of noncyclical bleeding, decrease the woman's risk of long-term complications from anovulation, and improve her overall quality of life. It is important for nurses to counsel patients that the treatment may initially cause heavy menstrual bleeding related to buildup of the endometrium. However, the bleeding should diminish over the course of 3 to 4 months.

Depending on the patient's age and physical findings, medications used include conjugated equine estrogens, low-dose combination oral contraceptives, a levonorgestrel intrauterine system (LNG-IUS), cyclical progestogens, iron supplementation, prostaglandin synthetase inhibitors (e.g., indomethacin [Indocin]), and NSAIDs (e.g., aspirin, ibuprofen, naproxen). Tranexamic acid (Lysteda), an oral nonhormonal, prothrombotic medication to treat heavy menstrual bleeding, works by stabilizing a protein that helps blood to clot. Because the use of this medication while taking hormonal contraceptives may increase the risk of blood clots, stroke, or heart attack, women using hormonal contraception should take tranexamic acid only if there is a strong medical need and the benefits outweigh the potential risks. The most common adverse effects of tranexamic acid are menstrual discomfort/cramps, headache, back pain, and nausea, and the medication is contraindicated in women who have active thromboembolic disease or a history of thrombosis or thromboembolism (ACOG, 2012a; Wilton, 2012).

Surgical procedures to treat abnormal uterine bleeding include dilation and curettage (D & C), endometrial ablation, and hysterectomy. These interventions are indicated for patients who fail to improve with medical therapy and who desire no future fertility. Women with significant acute bleeding may need a D & C for the immediate control of bleeding as well as for diagnosis. However, the beneficial effects associated with this surgical intervention are only temporary, and the D & C procedure is no longer the mainstay of treatment (ACOG, 2012a; Harmanli et al., 2012; Nelson & Baldwin, 2011).

A surgical alternative to hysterectomy is endometrial ablation, a procedure that uses a lighted viewing instrument (hysteroscope) and other instruments to destroy (ablate) the uterine lining. Depending on the method used, endometrial ablation may be performed in the physician office, outpatient facility, or hospital. The procedure may be done using a local or spinal anesthesia, although general anesthesia is sometimes used. Recovery following endometrial ablation generally ranges from a few days to a couple of weeks.

✿ Nursing Insight— *Understanding endometrial ablation*

The goal of endometrial ablation is to restore menses to normal or less. Endometrial ablation is used to control heavy, prolonged vaginal bleeding for the following circumstances: The bleeding has not responded to other treatments; childbearing is completed; the patient prefers not to have a hysterectomy to control the bleeding; or other medical problems prevent a hysterectomy. The five FDA-approved methods use a variety of energy sources to achieve endometrial destruction via hyperthermic or hypothermic methods, and each is designed to ablate down to the basal layer to prevent regeneration and subsequent menstrual flow. Hyperthermic endometrial ablation may be accomplished by laser beam (laser thermal ablation), electricity (electrothermal ablation), microwave (microwave endometrial ablation), or radiofrequency energy (radiofrequency ablation); hypothermic endometrial ablation is accomplished by freezing (cryoablation). With heat-based ablation (hyperthermia), the endometrium undergoes necrosis and then heals by scarring, which usually reduces or prevents uterine bleeding. Compared with hyperthermic ablation, cryoablation is less likely to stimulate the process of scar tissue formation and, owing to the anesthetic effect related to the cooling of tissues and nerves, may be less painful than the heat-based thermal ablation techniques. Regardless of the ablation method used, fertility is not preserved, although there is a remote possibility of pregnancy if a portion of the endometrium is left intact. Contraception is recommended for women who have not completed menopause (ACOG, 2013b; Auerbach, Duleba, & Whiteside, 2013; Comerford & Hurst, 2012; Macer, 2013).

Hysterectomy

A hysterectomy is a surgery to remove the uterus. After cesarean section, hysterectomy is the second most frequently performed major surgical procedure for women of reproductive age in the United States. Each year in this country, approximately 600,000 hysterectomies are performed, and an estimated 20 million women have had a hysterectomy. The three conditions most commonly associated with hysterectomy are uterine leiomyomata, endometriosis, and uterine prolapse. Other indications include cancer (i.e., uterine, ovarian, cervical, endometrial), adenomyosis, chronic pelvic pain, and abnormal vaginal bleeding (ACOG, 2009a; CDC, 2011b).

During the surgery, the whole uterus or a part of it may be removed. A *partial, subtotal,* or *supracervical* hysterectomy involves removal of the upper part of the uterus, leaving the cervix in place. A *total* hysterectomy removes the whole uterus and cervix, and a *radical* hysterectomy removes the whole uterus, along with the tissue on both sides of the cervix and the upper part of the vagina. This particular surgery is done for the most part when there is cancer present.

66What to say99 — *When explaining surgical approaches for hysterectomy*

Several different surgical approaches are used to perform removal of the uterus. To determine the most appropriate method, the physician assesses a number of factors, including the patient's health history, reason for the surgery, and personal preference. The nurse can explain the various procedures:

Abdominal hysterectomy: A 5- to 7-inch incision is made in the low abdomen, just above the pubic hairline. The incision may be in a vertical or horizontal direction. The uterus is removed through the incision. Recovery time varies from 4 to 6 weeks.

Vaginal hysterectomy: An incision is made in the vagina, and the uterus is removed through the vagina.

Laparoscopic hysterectomy: An instrument with a thin, lighted tube and small camera (laparoscope) is inserted into the abdomen to allow for visualization of the pelvic organs. Three or four small cuts are made in the abdomen for insertion of the laparoscope and other instruments. The uterus is divided into small segments and removed through the incisions.

Laparoscopically assisted vaginal hysterectomy (LAVH): The uterus is removed through the vagina, and the laparoscope is used to guide the procedure.

Robotic surgery: The doctor uses a special machine to perform the surgery as in laparoscopic surgery. This method is most often used when a patient has cancer or is very obese and vaginal surgery is considered unsafe.

Recovery from vaginal or laparoscopic surgery generally takes from 3 to 4 weeks. As with any surgical procedure, hysterectomy may be associated with complications (e.g., infection, venous thromboembolism, genitourinary and gastrointestinal tract injury, bleeding, nerve injury, vaginal cuff dehiscence), which vary based on route of surgery and surgical technique (Clarke-Pearson & Geller, 2013).

Prior to the surgery, a psychological assessment is an essential component of care. The nurse should ensure that the woman has an opportunity to consider the personal significance of the loss of her uterus, discuss misconceptions about the effects of the surgery, and ensure that she has an adequate support system for postoperative care and concerns. Recovery from a hysterectomy is a very personal experience that is shaped by a myriad of factors, such as the woman's age, her physical and emotional health, reason for the surgery, and type of surgery performed. The nurse can help to empower women facing uterine surgery by creating a therapeutic environment where the patient feels safe in sharing feelings and expressing concerns. Other nursing actions to help prepare the woman for the surgery and promote a healthy recovery include providing information, engaging the assistance of other health professionals, and making referrals when appropriate.

Now Can You— Discuss leiomyomas, abnormal uterine bleeding, and hysterectomy?

1. Identify common treatment modalities for leiomyomas, and develop a postoperative teaching plan for the woman undergoing a surgical intervention?
2. Differentiate between structural (PALM) and nonstructural causes (COEIN) of abnormal uterine bleeding?
3. Discuss the nurse's role when caring for the patient who will undergo a hysterectomy?

Ovarian Tumors

Because the ovary is composed of many different tissue types, growths or tumors involving the ovary may be of various types. Interestingly, more than 50 different types of ovarian tumors have been identified. Two of the most common types of ovarian tumors are follicular cysts and corpus luteum cysts, which are included in this discussion.

Nursing Insight— Understanding ovarian cysts

Ovarian cysts affect women of all ages; the vast majority of them are considered functional, or physiological. Most disappear within a few weeks without treatment. Ovarian cysts occur most often during the childbearing years and typically represent a normal process. A dermoid cyst is an abnormal cyst that usually affects younger women; it may range in size from 1 cm (less than a half inch) up to 45 cm (17 inches) in diameter. A dermoid cyst is usually a benign tumor (2% are malignant) sometimes referred to as a mature cystic teratoma. Originating from a totipotential germ cell (i.e., capable of developing into any variety of body cells), the cyst is similar to those present on skin tissue and can contain fat and occasionally bone, hair, and cartilage. A dermoid cyst can cause the ovary to twist ("torsion") and produce severe abdominal pain.

FOLLICULAR CYSTS

A follicular cyst is the most common growth that occurs on the ovary. It develops during the first half of the menstrual cycle, called the *follicular phase*. This type of ovarian cyst, termed a *functional* or *simple* cyst, forms when ovulation does not occur. Instead, the developing dominant follicle continues to grow and evolves into a large, fluid-filled cyst that contains a high concentration of estrogen. The follicular cyst can also form from one of the smaller follicles that failed to regress after another ovarian follicle gained dominance. Follicular cysts usually produce no symptoms and disappear spontaneously within a few months. However, approximately one-fourth of women with follicular cysts report symptoms such as pain or the sensation of a heavy, achy feeling in the pelvis.

The diagnosis is generally made on the basis of symptoms and bimanual examination. Ultrasonography may be used to confirm the findings and rule out pregnancy. Expectant management ("watch and wait") and a repeat examination in 6 to 10 weeks is the treatment of choice unless symptoms worsen. The majority of follicular cysts resolve after two to three menstrual cycles without intervention. On occasion, oral contraceptive pills are prescribed to hasten cyst resolution (ACOG, 2014).

CORPUS LUTEUM CYSTS

A corpus luteum cyst forms from the corpus luteum during the second half, or luteal phase, of the menstrual cycle. The woman with a corpus luteum cyst may experience menstrual irregularity (e.g., delayed menses), although most often, the cyst regresses and disappears spontaneously within one or two menstrual cycles. The cyst may, however, fill with fluid or blood and persist on the ovary. Less commonly, the cyst ruptures and can cause severe abdominal pain from the associated bleeding. When this occurs, surgical removal of the cyst may be necessary.

Polycystic Ovary Syndrome

Polycystic ovary syndrome (PCOS), also called Stein-Leventhal syndrome, is one of the most common endocrine disorders in reproductive-age women, affecting approximately 5% to 10% of women throughout the world. The disorder occurs when an endocrine imbalance results in elevated levels of estrogen, testosterone, and luteinizing hormone (LH) and a decreased secretion of follicle-stimulating hormone (FSH). Multiple follicular cysts develop on one or both ovaries and produce excessive amounts of estrogen. Clinical findings associated with PCOS include obesity, hirsutism, acne, and infertility. Menstrual irregularity, which occurs in approximately 75% of women with PCOS, may be the first presenting symptom suggestive of the disorder. Women with this condition often have insulin resistance and are at an increased risk for developing type 2 diabetes mellitus. There is also an increased risk for coronary artery disease, hypertension, cancer (e.g., endometrial, ovarian, breast), and dyslipidemia. PCOS is often diagnosed during adolescence, and the prevalence of the disorder in Mexican Americans is twice that of other ethnic groups (ACOG, 2009c; Divasta, 2013; MacKay & Woo, 2013; Nelson & Baldwin, 2011; Yawn, 2012).

Optimizing Outcomes— With lifestyle modifications to improve PCOS

Diet, exercise, and weight loss are considered the best first-line interventions to improve PCOS. An increase in exercise combined with dietary change has been shown to reduce diabetes risk comparable to or better than medication. Weight control improves many aspects of the condition, leading to more regular menstrual cycles, reduced androgen levels, lowered lipid levels, and better glucose metabolism. To achieve weight loss, a low-fat, high-fiber diet with low-glycemic-index carbohydrates is recommended. Typically, women with PCOS have unique challenges achieving and maintaining healthy weights. Because they consume less energy metabolizing their food, they often require a lower-calorie diet than other women to lose weight. Obese women with PCOS should follow a hypocaloric diet (500 kcal/day deficit) that reduces the glycemic load. Reducing alcohol consumption is another way to decrease caloric intake. Moderate physical activity combined with muscle-strengthening exercises improves insulin sensitivity and helps to limit the loss of lean muscle mass. Cognitive behavior therapy, which involves teaching problem-solving skills and enhancing and reframing perceptions, may be useful in helping women with PCOS to overcome the barriers to adopting lifestyle changes needed to improve health (ACOG, 2009c; Divasta, 2013; Smith & Taylor, 2011).

Where Research and Practice Meet: Quality of Life Among Young Women With PCOS

PCOS is increasingly being recognized as a chronic condition accompanied by a myriad of psychosocial issues, such as feelings of depression, isolation, anxiety, and frustration, and psychological distress and perceived diminished quality of life may well persist beyond medical treatment. Using personal, semistructured interviews, Weiss and Bulmer (2011) explored the psychosocial effects of living with PCOS among 12 young women aged 18 to 23 years. The participants' physical, social, and emotional challenges in dealing with PCOS were ongoing and distressing, and underscore the need for a holistic treatment approach that includes individualized psychosocial support.

Jones, Hall, Lashen, Balen, and Ledger (2011), who interviewed 15 young women (aged 17 to 21 years) diagnosed with PCOS to explore health-related quality of life (HRQoL), found that, overall, the chronic condition exerted a negative impact upon HRQoL, and weight problems (i.e., difficulties associated with managing/maintaining weight) and body perceptions were the most significant contributors to the reduced HRQoL. Based on their findings, the investigators concluded that among this young population, emotional and social functioning appeared to be most affected rather than areas of physical functioning, and health-care providers should be sensitive to the emotional impact of PCOS on adolescents' HRQoL and the potential for poor sexual health through risk-taking behaviors that may occur because of the potential loss of fertility.

Medical treatment of patients with PCOS usually depends on the presenting signs and symptoms. For women who are not attempting to conceive, combination low-dose hormonal contraceptives are the usual treatment because they inhibit LH and decrease testosterone levels. Oral contraceptives may also lessen acne and hirsutism. If pregnancy is desired, medications to induce ovulation, such as clomiphene citrate (Clomid), are usually prescribed. Oral antidiabetic medications for type 2 diabetes such as metformin hydrochloride (Glucophage) are used to lower insulin, testosterone, and glucose levels, which, in turn, can reduce symptoms of acne, hirsutism, abdominal obesity, and other symptoms associated with PCOS (ACOG, 2009c; Divasta, 2013; Mayhew, 2011; Yawn, 2012).

Nursing Insight— *Medication enhances ovulatory function in women with insulin resistance*

Owing to the fact that PCOS, one of the most common causes of infertility, is associated with insulin resistance, the use of insulin-lowering or insulin-sensitizing therapy may help to improve ovarian function and menstrual cyclicity. Myo-inositol, a dietary vitamin belonging to the B complex, has been shown to support and maintain menstrual cyclicity, oocyte quality, and ovulatory function through its effect on insulin receptor activity. Commercially available by its brand name Pregnitude, myo-inositol is an oral powder formulation mixed with water that combines 2 grams of myo-inositol with 200 micrograms of folic acid. Results from observational and controlled clinical investigations have shown that myo-inositol, an over-the-counter dietary supplement, improves ovarian function and ovulation induction in patients with oligomenorrhea or amenorrhea plus PCOS (Simon, Roseff, & Hait, 2012).

Nurses can counsel women with PCOS about their chronic disorder and the potential long-term effects on their health. A holistic approach to care encompasses a variety of lifestyle strategies, such as diet, exercise, and weight loss along with prescribed medications, when needed, to achieve good clinical outcomes and a better quality of life. Referrals for resources including cognitive behavior therapy, counseling for issues concerning body image and self-esteem, and support groups and nutritional information may be appropriate as well (Burton & Daley, 2011; Smith & Taylor, 2011). In some settings, an intervention called the group medical visit (GMV) has been shown to enhance care for women with chronic diseases such as PCOS. With this care delivery model, patients receive individualized care and counseling, as well as educational information and the opportunity to network with other women dealing with the same problems. GMV participants benefit from consistency in care and empowerment to facilitate symptom management and, it is hoped, prevent potentially adverse health consequences (Moore & Caldwell, 2011).

Ovarian Cancer

Ovarian cancer is the leading cause of gynecological deaths and the fourth most common cause of cancer deaths in women, resulting in 16,000 deaths annually. Ovarian cancer accounts for about 3% of all cancers in women, and a woman's risk of getting invasive ovarian cancer during her lifetime is approximately 1 in 72. Approximately one-half of women with ovarian cancer are 63 or older, and it is slightly more common in white women than in African American women. The American Cancer Society estimates that in 2013, about 22,240 women will receive a new diagnosis of ovarian cancer, and about 14,230 women will die of ovarian cancer (American Cancer Society [ACS], 2013).

Although the cause is unknown, there are identified risk factors, including increasing age (the highest incidence is between 60 and 64); nulliparity; pregnancy later in life; obesity (body mass index of at least 30); the presence of *BRCA1* and *BRCA2* genes; a personal history of breast cancer; and a family history of breast, ovarian, or colorectal cancer. Associative causes include the use of ovarian hyperstimulation medications prescribed for infertility; exposure to asbestos;

genital exposure to talcum powder; a diet high in fat, meat, and sweets; and childhood mumps infection. Pregnancy and oral contraceptive use provide some protection against ovarian cancer, and the use of postmenopausal estrogen may increase the risk (ACS, 2013; Cesario, 2010).

Unfortunately, the signs and symptoms of ovarian cancer are often vague until late in development. Although once termed a "silent killer," ovarian cancer should instead be considered a "whispering disease," whose symptoms must be listened to carefully by patients and providers alike. Ovarian cancer should be considered in any woman over age 40 who has complaints of vague abdominal or pelvic discomfort, pain, or enlargement; back pain; indigestion; inability to eat normally; feeling full after eating only a small amount; a sense of bloating; constipation; urinary incontinence; urinary frequency or urgency of recent onset; or unexplained weight loss. Ovarian cancer symptoms are likely to be progressive, persistent, frequent, and severe, and they are also more likely to occur in synchrony with other symptoms. Enlargement of the abdomen due to accumulation of fluid (ascites) is the most common sign. Because ovarian cancer is a rapidly growing neoplasm, the diagnosis is often not made until the cancer has metastasized (ACOG, 2011c; ACS, 2013; Cesario, 2010; Trouskova & Alexander, 2012).

Ovarian cancer is rarely diagnosed early. In fact, nearly 70% of women with ovarian cancer have already experienced metastatic spread outside of the pelvis by the time of the initial diagnosis. Methods for mass screening and early detection have not been successful, and currently an annual bimanual examination is recommended. Tests that are used most frequently to screen for ovarian cancer include transvaginal sonography, which can be used to determine the size, location, and quality (e.g., fluid filled, solid) of the mass, and serum CA-125 antigen levels (ACOG, 2011c; ACS, 2013; Rossi & Clarke-Pearson, 2011).

Optimizing Outcomes— Biomarkers for epithelial ovarian cancer

Cancer antigen 125 (CA-125) is a serum protein that is higher in many women with epithelial ovarian cancer. In premenopausal women with symptoms, a CA-125 measurement is frequently not useful because elevated levels of the protein are associated with a variety of common benign conditions (e.g., uterine leiomyomata, PID, endometriosis, pregnancy). In postmenopausal women with a pelvic mass, a CA-125 measurement may be helpful in predicting a higher likelihood of a malignant tumor than a benign tumor, although a normal CA-125 measurement alone does not rule out ovarian cancer. Human epididymis protein 4 (HE4) is a secreted glycoprotein expressed in normal glandular epithelium of the reproductive tract. HE4 has been validated as a serum tumor marker for epithelial ovarian cancer (EOC), and cleared by the FDA as a monitoring tool for patients diagnosed with EOC. A novel qualitative ovarian cancer blood test, called OVA1 Ovarian Triage Test, has also recently gained FDA approval. The OVA1 biomarker panel, which measures the serum levels of five potential biochemical markers for ovarian cancer, can help assess the likelihood of malignancy of an ovarian tumor before surgery and facilitate decisions about referral to a gynecological oncologist. The Risk of Ovarian Malignancy Algorithm

(ROMA) combines the results for ovarian markers CA-125 and HE4 with menopausal status to help predict the likelihood of malignancy in women with an adnexal mass and for whom surgery is planned. ROMA stratifies patients into a "high risk" or "low risk" category, and also provides individual results for both CA-125 and HE4. It should be noted that neither the OVA1 nor the HE4 is recommended or approved for use in the screening of asymptomatic women (ACOG, 2011c; ACS, 2013; Carter & Downs, 2011; Li, 2012).

A strong family history of breast cancer may be caused by an inherited mutation in the *BRCA1* or *BRCA2* gene. Because alterations in these genes have been detected in women with ovarian cancer, screening women with the *BRCA* mutations can be performed to determine whether they carry these genes. Interestingly, these mutations also increase the risks for primary peritoneal carcinoma and fallopian tube carcinoma. Furthermore, research has shown that the fimbriated end of the fallopian tube contains precursor lesions that lead to the development of ovarian cancers in both *BRCA*-positive and *BRCA*-negative populations. Based on this information, some experts suggest that offering patients a salpingectomy (removal of the fallopian tubes) during benign gynecological surgeries may provide an option for ovarian cancer prophylaxis for the general population (ACOG, 2009b, 2011c; ACS, 2013; Tellawi & Morozov, 2014).

Laparotomy is performed for surgical confirmation and clinical staging, which provides direction to the treatment and prognosis of the cancer. The preferred treatment for ovarian cancer is surgical removal and usually requires a hysterectomy with bilateral salpingo-oophorectomy. After surgery, chemotherapy (administered intravenously and intraperitoneally), sometimes combined with immunotherapy, is used to treat any remaining cancer. Radiation therapy may be used as a palliative measure, although it is not typically used as a treatment option for ovarian cancer (ACOG, 2008c; Carter & Downs, 2011).

🔘 Optimizing Outcomes— Enhancing ovarian cancer awareness

Nurses can help promote women's awareness and understanding of their bodies by empowering them with information about specific symptoms that may be associated with ovarian cancer. The Goff Symptom Index (Goff et al., 2007) was developed to aid in the early identification of women with potential ovarian cancer. The tool focuses on symptoms most often seen among women who were later diagnosed with ovarian cancer. The easy-to-administer symptom index includes the following symptoms: bloating, pelvic or abdominal pain, difficulty eating or feeling full quickly, and urinary urgency or frequency. Scientists note that the frequency and/or number of symptoms are correlated with the diagnosis of ovarian cancer, and women who experience any of these symptoms on a daily basis for more than a few weeks should be counseled to contact their women's health-care specialist. Recently, the Ovarian Cancer National Alliance issued the Interim Practice Guidance for the diagnosis of ovarian cancer. Posted online, these guidelines represent the first time that ovarian cancer diagnostic protocols have been made available to the public. In conjunction with the Gynecologic Cancer Foundation, a

🔘 Where Research and Practice Meet: Reporting of Ovarian Cancer Symptoms

It has been established that although many women with ovarian cancer experience symptoms before diagnosis, little is known about personal characteristics, medical conditions, or other habits that may influence the symptoms or how they are reported. Using the Goff Symptom Index (SI) and other screening tools, Lowe, Andersen, Kane, Robertson, and Goff (2013) explored various factors that may be associated with how a woman reports symptoms. The investigators found that certain characteristics including race (black women had a positive SI more often than did white or Asian women), number of gynecological conditions (women with multiple gynecological conditions were more likely to have a positive SI), and reason for health clinic visit (abdominal/pelvic pain and bloating) may influence which symptoms are reported and the specific pattern of reporting. Based on their findings, the investigators stressed the importance of the nursing role in routinely inquiring about ovarian cancer symptoms and in ensuring that symptoms that are new or frequent are investigated further.

Symptom Diary, designed to help women measure the persistency and severity of their symptoms, is also available at http://www.ovariancancer.org/diary (Ovarian Cancer National Alliance, 2013).

Endometrial Cancer

In the United States, cancer of the endometrium is the most common gynecological malignancy. According to estimates from the ACS (2013), for the year 2013, approximately 429,560 new cases of cancer of the uterine corpus (body) will be diagnosed. The estimates include both endometrial cancers and uterine sarcomas (which are rare and represent 2% of uterine body cancers). Most uterine malignancies arise within the inner lining of the uterus and are adenocarcinomas that develop from overgrowth (hyperplasia) of the endometrium. Uterine cancer is rarely found in women under age 40; approximately 70% of all cases are found in women in the 50 to 69 age group. However, certain conditions (e.g., chronic anovulation, diabetes, obesity, genetic predisposition) predispose some premenopausal women to excessive levels of circulating estrogen, increasing their risk for endometrial cancer. The average chance of a woman being diagnosed with endometrial cancer during her lifetime is about 1 in 38. Currently, there are more than 500,000 survivors of endometrial cancer living in this country. Interestingly, this cancer is more common in white women, but African American women are more likely to die of it (ACOG, 2005; ACS, 2013; Galic & Gupta, 2012; Leslie, Thiel, & Yang, 2012; Sorosky, 2012).

🌸 Nursing Insight— *Estrogen and endometrial cancer*

There is an established relationship between unopposed (i.e., absence of progesterone) exogenous estrogen and uterine cancer. Progesterone inhibits the growth of cells stimulated by estrogen and causes them to enter a more mature secretory state. Postmenopausal women who receive estrogen therapy without progesterone have much higher rates of uterine cancer.

Cultural Diversity: Endometrial Cancer in African American Women

The lifetime mortality risk for Caucasian women with uterine cancer is 2.8% (risk for disease) and 0.48% (risk for death), as compared with African American women, whose risk for developing this condition is 1.7% and whose risk for dying of the condition is 0.73%. The 5-year survival rate for white women older than 65 years is 80.8%; for African American women in the same age group, the 5-year survival rate is 53.3%. It is unclear whether the high mortality in black women is a result of delayed treatment, lack of access to care, or a higher likelihood of cancers with more serious prognostic characteristics. It is known, however, that of women with endometrial cancer, only 52% of black women older than 50 years have the condition confined to the uterus at the time of the original surgery, as compared with 73% of white women older than 50 years (ACOG, 2005; NCI, 2012).

The exact cause of uterine cancer is not known. However, risk factors have been established. These include unopposed estrogen therapy, nulliparity or low parity, early menarche (before age 12), late menopause (after age 55), therapy with tamoxifen (an antiestrogen medication used in the prevention and treatment of breast cancer), infertility, diabetes, gallbladder disease, PCOS, a history of ovarian granulosa-theca cell tumors, hypertension, diabetes mellitus, a high sugar, high-fat diet (which increases the levels of circulating estrogen), and obesity. Factors associated with a lower risk for endometrial cancer include multiparity, use of combination oral contraceptives, use of an intrauterine device, and menopausal estrogen therapy combined with progesterone therapy for women who have a uterus. A genetic syndrome known as Lynch syndrome (previously termed hereditary nonpolyposis colorectal cancer) has also been associated with both endometrial and ovarian cancer (ACOG, 2005; ACS, 2013; Sorosky, 2012; World Cancer Research Fund/American Institute for Cancer Research, 2013).

Nursing Insight— Lynch syndrome: a genetic cancer susceptibility syndrome

Lynch syndrome (LS), an autosomal-dominant condition, is a common genetic cancer susceptibility syndrome responsible for the majority of hereditary endometrial cancer and colorectal cancer. Women with LS have lifetime cancer risks of up to 80% for colorectal cancer (CRC), up to 71% for endometrial cancer (EC), and 12% for ovarian cancer. Patients with LS are also at high risk for stomach, pancreatic, biliary, renal pelvis, and brain cancers. When obtaining the family health history, it is essential that nurses inquire about the onset of cancer (in family members) at an early age—the average age of CRC onset for LS patients is 45, and EC onset is around age 50. Other "red flags" include CRC in two or more generations on the same side of the family, ovarian or gastric cancer at any age, and two or more individuals with any two Lynch spectrum cancers (Frieder, 2010; Frieder & Berlin, 2012).

Endometrial cancer is slow growing, and more than 75% of the neoplasms are adenocarcinomas that develop from endometrial hyperplasia. Most women are symptomatic in the early stages of this cancer, a factor that leads to early diagnosis and, frequently, successful treatment. There are no effective screening methods to detect endometrial cancer. Instead, women and their health-care providers must rely on signs and symptoms of the condition. For postmenopausal women, the cardinal symptom is vaginal bleeding; perimenopausal women may experience heavy or prolonged menstruation or spotting or bleeding between menses. Other symptoms for women in all age groups include pelvic pain, dyspareunia, and weight loss (ACOG, 2005; ACS, 2013; Sorosky, 2012).

Pelvic examination may reveal a uterine enlargement or mass. A patient who has abnormal vaginal bleeding should have an endometrial biopsy. Fractional curettage, a procedure that involves a scraping of the endocervix and the endometrium to obtain tissue for histological evaluation, may also be performed. Other diagnostic tests that may be conducted include hysteroscopy (examination of the uterus through an endoscope) and transvaginal ultrasound. If invasive endometrial cancer is present, systematic surgical staging is performed. The work-up may also include chest radiography, abdominal computed tomography (CT) scan, MRI, cystoscopy, proctoscopy, liver function tests, renal function tests, bone scans, and serum testing for the presence of cancer antigen 125 (CA-125, released by some endometrial and ovarian cancers) to determine the extent of metastasis (ACOG, 2005, 2009a, 2011a; ACS, 2013; Sorosky, 2012).

Endometrial cancer is staged based on its location and extension into surrounding tissue and distant metastases. Treatment involves total abdominal hysterectomy along with removal of the ovaries, fallopian tubes, and local lymph nodes. Following the surgery, radiation therapy, chemotherapy, or hormone therapy may be prescribed, depending on the clinical findings. When endometrial cancer is diagnosed and treated early, survival rates are good. For all cases of endometrial cancer, the relative 5-year survival rate is approximately 83%; for cancers treated at an earlier stage, the 5-year survival rate exceeds 92% (ACOG, 2005; ACS, 2013; Leslie et al., 2012; Sorosky, 2012).

Collaboration in Caring— Addressing sexual issues in women with gynecological cancer

A woman's sexual response is often affected by the myriad of physiological and psychological effects of cancer and cancer treatment. Physical factors include fatigue, pain, alopecia, weight change, loss of control over various bodily functions, and symptoms of menopause. Psychological effects on sexuality may stem from anxiety, depression, fear of dying or cancer recurrence, feelings of vulnerability and isolation, and, for many, the realization of an end to reproductive opportunity. It is important to establish communication about sexual issues early in the course of treatment; individualized interventions can help patients maintain their sexual quality of life after cancer. A multidisciplinary approach with a care team that includes psychologists or sex therapists with specialized training can be useful in addressing the various facets of sexual impairment in women after gynecological cancer (Ratner, Richter, Minkin, & Foran-Tuller, 2012).

Now Can You— Discuss ovarian tumors and endometrial cancer?

1. Differentiate between ovarian follicular cysts and corpus luteum cysts?

2. Develop a holistic nursing plan of care for a woman with a diagnosis of polycystic ovary syndrome?
3. Develop an ovarian cancer awareness educational program for women?
4. Discuss the major risk factors for endometrial cancer, and identify the primary presenting symptom?

Diseases of the Vulva

The external female genital organs, or vulva, include all visible structures that extend externally from the mons pubis to the perineum. The vulvar tissue is richly supplied with sweat and sebaceous glands, and some areas contain hair follicles as well. The vulvar region supports a moist environment that contains increased concentrations of skin bacteria.

Symptoms of vulvovaginal disorders are common, often chronic, and can significantly interfere with a woman's sexual function and sense of well-being. Obtaining a detailed health history is an essential tool in the patient assessment, and it is important to remember that systemic conditions such as Crohn's disease can cause vulvar symptoms. Vulvar pruritus, or itching, is the most frequent symptom, and women often delay evaluation because they self-treat with readily available vaginal preparations. Other commonly reported symptoms in the vulvar region include a sensation of burning, the presence of a lump or sore, vaginal discharge, a rash, and pain. Frequently encountered vulvar conditions include vaginal infections, Bartholin's gland abscess, parasites, molluscum contagiosum, and vulvar warts (ACOG, 2008b, 2011b).

INFECTION

Vaginal infections can produce vulvar symptoms. Candidiasis (yeast infection) often is associated with intense itching and tissue irritation. Women who are immunocompromised, diabetic, overweight, or receiving long-term antibiotic therapy are especially susceptible to vulvar yeast infections that may be resistant to treatment. Because the infection may stem from multiple types of yeasts or include bacterial organisms, it is important to perform an appropriate diagnostic evaluation (ACOG, 2008b).

BARTHOLIN'S GLAND ABSCESS

The Bartholin's glands, also known as the greater vestibular or vulvovaginal glands, are located deep within the posterior portion of the vestibule near the posterior vaginal introitus (Fig. 4-6).

A & P review **The Bartholin's Glands**

The vestibule is essentially an oval-shaped space enclosed by the labia minora. It contains openings to the urethra and vagina, the Skene's glands, and the Bartholin's glands. This area of a woman's anatomy is extremely sensitive to chemical irritants. The Bartholin's glands secrete a clear mucus that moistens and lubricates the vagina during sexual arousal. ◆

Bartholin's cysts are the most common benign lesions of the vulva. Obstruction of the Bartholin's gland duct leads to enlargement and formation of a cyst. The cyst may cause

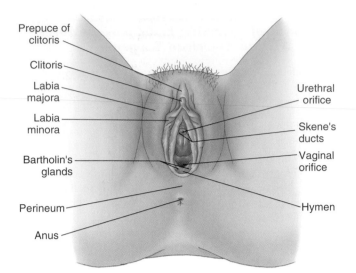

Figure 4-6 Female external genitalia. (Dillon, P.M. [2007]. *Nursing health assessment: A critical thinking approach* [2nd ed., p. 612]. Philadelphia, PA: F.A. Davis.)

no symptoms, but if it enlarges or becomes infected, the woman frequently experiences pain, dyspareunia, and an awareness of a tender mass in the area. When symptomatic, incision and drainage provide temporary relief. Because Bartholin's cysts tend to recur, a permanent opening for drainage may be recommended. Rarely, the abscess is caused by gonorrhea. Bartholin's abscesses are highly unusual in postmenopausal women and should be evaluated to rule out malignancy (ACOG, 2008b).

PARASITES

Lice or mites may infect the vulva. Intense itching of the skin that contains hair follicles is characteristic of infestation. Scabies, a dermatitis caused by the itch mite *Sarcoptes scabiei*, produces areas of excoriation composed of scaly papules and insect burrows. Scabies is transmitted by person-to-person contact or through infested bedding and clothing. The itching tends to worsen at night. Scabies spreads on the skin by fingernail contamination. Diagnosis is made by microscopic examination of skin scrapings to detect the presence of the mite, its eggs, or its excretions (Venes, 2013).

> ❋ *Nursing Insight— Formulating appropriate nursing diagnoses for patients with scabies*
>
> Nursing diagnoses for patients with scabies usually focus on Impaired Skin Integrity related to the presence of invasive parasites and the development of pruritus and Deficient Knowledge regarding the communicable nature of the infestation, possible complications, therapy, and self-care needs related to a lack of information or misinterpretation.

MOLLUSCUM CONTAGIOSUM (SEED WART)

Molluscum contagiosum is a rash composed of small, dome-shaped papules with a central crater filled with a cheesy (caseous) material (Fig. 4-7). The lesions of molluscum contagiosum are caused by a pox virus. In adults,

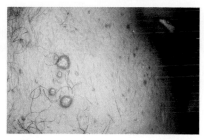

Figure 4-7 Molluscum contagiosum. (Venes, D. [Ed.]. [2013]. *Taber's cyclopedic medical dictionary* [22nd ed., p. 1530]. Philadelphia, PA: F.A. Davis.)

transmission is primarily sexual; in children, transmission is nonsexual and via fomites, substances that adhere to and transmit infection (Venes, 2013).

VULVAR CONDYLOMATA

A condyloma (plural: *condylomas, condylomata*) is a growth that resembles a wart on the skin or mucous membrane, usually of the genitals or anus. Vulvar condylomata, also known as *warts, genital warts, and venereal warts,* are caused by certain strains of the human papillomavirus, different from those that produce cervical lesions. Condylomata can appear as small, thickened growths or large cauliflowerlike masses on the vulva, along the perineum, or in and around the anus. The benign growths can be treated with chemicals, cryosurgery, electrosurgery, or laser vaporization. None of the treatments are fully successful, however, and recurrence is common. Despite removal of the lesions, surrounding tissues continue to harbor the human papillomavirus. Condylomata may be spread by physical contact with an area containing a wart, and the spread of a wart from one labium to the other by autoinoculation is possible (ACOG, 2008b; Venes, 2013). (See further discussion about human papillomavirus in Chapters 5 and 6.)

> ✿ *Nursing Insight— Premalignant and malignant vulvar lesions*
>
> Most vulvar cancer is squamous in origin. Because the vulva is covered with skin, any malignancy that appears elsewhere on the skin can also occur on the vulva. Vulvar intraepithelial neoplasia (VIN) is a cancer precursor often associated with human papillomavirus. The most common symptom of VIN is persistent itching; localized burning and/or skin thickening or discoloration (e.g., red, pink, lighter, or darker) in the affected area may also be present. Diagnosis is limited to visual assessment, and biopsy is indicated for any pigmented vulvar lesion. Treatment includes wide surgical excision (when cancer is suspected), laser ablation (when cancer is not suspected), and the application of topical imiquimod 5% (off-label use). Women with VIN are at risk of recurrent VIN and vulvar cancer throughout their lifetimes and should continue to receive monitoring. Immunization with the quadrivalent HPV vaccine (effective against HPV genotypes 6, 11, 16, and 18) has been shown to decrease the risk of VIN. Women who have a history of genital warts and who smoke have an increased risk of developing vulvar cancer. *Invasive vulvar cancer* is the presence of a malignant lesion that breaks through the cellular basement membrane. This type of cancer occurs most often in older (70+ years) women, and in the United States it is responsible

for 5% of all female genital malignancies (ACOG, 2011b; Hoffstetter, 2014).

Melanoma is the second most common type of invasive vulvar malignancy, but it is extremely rare, accounting for less than 5% of all vulvar cancers. Most melanomas are located on the labia minora or clitoris and are blue-black in color. They have a jagged or fuzzy border, and the lesions may be raised or ulcerated. Although the condition may affect women of all ages, vulvar melanoma is more common in older (70+ years) women, and more than 90% occur in white women. Biopsy is needed for diagnosis, and treatment involves surgical excision and in some situations inguinal lymphadenectomy (ACOG, 2008b; ACS, 2013).

Paget's disease is another rare neoplasm of the vulva. It also occurs more commonly in older (70+ years) women. Symptoms include intense vulvar itching and soreness, usually of long duration. Lesions of Paget's disease are thick, often leading to an impression of leukoplakia. The affected area may also be red, moist, and elevated; biopsy is necessary for diagnosis. Treatment consists of surgical excision (ACOG, 2008b; ACS, 2013).

VULVAR LICHEN SIMPLEX CHRONICUS, LICHEN SCLEROSUS, AND LICHEN PLANUS

Lichen simplex chronicus of the vulva is a chronic eczematous condition characterized by scaling and intense and unrelenting pruritus. It occurs primarily in mid- to late-adult life and represents an end-stage response to a wide variety of causative factors including environmental agents (e.g., heat, excessive sweating, irritation from clothing) and dermatological disease (e.g., candidiasis, lichen sclerosus). Lichen simplex chronicus affects quality of life including sexual and psychological well-being and has been associated with a number of psychological problems such as sleep disturbances, obsessive-compulsive disorder, anxiety, and depression. Treatment involves identification and elimination of the causative irritant/allergen; nighttime pruritus may be alleviated with oral amitriptyline, ice, and the topical application of high-potency corticosteroids (ACOG, 2008b; Krapf & Goldstein, 2012; Lipkin & Kwon, 2014).

Lichen sclerosus, an autoimmune inflammatory disorder of the skin, primarily affects women in the fifth to sixth decades of life, although it may occur at any age, including prepuberty. Patients most often complain of pruritus, burning, dyspareunia, tearing, and chronic vulvar pain. The skin typically appears thin, crinkled, and waxy, with porcelain-white papules and plaques—often described as a "cigarette paper" appearance. Progression of the disease results in scarring and narrowing of the introitus, fusion of the labia minora, fissures, and phimosis of the clitoral hood (Fig. 4-8). Treatment involves the topical application of a high-potency steroid ointment (ACOG, 2008b; Hoffstetter, 2014; Krapf & Goldstein, 2012; Lipkin & Kwon, 2014; Wedel & Johnson, 2014).

Lichen planus, an autoimmune inflammatory mucocutaneous disorder, affects approximately 1% of women, primarily during the third to sixth decades of life. Symptoms include pruritus, burning, dyspareunia, postcoital bleeding, and vaginal discharge. Lichen planus may markedly alter vulvovaginal anatomy, causing loss of the labia minora, narrowing of the introitus, and obliteration of the vagina, severely affecting sexual interaction. Initial treatment

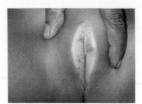

Figure 4-8 Lichen sclerosus. (Venes, D. [Ed.]. [2013]. *Taber's cyclopedic medical dictionary* [22nd ed., p. 1393]. Philadelphia, PA: F.A. Davis.)

involves the topical application of a high-potency steroid ointment; systemic treatment with an oral corticosteroid and surgical lysis of vulvovaginal adhesions may be necessary (ACOG, 2008b; Hoffstetter, 2014; Krapf & Goldstein, 2012; Lipkin & Kwon, 2014).

THE NURSE'S ROLE IN PROMOTING VULVAR HEALTH

Nurses should be aware of common vulvar irritants and allergens (Box 4-3) so that they can provide appropriate patient counseling and offer strategies for promoting and maintaining a healthy vulvar environment to reduce the risk of irritation and infection. Nurses can also teach women to wear cotton underwear, keep the vulvar area clean and dry, avoid douching, and perform monthly vulvar self-examination.

Box 4-3 **Common Vulvar Irritants and Allergens**

Adult or baby wipes

Antibiotics

Antiseptics (e.g., povidone-iodine, hexachlorophene)

Body fluids (e.g., semen, saliva)

Colored or scented toilet paper

Condoms (lubricant or spermicide containing)

Contraceptive creams, jellies, foams, nonoxynol-9, and lubricants

Douches

Dyes

Emollients (e.g., lanolin, jojoba oil, glycerin)

Heat

Laundry detergents, fabric softeners, and dryer sheets

Nickel (from piercings)

Nylon underwear

Rubber products (including latex)

Sanitary products, including tampons and pads

Soaps, bubble baths and salts, shampoos, and conditioners

Tea tree oil

Topical anesthetics (e.g., benzocaine, lidocaine, dibucaine)

Topical antibacterials (e.g., neomycin, bacitracin, polymyxin)

Topical antimycotics (e.g., imidazoles, nystatin)

Topical corticosteroids

Topical medications, including trichloroacetic acid, 5-fluorouracil, and podofilox or podophyllin

Vaginal hygiene products, including perfumes and deodorants

Sources: ACOG (2008b); Krapf & Goldstein (2012); Lipkin & Kwon (2014).

Family Teaching Guidelines...
Performing Vulvar Self-Examination

To prepare for vulvar self-examination, the woman places a flashlight and mirror within easy reach. She washes her hands, removes clothing from the waist down, and sits comfortably on the floor or bed, with a pillow support behind her back. The following steps should then be performed:

1. While bending her knees, she leans backward and allows her knees to fall slightly apart to expose the genital area. The mirror and flashlight should be positioned for optimal visualization.
2. External inspection of the genital area includes visualizing the labia, the clitoris, the urethral meatus, the vaginal opening, and the anal opening. Each area can be both looked at and touched gently with a finger, beginning with the mons pubis, which is the area above the vagina around the pubic bone where the pubic hair is located.
3. Using her fingers, the woman should gently spread the labia and inspect the vaginal vault. The vaginal walls should be pink and contain small folds or ridges called *rugae*.
4. The vaginal discharge should be evaluated at this time as well. Normal vaginal discharge is clear to cloudy and white, with a slightly acidic odor; it may be thick or thin, depending on the timing of the examination with regard to the menstrual cycle.
5. Findings that need to be reported to the health-care provider include the presence of thickening, ulcers, sores, or growths on the labia or vaginal walls; an unpleasant odor to the vaginal discharge, and changes in the color of the vulvar skin, such as whitening or an increase in skin pigmentation. Sores, redness, abnormal growths, malodorous or excessive vaginal discharge, and persistent itching may indicate irritation or infection; these symptoms should also be reported.

Vulvar self-examination should be performed once a month in between menstrual periods, or any time symptoms such as vulvar itching or pain, pain on penetration during sex, or vulvar lumps or thickening of the skin are noted.

Source: Vulvar Pain Society (2012).

 Now Can You— **Discuss conditions of the vulva?**

1. Describe signs, symptoms, and treatment modalities for a Bartholin's gland cyst?
2. Discuss signs and symptoms of vulvar carcinoma, and identify populations at greatest risk for development of this type of cancer?
3. Teach a patient how to perform vulvar self-examination?

Summary Points

◆ Menstrual disorders, such as amenorrhea, irregular bleeding, and dysmenorrhea, constitute some of the most common reproductive problems in women.

◆ Endometriosis is a chronic condition characterized by the presence of endometrial glands and tissue outside the uterus.

◆ Uterine leiomyomas are the most common solid pelvic tumors in women and the leading indication for hysterectomy.

◆ The acronym PALM-COEIN classifies uterine bleeding abnormalities by etiology and comprises two separate entities: structural abnormalities and nonstructural causes of abnormal uterine bleeding.

◆ Ovarian cysts affect women of all ages, although they occur most often during the childbearing years and typically represent a normal process.

◆ Polycystic ovary syndrome occurs when an endocrine imbalance results in elevated levels of estrogen, testosterone, and luteinizing hormone and a decreased secretion of follicle-stimulating hormone.

◆ Ovarian cancer is the leading cause of gynecological deaths and the fourth most common cause of cancer deaths in women.

◆ In the United States, cancer of the endometrium is the most common gynecological malignancy, and approximately 70% of all cases are found in women in the 50 to 69 age group.

◆ Nurses can promote vulvar health by teaching women about strategies such as the avoidance of common vulvar irritants and how to perform vulvar self-examination.

Review Questions

Multiple Choice

1. The nurse is aware that secondary amenorrhea may be caused by:
   A. Lactation
   B. Crohn's disease
   C. Congenital absence of the vagina
   D. Polycystic ovary syndrome

2. During patient teaching, the nurse explains that primary dysmenorrhea is related to:
   A. Pregnancy
   B. Leiomyoma
   C. Perimenopause
   D. Prostaglandins

3. When providing counseling for a patient with a diagnosis of endometriosis, the nurse explains that:
   A. Consuming a high-fat diet may help to minimize symptoms
   B. Medical treatment is designed to reduce the amount of estrogen in the body
   C. Laparoscopic surgical removal of the lesions results in a permanent cure
   D. Infertility is a rare complication of the condition

4. The nurse explains to a patient with a diagnosis of abnormal uterine bleeding that thermal endometrial ablation is a technique developed to:
   A. Restore fertility
   B. Destroy the uterine lining
   C. Treat uterine cancer
   D. Open blocked fallopian tubes

5. Nurses can teach women about strategies to promote vulvar health, such as:
   A. Performing monthly vulvar self-examination
   B. Using scented toilet paper
   C. Douching once a week
   D. Wearing synthetic underwear

REFERENCES

Altman, G., & Wolcyzk, M. (2010). Endometriosis: Overview and recommendations for primary care nurse practitioners. *The Journal for Nurse Practitioners—JNP, 6*(6), 427–434. doi:10.1016/j.nurpra.2009.07.0922

American Cancer Society (ACS). (2013). *Cancer topics.* Retrieved from http://www.cancer.org/cancer/index

American College of Obstetricians and Gynecologists (ACOG). (2005). Management of endometrial cancer. Practice Bulletin No. 65. (Reaffirmed 2011). *Obstetrics & Gynecology, 106*(8), 413–425.

American College of Obstetricians and Gynecologists (ACOG). (2006a). *Menstruation in girls and adolescents—using the menstrual cycle as a vital sign.* Committee Opinion No. 349. (Reaffirmed 2009). Washington, DC: Author.

American College of Obstetricians and Gynecologists (ACOG). (2006b). Vaginitis. Practice Bulletin No. 72. (Reaffirmed 2011). *Obstetrics and Gynecology, 107*(5), 1195–1206.

American College of Obstetricians and Gynecologists (ACOG). (2008a). Alternatives to hysterectomy in the management of leiomyomas. Practice Bulletin No. 96. (Reaffirmed 2012). *Obstetrics & Gynecology, 112*(8), 201–207.

American College of Obstetricians and Gynecologists (ACOG). (2008b). Diagnosis and management of vulvar skin disorders. Practice Bulletin No. 93. (Reaffirmed 2013). *Obstetrics & Gynecology, 111*(5), 1242–1253.

American College of Obstetricians and Gynecologists (ACOG). (2008c). Intraperitoneal chemotherapy for ovarian cancer. ACOG Committee Opinion No. 396. (Reaffirmed 2010). *Obstetrics and Gynecology, 111*(1), 249–251.

American College of Obstetricians and Gynecologists (ACOG). (2008d). Treatment of urinary tract infections in non-pregnant women. Practice Bulletin No. 91. (Reaffirmed 2012). *Obstetrics & Gynecology, 111*(3), 785–794.

American College of Obstetricians and Gynecologists (ACOG). (2009a). Choosing the route of hysterectomy for benign disease. ACOG Committee Opinion No. 444. (Reaffirmed 2012). *Obstetrics and Gynecology, 114*(11), 1156–1158.

American College of Obstetricians and Gynecologists (ACOG). (2009b). Hereditary breast and ovarian cancer syndrome. Practice Bulletin No. 103. (Reaffirmed 2011). *Obstetrics & Gynecology, 113*(4), 957–966.

American College of Obstetricians and Gynecologists (ACOG). (2009c). Polycystic ovary syndrome. Practice Bulletin No. 108. (Reaffirmed 2011). *Obstetrics and Gynecology, 114*(10), 936–949.

American College of Obstetricians and Gynecologists (ACOG). (2010). Management of endometriosis. Practice Bulletin No. 114. (Reaffirmed 2013). *Obstetrics & Gynecology, 116*(1), 223–236.

American College of Obstetricians and Gynecologists (ACOG). (2011a). Hysteroscopy. Technology Assessment No. 7. *Obstetrics & Gynecology, 117*(6), 1486–1491.

American College of Obstetricians and Gynecologists (ACOG). (2011b). Management of vulvar intraepithelial neoplasia. Committee Opinion No. 509. *Obstetrics and Gynecology, 118*(5), 1192–1194.

American College of Obstetricians and Gynecologists (ACOG). (2011c). The role of the obstetrician–gynecologist in the early detection of epithelial ovarian cancer. ACOG Committee Opinion No. 477. *Obstetrics & Gynecology, 117*(3), 742–746.

American College of Obstetricians and Gynecologists (ACOG). (2012a). Diagnosis of abnormal uterine bleeding in reproductive-aged women. Practice Bulletin No. 128. *Obstetrics & Gynecology, 120*(7), 197–206.

American College of Obstetricians and Gynecologists (ACOG). (2012b). Sonohysterography. Technology Assessment No. 8. *Obstetrics & Gynecology, 119*(6), 1325–1328.

American College of Obstetricians and Gynecologists (ACOG). (2012c). Well-woman visit. Committee Opinion No. 534. *Obstetrics and Gynecology, 120*(8), 421–424.

American College of Obstetricians and Gynecologists (ACOG). (2013a). Management of abnormal uterine bleeding associated with ovulatory dysfunction. Practice Bulletin No. 136. *Obstetrics & Gynecology, 122*(1), 176–186.

American College of Obstetricians and Gynecologists (ACOG). (2013b). Management of acute abnormal uterine bleeding in nonpregnant reproductive-aged women. Committee Opinion No. 557. *Obstetrics & Gynecology, 121*(4), 891–896.

American College of Obstetricians and Gynecologists (ACOG). (2013c). Von Willebrand disease in women. Committee Opinion No. 580. *Obstetrics & Gynecology, 122*(6), 1368–1373.

American College of Obstetricians and Gynecologists (ACOG). (2014). *Ovarian cysts.* Frequently Asked Questions – FAQ 075. Washington, DC: Author.

American Society for Reproductive Medicine (ASRM). (2012). Endometriosis and infertility. Retrieved from http://asrm.org/Endometriosis_and_Infertility_Can_Surgery_Help/

Auerbach, R.D., Duleba, A.J., & Whiteside, D.C. (2013). Endometrial ablation: The facts. *Contemporary OB/GYN, 58*(Suppl. 2), 1–8.

Billhult, A., & Stener-Victorin, E. (2012). Acupuncture with manual and low frequency electrical stimulation as experienced by women with polycystic ovary syndrome: A qualitative study. *BMC Complementary and Alternative Medicine, 12*(32), 1–6.

Bulechek, G.M., Butcher, H.K., & Dochterman, J.M., & Wagner, C. (2013). *Nursing interventions classification (NIC)* (6th ed.). St. Louis, MO: Elsevier Mosby.

Burton, M.E., & Daley, A.M. (2011). Health-risk counseling for adolescents with polycystic ovary syndrome. *The American Journal for Nurse Practitioners, 15*(3/4), 51–60.

Carter, J.S., & Downs, L.S., Jr. (2011). Ovarian cancer tests and treatment. *The Female Patient, 36*(4), 30–35.

Centers for Disease Control and Prevention (CDC). (2011a). *Sexually transmitted diseases treatment guidelines.* Retrieved from http://www.cdc.gov/std/treatment/2010/vaginal-discharge.htm#a1

Centers for Disease Control and Prevention (CDC). (2011b). *Women's reproductive health: Hysterectomy.* Retrieved from http://www.cdc.gov/reproductivehealth/WomensRH/Hysterectomy.htm

Cesario, S. (2010). Advances in the early detection of ovarian cancer. *Nursing for Women's Health, 14*(3), 223–234. doi:10.1111/j.1751-486X.2010.01543.x

Clarke-Pearson, D.L., & Geller, E.J. (2013). Complications of hysterectomy. *Obstetrics & Gynecology, 121*(3), 654–673. doi:10.1097/AOG.0b013e3182841594

Comerford, K.P., & Hurst, B.S. (2012). Alternatives to hysterectomy for symptomatic uterine myomas. *The Female Patient, 37*(8), 29–38.

Coughlin, G., & Secor, M. (2010). Bacterial vaginosis: Update on evidence-based care. *Advance for Nurse Practitioners, 18*(1), 41–45.

Divasta, A. (2013). PCOS in adolescents: Beyond the reproductive implications. *Contemporary OB/GYN, 58*(12), 63–66.

Dominguez, L. (2012). Heavy menstrual bleeding: Treating with tranexamic acid. *The American Journal for Nurse Practitioners, 16*(5/6), 6–10.

Dura, M., & Baresic, D. (2011). Respect yourself, protect yourself. *Nursing for Women's Health, 15*(6), 522–528. doi:10.1111/j.1751-486X.2011.01684.x

Eckert, L.O., & Lentz, G.M. (2012). Infections of the lower genital tract: Vulva, vagina, cervix, toxic shock syndrome, endometritis, and salpingitis. In R.A. Lobo, G.M. Lentz, D.M. Gershenson, & V.L. Katz (Eds.), *Comprehensive gynecology* (6th ed., pp. 519–560). Philadelphia, PA: Mosby.

Falcone, T., & Lebovic, D.I. (2011). Clinical management of endometriosis. *Obstetrics & Gynecology, 118*(3), 691–705. doi:10.1097/AOG.0b013e31822adfd1

Falcone, T., & Parker, W.H. (2013). Surgical management of leiomyomas for fertility or uterine preservation. *Obstetrics & Gynecology, 121*(4), 856–868. doi:10.1097/AOG.0b013e3182888478

Flower, A., Liu, J.P., Chen, S., Lewith, G., Little, P., & Li, Q. (2012). Chinese herbal medicine for endometriosis. *Cochrane Database of Systematic Reviews, 5,* CD006568. doi:10.1002/14651858.CD006568.pub3

Flyckt, R., & Falcone, T. (2011). Myomectomy: Surgical approaches. *The Female Patient, 36*(12), 24–32.

Frieder, R.P. (2010). Lynch syndrome: A gynecologic condition. *The Female Patient, 35*(Suppl. 10), 1–8.

Frieder, R.P., & Berlin, S.M. (2012). Hereditary cancer risk assessment in obstetrics and gynecology: The evolving standard of care. *The Female Patient, 37*(Suppl. 10), 1–6.

Galic, V., & Gupta, D. (2012). Fertility-sparing management of endometrial carcinoma. *The Female Patient, 37*(6), 39–47.

Garcia, A. (2013). Minimally invasive gynecology. *OBG Management, 25*(4), 33–40.

Garza-Cavazos, A., & Loret de Mola, R. (2012). Abnormal uterine bleeding: New definitions and contemporary terminology. *The Female Patient, 37*(7), 27–36.

Goff, B., Mandel, L., Drescher, C., Urban, N., Gough, S., Schurman, K., . . . & Andersen, M. (2007). Development of an ovarian cancer symptom index. *Cancer, 109*(2), 221–227. doi:10.1002/cncr.22371

Gupta, J.K., Sinha, A., Lumsden, M.A., & Hickey, M. (2012). Uterine artery embolization for symptomatic uterine fibroids. *Cochrane Database of Systematic Reviews, 5,* CD005073. doi:10.1002/14651858.CD005073.pub3

Gura, M., & Baresic, D. (2011). Respect yourself, protect yourself. An educational campaign about vaginitis in the Dominican Republic. *Nursing for Women's Health, 15*(6), 522–528. doi: 10.1111/j.1751-486X.2011.01684.x

Halloran, L. (2011). Management of abnormal vaginal bleeding. *The Journal for Nurse Practitioner—JNP, 7*(6), 523–524.

Harmanli, O., Wheeler, T.L., Matteson, K.A., Abed, H., Sung, V.W., Rahn, D.D., . . . Balk, E.M. (2012). Evidence-based recommendations for abnormal uterine bleeding. *The Female Patient, 37*(10), 28–32.

Hoffstetter, S. (2014). Diagnosing diseases of the vulva. *The Clinical Advisor, 17*(4), 62–71.

Jacobs, A.M. (2012). Oligomenorrhea in the adolescent. *The Female Patient, 37*(7), 18–24.

Johns Hopkins University. (2011). Bacterial vaginosis. Retrieved from http://iwantthekit.org/female/other_bv.html

Jones, G.L., Hall, J.M., Lashen, H.L., Balen, A.H., & Ledger, W.L. (2011). Health-related quality of life among adolescents with polycystic ovary syndrome. *Journal of Obstetric, Gynecologic & Neonatal Nursing, 40*(5), 577–588. doi:10.1111/j.1552-6909.2011.01279.x

Kaatz, J., Solari-Twadell, A., Cameron, J., & Schultz, R. (2010). Coping with endometriosis. *Journal of Obstetric, Gynecologic & Neonatal Nursing, 39*(2), 220–226. doi:10.1111/j.1552-6909.2010.0110.x

Krapf, J.M., & Goldstein, A. (2012). The vulvar dermatoses. *The Female Patient, 37*(4), 28–33.

Lasco, A., Catalano, A., & Benvenga, S. (2012). Improvement of primary dysmenorrhea caused by a single oral dose of vitamin D: Results of a randomized, double-blind, placebo-controlled study. *Archives of Internal Medicine, 172*(9), 366–367.

Laughlin, S.K., & Stewart, E.A. (2011). Uterine leiomyomas: Individualizing the approach to a heterogeneous condition. *Obstetrics & Gynecology, 117*(2), 396–403. doi:10.1097/AOG.0b013e31820780e3

Leslie, K.K., Thiel, K.W., & Yang, S. (2012). Endometrial cancer: Potential treatment and prevention with progestin-containing intrauterine devices. *Obstetrics & Gynecology, 119*(2), 419–420.

Li, A.J. (2012). New biomarkers for ovarian cancer. *Contemporary OB-GYN, 57*(4), 28–34.

Lipkin, D., & Kwon, Y. (2014). Therapies and nursing care of women with vulvar dermatologic disorders. *Journal of Obstetric, Gynecologic & Neonatal Nursing, 43*(2), 246–252. doi:10.1111/1552-6909.12286

Lowe, K.A., Andersen, M.R., Kane, J.C., Robertson, M.D., & Goff, B.A. (2013). Effects of demographics and over-the-counter analgesics on ovarian cancer symptoms. *The Journal for Nurse Practitioners, 9*(1), 28–33.

Macer, J.A. (2013). For uterine-sparing fibroid treatment, consider laparoscopic ultrasound-guided radiofrequency ablation. *OBG Management, 25*(11), 50–54.

MacKay, H.T., & Woo, J. (2013). Gynecologic disorders. In M. Papadakis, S.J. McPhee, & M.W. Rabow (Eds.), *Current medical diagnosis & treatment* (52nd ed., pp. 747–780). New York, NY: McGraw-Hill Medical.

Marazzo, J.M., & Cates, W., Jr. (2011). Reproductive tract infections, including HIV and other sexually transmitted infections. In R.A. Hatcher, J. Trussell, A.L. Nelson, W. Cates, D. Kowal, & M.S. Policar (Eds.), *Contraceptive technology* (20th ed., pp. 571–620). Decatur, GA: Bridging the Gap Communications.

Matteson, K., Rahn, D., Wheeler, T., Casiano, E., Siddiqui, N., Harvie, H., . . . & Sung, V. (2013). Nonsurgical management of heavy menstrual bleeding. *Obstetrics & Gynecology, 121*(3), 632–643. doi:10.1097/AOG.0b013e3182839e0e

Mayhew, M.S. (2012). Treatment for polycystic ovary syndrome. *The Journal for Nurse Practitioners—JNP, 7*(6), 517–518.

Minkin, M.J. (2011). Urinary tract infection 101: Diagnosis and therapy. *The Female Patient, 36*(10), 14–18.

Moore, A. (2013). Heavy menstrual bleeding: Evaluation and treatment strategies. *Advance for NPs & PAs, 4*(1), 21–23.

Moore, A., & Caldwell, J. (2011). The importance of collaboration in treating chronic disease: A focus on PCOS and group medical visits. *Women's Health Care: A Practical Journal for Nurse Practitioners, 10*(9), 10–18.

Moorhead, S., Johnson, M., Maas, M.L., & Swanson, E. (2013). *Nursing outcomes classification (NOC)* (5th ed.). St. Louis, MO: Elsevier Mosby.

Munro, M.G., Critchley, H.O., Broder, M.S., & Fraser, I.S. (2011). FIGO classification system (PALM-COEIN) for causes of abnormal uterine bleeding in nongravid women of reproductive age. FIGO Working Group on Menstrual Disorders. *International Journal of Gynaecology and Obstetrics, 113*(3), 3–13.

National Cancer Institute (NCI). (2011). Diethylstilbestrol (DES) and cancer. Retrieved from http://www.cancer.gov/cancertopics/factsheet/Risk/DES

National Cancer Institute (NCI). (2012). SEER stat fact sheets: Corpus and uterus. Retrieved from http://seer.cancer.gov/statfacts/html/corp.html

National Cancer Institute (NCI). (2013). *General information about vaginal cancer.* Retrieved from http://www.cancer.gov/cancertopics/pdq/treatment/vaginal/HealthProfessional

Neal, D.D., Formyduval, A.M., & Taylor, J.S. (2010). HER LIFESTYLE: A mnemonic for addressing polycystic ovary syndrome in adolescents. *Nursing for Women's Health, 13*(6), 473–478

Nelson, A.L., & Baldwin, S. (2011). Menstrual disorders. In R.A. Hatcher, J. Trussell, A.L. Nelson, W. Cates, D. Kowal, & M.S. Policar (Eds.), *Contraceptive technology* (20th ed., pp. 533–570). Decatur, GA: Bridging the Gap Communications.

Nosti, P.A., Arnold, K.C., & Iglesia, C.B. (2013). Have you tried these innovative alternatives to antibiotics for UTI prevention? *OBG Management, 25*(2), 17–26.

Nyirjesy, P., Robinson, J., Mathew, L., Lev-Sagie, A., Reyes, I., & Culhane, J. (2011). Alternative therapies in women with chronic vaginitis. *Obstetrics & Gynecology, 117*(4), 856–861. doi:10.1097/AOG.0b013e31820b07d5

Ovarian Cancer National Alliance. (2013). *Symptom diary and practice guidance.* Retrieved from http://www.ovariancancer.org/diary/

Perriera, L.K., & Greenfield, M. (2011). OC therapy in teens. *Contemporary OB/GYN, 56*(5), 40–47.

Ratner, E.S., Richter, C.E., Minkin, M.J., & Foran-Tuller, K.A. (2012). How to talk about sexual issues with cancer patients. *Contemporary OB-GYN, 57*(5), 40–50.

Robinson, C., & Wiczyk, H. (2011). Treating common gynecologic conditions with acupuncture. *The Female Patient, 36*(5), 32–38.

Rossi, E., & Clarke-Pearson, D.L. (2011). Screening for ovarian cancer in midlife women. *The Female Patient, 36*(9), 37–40.

Rubin, R.N. (2013). Young woman with dysuria and increased frequency and urgency. *Consultant, 53*(1), 37–38.

Rutecki, G.W. (2012). Vitamin D as a contemporary panacea. *Consultant, 52*(5), 346.

Rydz, N., & Jamieson, M.A. (2013). Managing heavy menstrual bleeding in adolescents. *Contemporary OB/GYN, 58*(7), 49–52.

Sampson, J.A. (1940). The development of the implantation theory for the origin of peritoneal endometriosis. *American Journal of Obstetrics and Gynecology, 40*(6), 549–557.

Schwartz, J., & Gabelnick, H.L. (2011). Contraceptive research and development. In R.A. Hatcher, J.Trussell, A.L. Nelson, W. Cates, D. Kowal, , & M.S. Policar (Eds.), *Contraceptive technology* (20th ed., pp. 513–532). Decatur, GA: Bridging the Gap Communications.

Sego, S. (2012). Acupuncture. *The Clinical Advisor, 15*(7), 51–52.

Simon, J.A., Roseff, S., & Hait, H. (2012). New options for supporting women having difficulty conceiving. *The Female Patient, 37*(Suppl. 4), 1–6.

Smith, J.W., & Taylor, J.S. (2011). Polycystic ovary syndrome. *Nursing for Women's Health, 15*(95), 404–411. doi:10.1111/j.1751-486X.2011.01664.x

Smith, O.W. (1948). Diethylstilbestrol in the prevention and treatment of complications of pregnancy. *American Journal of Obstetrics and Gynecology, 56*(3), 821–834.

Sorosky, J.I. (2012). Endometrial cancer. *Obstetrics & Gynecology, 120*(2), 383–398. doi:10.1097/AOG.0b013e3182605bf1

Speroff, L., & Fritz, M.A. (2011). *Clinical gynecologic endocrinology and infertility* (8th ed.). Philadelphia, PA: Lippincott Williams & Wilkins.

Tellawi, A.R., & Morozov, V.V. (2014). Prophylactic salpingectomy: The future of ovarian cancer prevention? *Contemporary OB/GYN, 59*(3), 46–65.

Trouskova, O., & Alexander, B. (2012). Early detection of ovarian cancer. *Advance for NPs & PAs, 3*(1), 21–25.

Tulandi, T., & Salamah, K. (2010). Fertility and uterine artery embolization. *Obstetrics & Gynecology, 115*(4), 847–860.

Vallerand, A., & Sanoski, C. (2013). *Davis's drug guide for nurses* (13th ed.). Philadelphia, PA: F.A. Davis.

Venes, D. (2013). *Taber's cyclopedic medical dictionary* (22nd ed.). Philadelphia, PA: F.A. Davis.

Vulval Pain Society. (2012). *How to perform a vulval self-exam.* Retrieved from http://vulvalpainsociety.org/index.php?page=self-examination

Waldman, J. (2012). NuSwab VG: A new diagnostic approach to vaginitis. *The Female Patient, 37*(Suppl. 5), 1–4.

Wedel, N., & Johnson, L. (2014). Vulvar lichen sclerosus: Diagnosis and management. *The Journal for Nurse Practitioners, 10*(1), 42–48.

Weiss, T.R., & Bulmer, S.M. (2011). Young women's experiences living with polycystic ovary syndrome. *Journal of Obstetric, Gynecologic & Neonatal Nursing, 40*(6), 709–718. doi:10.1111/j.1552-6909.2011.01299.x

Wilton, J.M. (2012). Tranexamic acid: A new option for heavy menstrual bleeding. *Nursing for Women's Health, 16*(2), 146–150. doi:10.1111/j.1751-486X.2012.01720.x

Woo, P., & McEneaney, J. (2010). New strategies to treat primary dysmenorrhea. *The Clinical Advisor, 13*(11), 43–49.

World Cancer Research Fund/American Institute for Cancer Research. (2013). Continuous project update report. Food, nutrition, physical activity, and the prevention of endometrial cancer. Retrieved from http://www.dietandcancerreport.org/

Wortman, M. (2012). Hysteroscopic myomectomy: Pearls and pitfalls from 24 years of practice. *Contemporary OB/GYN, 57*(8), 26–31.

Xu, F., Stoner, B.P., Taylor, S.N., Mena, L., Tian, L.H., Papp, J., . . . Markowitz, L.E. (2011). Use of home-obtained vaginal swabs to facilitate re-screening for *Chlamydia trachomatis* infections: Two randomized controlled trials. *Obstetrics & Gynecology, 118*(2, Pt. 1), 231–239. doi:10.1097/AOG.0b013e3182246a83

Yawn, V. (2012). Polycystic ovarian syndrome. *Advance for NPs & PAs, 13*(7), 11–15.

CONCEPT MAP

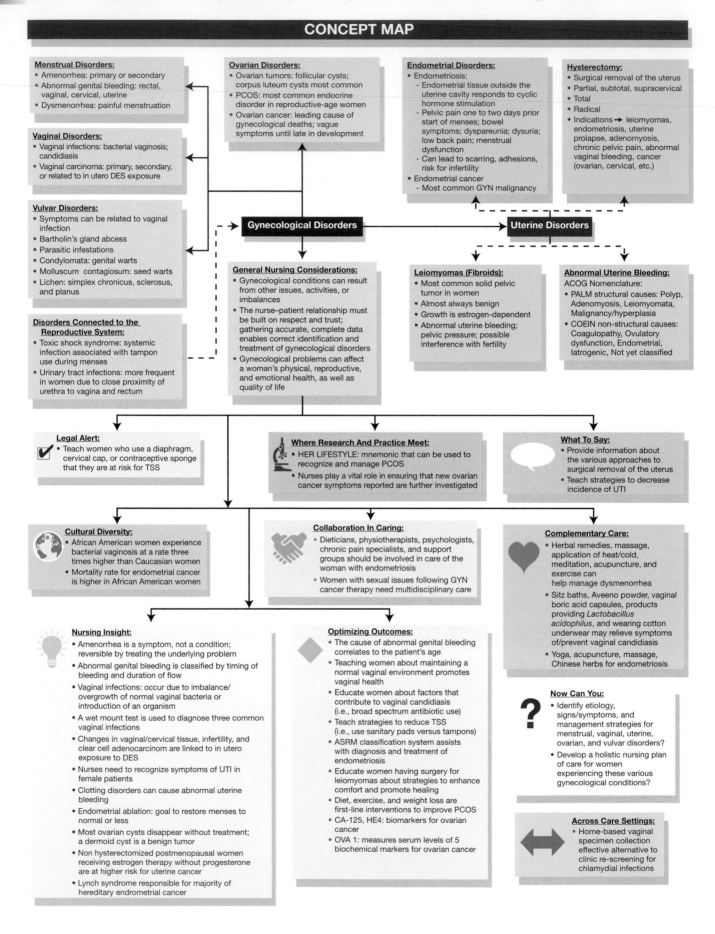

Menstrual Disorders:
- Amenorrhea: primary or secondary
- Abnormal genital bleeding: rectal, vaginal, cervical, uterine
- Dysmenorrhea: painful menstruation

Vaginal Disorders:
- Vaginal infections: bacterial vaginosis; candidiasis
- Vaginal carcinoma: primary, secondary, or related to in utero DES exposure

Vulvar Disorders:
- Symptoms can be related to vaginal infection
- Bartholin's gland abcess
- Parasitic infestations
- Condylomata: genital warts
- Molluscum contagiosum: seed warts
- Lichen: simplex chronicus, sclerosus, and planus

Disorders Connected to the Reproductive System:
- Toxic shock syndrome: systemic infection associated with tampon use during menses
- Urinary tract infections: more frequent in women due to close proximity of urethra to vagina and rectum

Ovarian Disorders:
- Ovarian tumors: follicular cysts; corpus luteum cysts most common
- PCOS: most common endocrine disorder in reproductive-age women
- Ovarian cancer: leading cause of gynecological deaths; vague symptoms until late in development

Endometrial Disorders:
- Endometriosis:
  - Endometrial tissue outside the uterine cavity responds to cyclic hormone stimulation
  - Pelvic pain one to two days prior start of menses; bowel symptoms; dyspareunia; dysuria; low back pain; menstrual dysfunction
  - Can lead to scarring, adhesions, risk for infertility
- Endometrial cancer
  - Most common GYN malignancy

Hysterectomy:
- Surgical removal of the uterus
- Partial, subtotal, supracervical
- Total
- Radical
- Indications → leiomyomas, endometriosis, uterine prolapse, adenomyosis, chronic pelvic pain, abnormal vaginal bleeding, cancer (ovarian, cervical, etc.)

Gynecological Disorders

Uterine Disorders

General Nursing Considerations:
- Gynecological conditions can result from other issues, activities, or imbalances
- The nurse–patient relationship must be built on respect and trust; gathering accurate, complete data enables correct identification and treatment of gynecological disorders
- Gynecological problems can affect a woman's physical, reproductive, and emotional health, as well as quality of life

Leiomyomas (Fibroids):
- Most common solid pelvic tumor in women
- Almost always benign
- Growth is estrogen-dependent
- Abnormal uterine bleeding; pelvic pressure; possible interference with fertility

Abnormal Uterine Bleeding:
ACOG Nomenclature:
- PALM structural causes: Polyp, Adenomyosis, Leiomyomata, Malignancy/hyperplasia
- COEIN non-structural causes: Coagulopathy, Ovulatory dysfunction, Endometrial, Iatrogenic, Not yet classified

Legal Alert:
- Teach women who use a diaphragm, cervical cap, or contraceptive sponge that they are at risk for TSS

Where Research And Practice Meet:
- HER LIFESTYLE: mnemonic that can be used to recognize and manage PCOS
- Nurses play a vital role in ensuring that new ovarian cancer symptoms reported are further investigated

What To Say:
- Provide information about the various approaches to surgical removal of the uterus
- Teach strategies to decrease incidence of UTI

Cultural Diversity:
- African American women experience bacterial vaginosis at a rate three times higher than Caucasian women
- Mortality rate for endometrial cancer is higher in African American women

Collaboration In Caring:
- Dieticians, physiotherapists, psychologists, chronic pain specialists, and support groups should be involved in care of the woman with endometriosis
- Women with sexual issues following GYN cancer therapy need multidisciplinary care

Complementary Care:
- Herbal remedies, massage, application of heat/cold, meditation, acupuncture, and exercise can help manage dysmenorrhea
- Sitz baths, Aveeno powder, vaginal boric acid capsules, products providing *Lactobacillus acidophilus*, and wearing cotton underwear may relieve symptoms of/prevent vaginal candidiasis
- Yoga, acupuncture, massage, Chinese herbs for endometriosis

Nursing Insight:
- Amenorrhea is a symptom, not a condition; reversible by treating the underlying problem
- Abnormal genital bleeding is classified by timing of bleeding and duration of flow
- Vaginal infections: occur due to imbalance/overgrowth of normal vaginal bacteria or introduction of an organism
- A wet mount test is used to diagnose three common vaginal infections
- Changes in vaginal/cervical tissue, infertility, and clear cell adenocarcinom are linked to in utero exposure to DES
- Nurses need to recognize symptoms of UTI in female patients
- Clotting disorders can cause abnormal uterine bleeding
- Endometrial ablation: goal to restore menses to normal or less
- Most ovarian cysts disappear without treatment; a dermoid cyst is a benign tumor
- Non hysterectomized postmenopausal women receiving estrogen therapy without progesterone are at higher risk for uterine cancer
- Lynch syndrome responsible for majority of hereditary endometrial cancer

Optimizing Outcomes:
- The cause of abnormal genital bleeding correlates to the patient's age
- Teaching women about maintaining a normal vaginal environment promotes vaginal health
- Educate women about factors that contribute to vaginal candidiasis (i.e., broad spectrum antibiotic use)
- Teach strategies to reduce TSS (i.e., use sanitary pads versus tampons)
- ASRM classification system assists with diagnosis and treatment of endometriosis
- Educate women having surgery for leiomyomas about strategies to enhance comfort and promote healing
- Diet, exercise, and weight loss are first-line interventions to improve PCOS
- CA-125, HE4: biomarkers for ovarian cancer
- OVA 1: measures serum levels of 5 biochemical markers for ovarian cancer

Now Can You:
- Identify etiology, signs/symptoms, and management strategies for menstrual, vaginal, uterine, ovarian, and vulvar disorders?
- Develop a holistic nursing plan of care for women experiencing these various gynecological conditions?

Across Care Settings:
- Home-based vaginal specimen collection effective alternative to clinic re-screening for chlamydial infections

Promoting Reproductive Health Through an Understanding of Sexually Transmitted Diseases

We may run, walk, stumble, drive, or fly, but let us never lose sight of the reason for the journey, or miss a chance to see a rainbow on the way.

—Gloria Gaither

LEARNING TARGETS *At the completion of this chapter, the student will be able to:*

◆ Discuss signs and symptoms, modes of transmission, and treatment options for the most common sexually transmitted diseases (STDs).

◆ Identify various safer sex strategies.

◆ Describe the nurse's role in STD counseling and education.

PICO(T) Questions

The intent of Evidence-Based Practice (EBP) is to provide nursing care that integrates the best available evidence. An initial step in EBP is to write a PICO(T) question that effectively guides the research. A PICO(T) question is an acronym that stands for population (P), intervention or issue (I), comparison of interest (C), outcome (O), and time frame (T). Depending on the question, all or some of the question components are used in the research process. Use these

PICO(T) questions to spark your thinking as you read the chapter.

1. Is the (I) incidence of sexually transmitted diseases (O) lower among (P) high school students who receive education on prevention of STDs than (C) among high school students who do not receive education on prevention?

2. What are the (O) most important prevention (I) strategies nurses should teach (P) people at risk of becoming infected with hepatitis B?

Evidence-Based Practice

Fine, D., Thomas, K.K., Nakatsukasa-Ono, W., & Marrazzo, J. (2012). Chlamydia positivity in women screened in family planning clinics: Racial/ethnic differences and trends in the Northwest U.S., 1997–2006. *Public Health Reports, 127*(1), 38–51.

The purpose of this study was to examine trends, individual-level risk factors, and population-level, area-based socioeconomic measures of women infected with *Chlamydia trachomatis* (Chlamydia). Chlamydia surveillance and prevalence monitoring has revealed differences in sexually transmitted disease (STD) rates by age, gender, socioeconomic levels, and racial/ethnic groups, and at the regional, state, and local levels. A regional monitoring system for the states of Alaska, Idaho, Oregon, and Washington (U.S. Public Health Service [PHS] Region X) was put into place in 1988 to monitor screening and treatment for Chlamydia within this

region. Chlamydia screening was recommended for all female clients younger than 25 years of age who were seen in family planning clinics. Data from system monitoring estimated a 60% decline in Chlamydia for clients aged 15 to 24, although disease estimates by race/ethnicity rates increased. In 1996, the Chlamydia rate for black clients was 62% higher than for white clients; between 1997 and 2004, overall positive Chlamydia rates increased.

Recent research has focused on racial/ethnic population disparities and included social determinants, such as poverty, crime,

(continued)

Evidence-Based Practice (continued)

health-care access, sexual partnerships, and high-risk behaviors. Previous studies have also linked socioeconomic conditions and population density to racial/ethnic differences in STD rates. The authors note that prevalence monitoring does not capture data on social determinants, sexual networks, or individuals' household socioeconomic position. The authors proposed to assess the relationship among individual risk factors, population-level social determinants, and Chlamydia rates in women aged 15 to 24 years who were attending family planning clinics in the four-state region.

Data used in this study included demographic and Chlamydia test results obtained from 667,223 women aged 15 to 24 years screened in 201 family planning clinics in the Region X ZIP codes. Data collection information included race/ethnicity (75% white; 5% Hispanic; 4% black; 4% Asian/Pacific Islander; 1% American Indian/Alaska Native; 1% "other"), age (ages 15 to 17, 21%; ages 18 to 19, 25%; ages 20 to 24, 53%), ZIP code, specimen collection date, incidence of a Chlamydia infection within the past year, experience of having a partner with Chlamydia as reason for the clinic visit, behavioral risks in the past 60 days, condom use, clinical findings consistent with an STD, and diagnostic test type and results.

Behavioral risks included the following: a new sexual partner; multiple partners; or a symptomatic partner. Eighty-nine percent reported no more than one sex partner in the past 60 days, 77% reported no new sex partner in the past 60 days, 90% reported no symptomatic sex partner in the past 60 days, 72% reported no condom use with the last sex, and 94% reported no positive Chlamydia test in the past year. Other data included the following: racial/ethnic groups with a median household income in the lowest quintile: 8% white, 7% black, 15% American Indian/Alaska Native, 5% Asian/Pacific Islander, 11% Hispanic; racial/ethnic groups with no high school diploma aged older than 25: 14% white, 15% black, 24% American Indian/Alaska Native, 22% Asian/Pacific Islander, 41% Hispanic.

Data analysis revealed the following: positive Chlamydia rates—Hispanic (4%), whites (4.8%), Asian/Pacific Islanders (6%), Native Americans/Alaska Natives (7%), and blacks (10.3%). The relation of population-level socioeconomic status to Chlamydia rates, sexual risk behaviors, and clinical signs of infection was not found to be significant. Racial and ethnic population area-based socioeconomic measures were found to be associated with STDs in black and Hispanic clients. The rate of infection increase among black women living in areas with a greater than 40% minority population demonstrated a 48% increase, as compared with black women living in an area with less than 5% racial minority residents. The rate of increase among Hispanic women living in areas with a greater than 25% Hispanic population demonstrated a 40% increase, as compared with Hispanic women living in an area with less than 5% racial minority residents. Chlamydia rates of white women living in areas with more racially and ethnically diverse populations did not show a significant increase. High rates of Chlamydia were also found among black, American Indian, and Alaska Native women without any significant risk factors. Overall, positive Chlamydia rates were higher among adolescents, women reporting high-risk behaviors, women with STDs, women who reported a Chlamydial infection in the past year, and women with known contact to someone diagnosed with Chlamydia. As expected, Chlamydia rates were lower in women who reported condom use at the last sexual intercourse. Sixty-two percent of Hispanic women and 44% of black women reported no individual-level risk factors.

Based on their findings, the researchers concluded that differences in racial/ethnic Chlamydia rates persisted over time and were not mitigated by adjustments for socioeconomic position or race/ethnicity.

1. How is this information useful to clinical nursing practice?
2. Based on these findings, what are implications for further research?

Introduction

This chapter focuses on sexually transmitted diseases (STDs). Information regarding signs, symptoms, modes of transmission, and treatment options for various STDs is presented, along with a discussion of the nurse's role in promoting reproductive health. STDs encompass more than 25 infectious organisms that cause reproductive tract infections that are primarily transmitted by close, intimate contact. Nurses are perfectly situated to provide evidence-based, culturally sensitive STD counseling and education that facilitates understanding of these potentially lethal health threats and empowers women to make informed choices in their intimate relationships.

In many clinical settings, the terms *sexually transmitted disease* and *sexually transmitted infection* are used interchangeably. "Sexually transmitted disease" is the accepted subject heading in the PubMed database, and *STD* is also the term used by the Centers for Disease Control and Prevention (CDC). According to the CDC (2010), an important component of STD health care is that providers use language that is understandable to patients. Owing to the fact that stigma associated with an STD can be a barrier to appropriate diagnosis and treatment (Royer & Cerf, 2009), some clinicians use the term *STI* instead of *STD* because discussing an infection with a patient may be less embarrassing than discussing a disease (Marrazzo & Cates, 2011).

In addition to the short-term emotional and physical distress usually associated with a reproductive tract infection, many serious long-term effects may also result from many of the STDs. Potential complications include fallopian tube blockage with resultant infertility, an increased risk of ectopic pregnancy, chronic pelvic pain, an increased risk of liver cancer and serious liver disease, and death. Women suffer more long-term reproductive consequences from STDs than do men, and women are more

Where Research and Practice Meet:
Exploring Young Women's Beliefs About the Terms Sexually Transmitted Disease and Sexually Transmitted Infection

It is unknown whether patients understand what their health-care provider means when using the terms *sexually transmitted disease* and *sexually transmitted infection,* and recent research suggests that some female patients may be more familiar with the terms *sexually transmitted disease,* or *STD.*

Royer and Cerf (2009) conducted a survey to determine whether young women differentiate between the terms *sexually transmitted disease* and *sexually transmitted infection* and, if so, whether their reasons were consistent with those of health-care providers. A total of 302 women aged 18 to 24 years completed a survey that measured beliefs about STDs and whether they considered the terms *sexually transmitted disease* and *sexually transmitted infection* to be interchangeable. Fifty-seven percent responded that *sexually transmitted disease* and *sexually transmitted infection* do not mean the same thing; 28% believed that *STD* and *STI* do mean the same thing; and 15% responded that they did not know. The investigators concluded that although a majority of the young women do differentiate between the two terms, their rationale for doing so is not consistent with the rationale used by health-care providers. Based on the findings, the researchers suggested that professionals clarify their use of the terms *sexually transmitted disease* and *sexually transmitted infection* when talking with patients as a strategy to improve health communication and to improve STD health care.

likely than men to acquire an infection from any single sexual encounter. Unfortunately, owing to the asymptomatic nature of many STDs, treatment is often delayed, and this factor increases the likelihood of more serious long-term consequences.

The incidence of several STDs has increased over the past few years. In late 2012, the CDC (2012b) released STD surveillance data for the year 2011. According to the findings, Chlamydia remains the most commonly reported infectious disease in the United States. The rate of this infection has increased by 8% as compared with the 2010 data; however, it is important to note that the increase could be related to factors such as improved screening methods and testing. During the period 1991 to 2011, the rate of reported chlamydial infection increased from 179.7 to 457.6 cases per 100,000 population. Gonorrhea is the second most commonly reported notifiable disease in the United States. (A notifiable or "reportable" disease is one that must be reported to public health authorities at the time of diagnosis because it is potentially dangerous to human or animal health.) During the period 1975 to 1997, the national gonorrhea rate declined 74%, and decreased further to 98.1 cases per 100,000 population in 2009. However, the rate increased in 2010 and again in 2011 to 104.2 per 100,000 population. The increase in gonorrhea rates during 2010–2011 was observed among both men and women, among all racial/ethnic groups, and in all regions of the United States. Similarly to Chlamydia, gonorrhea continues to be underdiagnosed and underreported. Cases of syphilis have also increased in recent years, with an increase of 18%, as compared with the 2007 data. Interestingly, at one point, this disease was once on the verge of elimination, but there have been increasing numbers of reported cases since 2001. Much of the increase has occurred among men who have

sex with men and is attributed to increased rates of unsafe sexual practices (CDC, 2012b).

In February 2013, the CDC published two analyses to allow an in-depth look at the huge human and economic burden of STDs in the United States. According to the latest estimates, at present there are about 20 million new infections in the United States each year, costing the health-care system close to $16 billion in direct medical costs alone. Nearly one-half of all new STDs occur among young men and women, although they represent only 25% of the sexually experienced population. The complete report may be accessed at http://www.cdc.gov/std/stats/STI-Estimates-Fact-Sheet-Feb-2013.pdf.

Nursing Insight— *The National Health Initiative addresses sexually transmitted diseases*

Several Healthy People 2020 National Health Goals specifically focus on STDs:

- Reduce the proportion of females aged 15 to 24 years who attended family planning clinics in the past 12 months and tested positive for *Chlamydia trachomatis* infections from a baseline of 7.4% to a target of 6.7%.
- Reduce gonorrhea rates among females aged 15 to 44 years from 279.9 new cases of gonorrhea per 100,000 females to 251.9 new cases per 100,000 population.
- Reduce sustained domestic transmission of primary and secondary syphilis among females from 1.4 new cases per 100,000 females to 1.3 new cases per 100,000 population.
- Reduce the proportion of young adults with genital herpes infection due to herpes simplex type 2 from a baseline of 10.5% to a target of 9.5%.
- Reduce the proportion of females aged 15 to 44 years who have ever required treatment for pelvic inflammatory disease from a baseline of 4.2% to a target of 3.8% (U.S. Department of Health and Human Services [USDHHS], 2013).

Nurses can help the nation to meet these goals by providing education about methods of preventing STDs and information about how to recognize the signs and symptoms of these illnesses. Nurses can design studies and engage in research to provide evidence-based practice strategies for issues such as teaching women about safer sex practices, teaching youth about the methods of transmission of infection and the long-term consequences of the diseases, and providing ways that health professionals can increase STD awareness in their practice settings.

Optimizing Outcomes— **Including seniors in STD counseling and screening**

Over the past decade, the prevalence of HIV and STDs among older adults has risen steadily. Unfortunately, prevailing societal perceptions often incorrectly view senior citizens as sexually inactive. In actuality, older adults engage in more sexual activity than previously believed. It is important that nurses who work with women across the life span routinely include sexual health assessments during the physical health evaluation, offer STD information and counseling when appropriate, and conduct STD screening when indicated (Maes & Louis, 2011; Stewart & Graham, 2013; Taylor & Gosney, 2011; Taylor & James, 2012).

HIV/AIDS

In the years since acute HIV infection was first described, research has identified the cellular mechanisms that accompany its clinical presentation. HIV most commonly enters the host through percutaneous or genital routes. Once the virus has penetrated the mucosal epithelium, it infects macrophages, CD4+ T cells, and dendritic cells and spreads to the systemic lymph nodes within 2 days after infection. Within 3 days, it is detectable in the plasma. Plasma viremia then results in dissemination to various body organs, including the brain and spleen (Kahn & Walker, 1998).

Infection with HIV leads to a progressive disease that results in AIDS. The AIDS epidemic has in some way touched everyone's life, and the health profession has been affected profoundly. However, many individuals living in the United States remain ignorant of the fact that AIDS affects men, women, and children and has reached epidemic proportions in many areas.

In this country, more and more young people, especially women, are contracting HIV. Individuals between the ages of 13 and 24 represent more than one-fourth of new HIV infections each year and most of them are unaware they are infected, according to a *Vital Signs* report from the CDC, available at www.cdc.gov/vitalsigns/HIVAmongYouth/index.html. Most women are infected during sex with an HIV-infected man or while using HIV-contaminated syringes for the injection of drugs such as heroin, cocaine, and amphetamines. According to the CDC (2013b), approximately 49,273 individuals were newly infected with HIV in 2011, and in that same year, an estimated 32,052 people were diagnosed with AIDS. An estimated 1,148,200 persons aged 13 years and older are living with HIV infection, including 207,600 (18.1%) who are unaware of their infection. Although the annual number of new HIV infections has remained relatively stable, the present pace of new infections underscores the need to keep HIV prevention at the top of the public health agenda. In the United States, women aged 15 to 44 years represent one of the fastest growing segments of the epidemic. It is important to note that women are more likely than men to acquire HIV at any one contact (CDC, 2013b). Because HIV infection can remain asymptomatic for years, infected women can unknowingly harbor and transmit the virus. Women who are infected with HIV have special gynecological health needs that must be assessed and addressed (Marrazzo & Cates, 2011).

Cultural Diversity: HIV Disparities in the United States

According to the CDC (2013b), women account for 25% of people living with HIV in the United States. African American women and Latinas are disproportionately affected by HIV infection compared with women of other races/ethnicities. In 2010, the rate of new infections (per 100,000 population) among African American women was 20 times that of white women and the rate among Hispanic women was four times the rate of white women. However, the number of new infections among African American women in 2010 (6,100) represented a decrease of 21% since 2008, when the rate was 7,700. Young women aged 25 to 44 accounted for the majority of new HIV infections among U.S. women in 2010. Current estimates are that 1 in 32 African American women and 1 in 106 Hispanic women will acquire HIV infection in their lifetimes, compared with 1 in 562 white women. In 2012, the CDC launched the *Take Charge, Take the Test* campaign to increase HIV testing and awareness among African American women. The campaign features advertising, a Web site, and community outreach (CDC, 2013b).

Today, AIDS is the leading cause of death among young women in most of the world. The ratio of infected men and women worldwide approaches 1:1. Both sexual activity and IV drug use play major roles in current transmission statistics.

RISK FACTORS

Lifestyle behaviors that place a woman at risk for contracting HIV are listed in Box 5-1. When obtaining the patient history, it is important to routinely inquire about symptoms that may be associated with HIV. Although primary HIV infection is typically asymptomatic, women may describe nonspecific flu-like discomforts such as fever, headache, night sweats, malaise, muscle aches, nausea, diarrhea, weight loss, sore throat, skin rash, and lymphadenopathy (Marrazzo & Cates, 2011).

Across Care Settings: Socioeconomic HIV risk factors reach across communities

A number of socioeconomic factors also affect HIV risk. *Poverty,* for example, can limit access to health care, HIV testing, and medications that can lower serum HIV levels and help prevent transmission. Also, individuals who cannot afford basic necessities may be confronted with circumstances that increase their HIV risk. *Discrimination, stigma, and homophobia* may discourage individuals from seeking testing, prevention, and treatment services. As the *prevalence of HIV and other STDs in a community* increases, so does an individual's risk of infection with each sexual encounter, especially if, within those communities, people select partners who are from the same ethnicity. In any community, *higher rates of undiagnosed/untreated STDs* can increase the risk of both acquiring and transmitting HIV and *higher rates of incarceration among men* can disrupt social and sexual networks and decrease the number of available partners for women, fueling the spread of HIV (CDC, 2013b).

Box 5-1 Risk Factors for HIV Infection

- Current or past history of drug use, especially IV drug use
- History of prostitution
- Frequent sexual intercourse with multiple partners
- Engaging in sexual intercourse under the influence of drugs
- Engaging in sexual intercourse with men who also have sex with men
- Residing in an area with a high prevalence of HIV infection (e.g., rural South and Northeast United States)
- Having received a blood transfusion or blood products before 1985

Source: CDC (2013b).

DETECTION, TESTING, AND DOCUMENTATION

Detecting HIV is a primary step in prevention of the virus. The CDC (2006) recommends opt-out HIV testing for all patients in all health-care settings, including pregnant women. (*Opt-out testing* is defined as performing HIV screening after notifying the patient that the test will be performed and that the patient may elect to decline or defer testing. Assent is inferred unless the patient declines testing. *Opt-in testing* means that testing is offered and the patient is required to actively give permission before it can occur.) Studies show that the opt-out approach increases the testing rates among pregnant women (thereby increasing the number of pregnant women who know their HIV status), increases the number of HIV-infected women who are offered treatment, and reduces maternal HIV transmission.

The American College of Obstetricians and Gynecologists (ACOG) supports routine screening for women aged 19 to 64 years and targeted screening for women with risk factors outside of that age range (e.g., sexually active adolescents younger than 19 years). ACOG recommends a combination of testing, education, and brief behavioral interventions to reduce the rate of HIV infection. Additional approaches include early recognition of positive HIV testing results, safe sex practices, and training of office personnel in risk reduction interventions (ACOG, 2010a, 2012). In 2013, the U.S. Preventive Services Task Force (USPSTF) published a recommendation that clinicians screen for HIV infection in adolescents and adults aged 15 to 65 years. Younger adolescents and older adults who are at increased risk should also be screened. The latest guidelines are aimed at improving access to HIV testing across the country and increasing the number of individuals who are tested each year. It is estimated that up to 25% of persons infected with HIV are unaware of their status, and universal testing may identify more of them (ACOG, 2010a; CDC, 2013b).

Optimizing Outcomes— With CDC-endorsed HIV testing

The CDC (2006) has published the following recommendations for HIV testing:

Patients in all health-care settings:

- Perform HIV screening on every patient after informing the patient that testing will be performed unless the patient declines (opt-out testing).
- Screen patients at highest risk for HIV at least annually.
- General consent for medical care should be sufficient to encompass consent for HIV testing; no separate written consent should be required.
- Prevention counseling should not be required with HIV testing.

Pregnant women:

- Include HIV screen in routine prenatal testing for all pregnant women.
- Screening should be on an opt-out basis.
- General consent for medical care should be sufficient to encompass consent for HIV testing; no separate written consent should be required.
- Repeat HIV testing in the third trimester is recommended.

It is important for the nurse to assess the patient's level of understanding to ensure that she is aware of the legal, emotional, and medical implications of a positive or negative HIV test before she takes the test. Pregnancy is not encouraged for women who are HIV positive; contraceptive counseling should be offered to HIV-positive women who do not desire pregnancy. Post-test counseling centers on telling the patient her test results, explaining the meaning of the results, and reinforcing infection prevention measures. Women should be advised that if they have been exposed in the past 6 months, they should be retested. All pre- and posttest counseling should be documented on the patient's chart.

legal alert— Conforming to HIPAA regulations

If the HIV test results are to be placed on the patient's medical record, they are then available to everyone who accesses the chart. The patient must be advised of this policy before testing. Health-care facilities must have policies in place to safeguard patient information from inadvertent or inappropriate breaches of confidentiality. In some clinical settings, HIV-related information is maintained in a separate chart and a code is assigned for HIV test results. In other facilities, HIV-related information is removed from the medical record before it is released. Federal regulations set forth in the Health Insurance Portability and Accountability Act (HIPAA) also provide specific rules for what information may be shared with other practitioners and agencies with and without an individual's permission. Results of HIV testing may need to be recorded and stored in a certain way. It is incumbent upon nurses to be familiar with the legal requirements that exist in the particular practice setting. Also, many states require reporting when HIV is detected; state-specific information is available at http://www.cdc.gov/hiv/law/states/testing.htm (Marrazzo & Cates, 2011).

HIV infection is usually diagnosed via the HIV-1 and HIV-2 antibody tests. A schema for HIV screening in women is presented in Figure 5-1. Antibody testing is first performed with a sensitive screening test such as the enzyme-linked immunoassay (ELISA) (also called enzyme immunoassay [EIA]), which detects serum antibodies to HIV. Reactive screening tests are then confirmed by an additional test such as the Western blot or, less commonly, an immunofluorescence assay (IFA). If a positive antibody test is confirmed by a supplemental test, the woman is infected with HIV and is capable of infecting others. These diagnostic tests are very reliable; false-positive and false-negative results are rare. In general, seroconversion for HIV in adolescents and adults occurs from 6 to 12 weeks after transmission of the virus; HIV antibodies are detectable in at least 95% of patients within 3 months after infection (CDC, 2006).

Methods of rapid testing for HIV antibodies use a blood sample obtained by finger stick, venipuncture, or an oral fluid sample. The rapid tests can help to reduce unrecognized infections by improving access to testing in both clinical and nonclinical settings and increase the proportion of those tested who learn their results. Rapid testing facilitates patients receiving their test results the same day, usually at the encounter where the test specimen was collected. Like the conventional HIV EIAs, the rapid HIV tests are screening tests that require confirmation if reactive. Although false negatives are rare, they may occur in an individual who has been acutely infected but who has not yet developed HIV antibodies. All of the rapid tests are interpreted visually and require no instrumentation (CDC, 2013b).

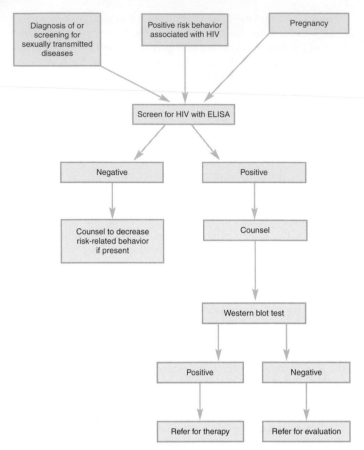

Figure 5-1 Screening for HIV in women.

Nursing Insight— *Home testing for HIV*

Patients who are reluctant to visit a care provider for testing can purchase a home collection kit at a pharmacy and collect their own finger-prick blood sample. The sample is then mailed to a laboratory and the patient may call for anonymous results and telephone counseling a few days later. An FDA-approved over-the-counter rapid HIV test kit for home use is also available. Individuals can perform this test at home by swabbing the upper and lower gums inside the mouth to collect an oral fluid sample. After placing the sample into the vial, the test results are available within 20 to 40 minutes (Marrazzo & Cates, 2011).

Currently, no cure is available for HIV. Current standard of care for HIV is highly active antiretroviral therapy (HAART), a combination of oral antiretroviral agents that inhibit different targets of the virus. The use of antiretroviral agents has been demonstrated to be effective in maintaining the health of HIV-positive women and in reducing or preventing the perinatal transmission of the virus. The primary goals of antiretrovirus therapy are to improve and/or preserve immune function and to reduce HIV-associated morbidity and mortality. Antiretrovirals reduce the amount of HIV the body generates, allowing the immune system to be restored, and reducing or preventing the risk of HIV transmission (Kurtyka, 2012; USDHHS Panel on Antiretroviral Guidelines for Adults and Adolescents, 2011). A number of opportunistic infections often accompany HIV infection. Information and current guidelines about management are available at the CDC AIDS Prevention hotline (1-800-CDC-INFO [232-4636]) and at its Web site, http://www.cdc.gov/hiv/.

SPECIAL CONCERNS FOR HIV-POSITIVE WOMEN

Women who are HIV positive may experience a number of psychosocial issues. They are often primary caregivers who bear the burden of responsibility for the care of their children. The illness presents major challenges in keeping appointments, receiving adequate rest, and complying with medication regimens. Other immediate needs may involve housing and financial difficulties, and in many situations, other family members are infected as well.

Gynecological problems are also a major concern. Owing to the immunocompromised state, vulvovaginal candidiasis, genital warts caused by human papillomavirus (HPV), and genital herpes lesions are more common and more severe in HIV-infected women. Menstrual problems such as heavy bleeding may require hormonal intervention to address the anemia and lessen the discomfort. However, because the relationship between HIV and menstrual disruption is unclear, all menstrual irregularities should be investigated (ACOG, 2010a; Marrazzo & Cates, 2011).

Across Care Settings: Reducing HIV-related occupational risks for health-care providers

There are three routes of transmission for HIV: direct sexual contact; perinatal transmission from the HIV-infected mother to her fetus or newborn; and direct inoculation with contaminated blood products, needles, or syringes. All health-care providers who may come in contact with contaminated blood products, needles, or syringes in any acute care, long-term care, or home care setting are at risk for occupational exposure to HIV. To address this risk, the CDC developed standard precautions, a set of principles to be used in the care of all patients at all times. To minimize personal risk, all health-care workers should consistently comply with the precautions.

Now Can You— Discuss aspects of HIV infection?

1. Identify six risk factors for HIV infection?
2. Describe what is meant by "opt-out" HIV testing recommended by the CDC?
3. Discuss special concerns for HIV-positive women?

Chlamydia Trachomatis

Chlamydia trachomatis infection is the most common bacterial sexually transmitted disease in the United States and the leading cause of preventable infertility and ectopic pregnancy. Other potential complications include pelvic inflammatory disease (PID) and Fitz-Hugh-Curtis syndrome (infection of the liver capsule with adhesion formation on the anterior abdominal wall). More than 1.4 million cases were reported to the CDC in 2011, and more than half occurred in women 15 to 24 years old. The reported rate of Chlamydia infection for women substantially exceeds the rate for men, primarily due to increased detection of asymptomatic infection in women through screening. It is estimated that 1 in 10 adolescent girls tested for Chlamydia is infected. Teenage girls tend to have the highest rates of Chlamydial infection. *C. trachomatis* is widespread geographically and is highly prevalent among economically disadvantaged young women (CDC, 2012b; Kapur & Effron, 2011; Marrazzo & Cates, 2011; Turner, 2012). (See the Evidence-Based Practice feature at the beginning of the chapter.)

Optimizing Outcomes— Teaching patients about STD prevention

Chlamydia can be transmitted during vaginal, anal, or oral sex and has been referred to as a "silent" disease because women are often unaware that they are infected. Nurses can teach patients about strategies to prevent or decrease the transmission of Chlamydia and other STDs: practicing abstinence from sexual intercourse or sharing a mutually monogamous relationship with a partner who has been tested and is known to be uninfected and correctly and consistently using latex condoms, and avoiding condoms lubricated with the spermicide nonoxynol-9 (N-9), an agent that has been associated with disruption of the genital epithelium, which may increase the risk for the transmission of infection (Fantasia, Fontenot, Sutherland, & Harris, 2011).

The majority (75%) of Chlamydial infections are asymptomatic, especially in women. Only about 30% of those infected have a mucopurulent cervical discharge; other symptoms include spotting or postcoital bleeding and dysuria. Infected women who use oral contraceptives may report breakthrough bleeding. Chlamydia infection of the cervix causes inflammation that produces microscopic ulcerations, which may increase the risk for contracting HIV (CDC, 2012b; Marrazzo & Cates, 2013).

The CDC and the U.S. Preventive Services Task Force (USPSTF) recommend annual screening for Chlamydia in all sexually active women aged 25 years and younger. Chlamydia infection can be diagnosed using several different testing methods, such as culture, direct immunofluorescence, nucleic acid hybridization, and EIA, all of which require a pelvic examination to collect cervical epithelial cells. The nucleic acid amplification test (NAAT), which can detect Chlamydia from a cervical or vaginal swab (self- or clinician-collected) or urine sample (using a "clean-catch method"), is considered to be the most sensitive and specific test (CDC, 2012b, 2014; Roberts, Sheffield, McIntire, & Alexander, 2011; USPSTF, 2008).

Optimizing Outcomes— Recognizing and addressing barriers to screening for Chlamydia

Although Chlamydia screening is considered a priority preventive service, it remains underutilized by health-care providers. Barriers to screening include a lack of awareness that patients are sexually active and at risk for STDs, inaccessibility to screening kits, a lack of reimbursement for the time required to conduct patient testing and counseling, and a lack of knowledge that screening can be performed without a pelvic examination. Strategies to change provider behavior include the use of computerized reminders, simplified request forms, placement of Chlamydia collection swabs alongside Pap test collection materials, and the practice of performing routine Chlamydia screening with other laboratory testing (CDC, 2012b; McNulty et al., 2013; McNulty et al., 2010).

Where Research and Practice Meet:
Improving Chlamydia Screening and Rescreening

Kettinger (2012) described a clinical practice intervention to increase routine screening rates in a woman's health primary care setting. The preventive care–focused goal setting/assessment/plan/start-up (GAPS) model, a four-step continuous quality improvement method, was applied in a university faculty outpatient women's health clinical practice. Providers and nursing staff engaged in the following activities: set goals to achieve routine Chlamydia screening; assessed current screening rates and clinic processes; developed a plan to modify existing screening practices; and provided support for providers' improved practices. Following the intervention, Chlamydia screening rates increased from 53.4% to 76.1%, findings that suggest that a combination of education, provider feedback, and clinic prompts (i.e., screening packets with neon orange "flags") can influence Chlamydia screening behavior among providers.

Xu and colleagues (2011) conducted two randomized trials to determine whether the use of home-based, self-obtained vaginal swabs among women who were treated for Chlamydia infection would increase rescreening rates in comparison with clinic-based rescreening. Their findings suggested that in the STD and family planning clinics, use of the home-based, self-obtained vaginal swabs resulted in significant increases in rescreening rates compared with rescreening in the clinic. The researchers concluded that home-based specimen collection can serve as an effective alternative to clinic-based rescreening for Chlamydia infection in women.

Unlike viruses, the Chlamydia bacterium is susceptible to antibiotics. The recommended antibiotic regimens for treatment of *C. trachomatis* are azithromycin (Zithromax) 1 g orally, given in a single dose (preferred), *or* doxycycline (Doxycin) 100 mg orally twice a day for 7 days. Alternative regimens are erythromycin base (E-Mycin) 500 mg orally four times a day for 7 days *or* erythromycin ethylsuccinate (E.E.S.) 800 mg orally four times a day for 7 days *or* levofloxacin (Levaquin) 500 mg orally once daily for 7 days *or* ofloxacin (Floxin) 300 mg orally two times a day for 7 days. The erythromycin-based regimens are frequently associated with gastrointestinal side effects that can lead to noncompliance and should be used as a second-line therapy. Although levofloxacin and ofloxacin are effective treatment alternatives, these agents are more expensive and offer no advantage in the dosage regimen. The CDC recommends treating all sex partners of those who test positive for Chlamydia. Also, owing to the fact that coinfection with *C. trachomatis* frequently occurs among patients who have gonococcal infection, presumptive treatment of such patients for Chlamydia is also recommended. To enhance compliance with recommended treatment, the CDC urges health-care providers to dispense medications on site and observe ingestion of the first dose. Also, persons treated for Chlamydia should be instructed to abstain from sexual intercourse for 7 days after single-dose therapy or until completion of a 7-day regimen and abstain from sexual intercourse until all sex partners have been treated (CDC, 2012b; Marrazzo & Cates, 2013).

Optimizing Outcomes— Expedited partner therapy

Expedited partner therapy (EPT), also known as patient-delivered partner therapy (PDPT), is the practice of treating sex partner(s) of patients with an STD without health-care practitioner evaluation or professional prevention counseling. This approach involves delivering a prescription (written in the partner's name) of the medication; informing the partner(s) of the infection; and providing them with written materials about treatment instructions, appropriate warnings, and the importance of seeking evaluation for any symptoms suggestive of complications. EPT, which can decrease reinfection rates (e.g., gonorrhea, Chlamydia) compared with standard partner referrals for examination and treatment, is endorsed by many professional organizations including the American Medical Association, the American Academy of Pediatrics, the American Bar Association, and the American College of Obstetricians and Gynecologists (ACOG, 2011a; CDC, 2011; Wysocki & Woodward, 2010). EPT may be prohibited in some states; state-specific information can be obtained by visiting the CDC Web site at www.cdc.gov/std/ept.

Gonorrhea

Gonorrhea is caused by the gram-negative intracellular diplococcal bacterium *Neisseria gonorrhoeae*. Approximately 700,000 new cases of gonorrhea occur each year, making it the second most commonly reported bacterial STD in the United States. Similar to Chlamydia, gonorrhea is prevalent in the adolescent population and disproportionately affects minority groups. The rate of gonorrheal infections in African American women aged 15 to 19 is 15.9 times higher than in Caucasian women in the same age group (CDC, 2012b; Marrazzo & Cates, 2013).

Nursing Insight— *The magnitude of chlamydial and gonorrheal infections in young women*

Chlamydia and gonorrhea are the two most commonly reported infectious diseases in the United States. Adolescent girls and young women are especially hard hit by these two diseases. According to the CDC (2012b), estimates suggest that young people aged 15 to 24 acquire close to one-half of all new STDs. During 2010–2011, rates of reported chlamydial infection increased 3.5% for females aged 15 to 19 years and 10.5% for those aged 20 to 24 years. In 2011, women aged 15 to 19 years had the second highest rate of gonorrhea compared with any other age or sex group, and women aged 20 to 24 years had the highest rate of gonorrhea compared with any other age or sex group. Because patients with gonorrhea are often coinfected with chlamydia, dual treatment is indicated (CDC, 2012b).

In men, symptoms usually consist of dysuria and penile discharge. Women, however, are commonly asymptomatic. When present, symptoms are frequently less specific than in males but may include abnormal vaginal discharge, irregular menses, postcoital bleeding, low backache, and urinary frequency and dysuria.

The USPSTF recommends targeted screening of young women (25 years or younger) at increased risk for infection (e.g., women with previous gonorrhea infection, other STDs, new or multiple sex partners, and inconsistent condom use, those who engage in commercial sex work and drug use, women in certain demographic groups, those living in communities with a high prevalence of disease); the CDC supports these recommendations. Gonorrhea is most often tested through government screening programs; gonorrhea and Chlamydia testing are often performed together (CDC, 2012b, 2014; USPSTF, 2008). Testing methods include culture, nucleic acid hybridization, and NAAT. Either cervical swab or urine can be used as the specimen for NAAT.

The recommended treatment regimen for uncomplicated gonococcal infection of the cervix is ceftriaxone (Rocephin) 250 mg in a single intramuscular dose *plus* azithromycin 1 g orally in a single dose *or* doxycycline 100 mg orally twice daily for 7 days. If ceftriaxone is not available, the alternative treatment regimen is cefixime (Suprax) 400 mg in a single oral dose *plus* azithromycin 1 g orally in a single dose *or* doxycycline 100 mg orally twice daily for 7 days plus a test-of-cure in 1 week. If the patient has a severe cephalosporin allergy, the recommended therapy is azithromycin 2 g in a single oral dose *plus* a test-of-cure in 1 week (CDC, 2012b; Marrazzo & Cates, 2011). Prophylactic treatment for Chlamydia is given concurrently with gonorrhea treatment. Sex partners also require treatment. Health professionals should consult the CDC's Web site (http://www.cdc.gov/std /treatment) for frequent updates regarding treatment recommendations.

⑤ Optimizing Outcomes— With home screening for _C. trachomatis_ and _N. gonorrhoeae_

Graseck, Secura, Allsworth, Madden, and Peipert (2010) conducted a study to compare the acceptability of home screening with clinic-based screening for two STDs (_C. trachomatis_ and _N. gonorrhoeae_). In a telephone interview, women (aged 14–45 years) were given a choice of no-cost screening with vaginal swabs for self-collection mailed to their home (detailed instructions and a pread-dressed and stamped specimen mailer were included in the kit) or screening that was available without an appointment at area family planning clinics. The participants were much more likely to choose to screen for STDs at home than at a clinic or with their own medical provider. The researchers concluded that future interventions to increase screening rates in young women should consider alternative screening strategies such as home-based or patient-controlled testing.

Pelvic inflammatory disease (PID) develops in up to 40% of untreated women with cervical gonorrhea and may progress to a systemic infection. Because gonorrhea can be transmitted by vaginal, oral, or anal sex, patients with gonorrhea who have oral sex should be evaluated and treated for pharyngeal gonorrhea as necessary. Rectal testing for Chlamydia and gonorrhea may improve case finding for both STDs; research conducted by Barry, Kent, Philip, and Klausner (2010) revealed that among women, rectal infections were as common as genital infections. Maternal transfer of both gonorrhea and Chlamydia may occur during childbirth, causing neonatal eye infection (ophthalmia neonatorum), scalp abscess at the site of fetal monitors, rhinitis, or anorectal infection. All infected individuals who remain untreated are at risk for disseminated gonococcal infection (Marrazzo & Cates, 2011).

Trichomoniasis

Caused by the protozoan _Trichomonas vaginalis_, trichomoniasis is the most common curable STD in the United States. An estimated 7.4 million new cases occur in this country each year. Risk factors include multiple sexual partners, previous history of STDs, prostitution, and substance abuse. Infection with trichomoniasis has been shown to increase the risk of HIV transmission. Although infection with _T. vaginalis_ may be asymptomatic, it often produces a profuse frothy gray or yellow-green vaginal discharge with a foul odor. Erythema, edema, and pruritus of the external genitalia may be present, and the patient may report dysuria and dyspareunia. Upon examination, small red ulcerations in the vagina or on the cervix ("strawberry cervix") may be observed. The pH of the vaginal discharge is usually higher (more alkaline) than normal (CDC, 2013c; Marrazzo & Cates, 2011; Schwebke, 2012).

Microscopic evaluation is used to confirm trichomoniasis. Microscopic examination of the vaginal secretions on a wet-prep reveals the motile trichomonad parasites (Fig. 5-2). _T. vaginalis_ can also be detected by culture, or by a Trichomonas Rapid Test (results available in 20 minutes), a DNA hybridization probe test (Affirm VPIII) (results available

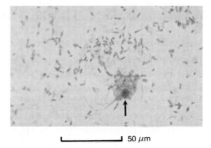

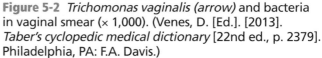

Figure 5-2 _Trichomonas vaginalis (arrow)_ and bacteria in vaginal smear (× 1,000). (Venes, D. [Ed.]. [2013]. _Taber's cyclopedic medical dictionary_ [22nd ed., p. 2379]. Philadelphia, PA: F.A. Davis.)

in 50 minutes), or a nucleic acid amplification test (APTIMA TV) (results available in 24 hours) (CDC, 2012b; Chapin, 2013; Schwebke, 2012, 2013).

🌸 Nursing Insight— _The vaginal wet mount_

A wet mount, also known as a "wet-prep" or "wet smear," is frequently used in the clinical setting to diagnose three of the most common vaginal infections: bacterial vaginosis, trichomoniasis, and yeast (candidiasis). To perform this test, the clinician inserts a speculum and uses a moist cotton swab to take a sample of the discharge from the posterior vaginal fornix. The discharge is then placed on a glass slide and viewed under a microscope. Alternately, a dry swab may be used: The sample is placed in 1 mL of saline, mixed, and placed on a slide, or a drop of saline is placed on a slide and the sample is added to it.

The slide may be warmed briefly (to increase motility of the trichomonads). A cover slip is then applied and the slide is promptly viewed.

Metronidazole (Flagyl), the medication of choice for trichomoniasis, is associated with a 95% cure rate. Metronidazole may be administered as a single dose—2 g orally—or 500 mg orally twice daily for 7 days. Alternately, tinidazole (Tindamax) 2 g orally as a single dose may be used, and this medication is recommended for the treatment of metronidazole-resistant _T. vaginalis_ infections. Partners should be simultaneously treated, and patients should be counseled to use condoms to prevent future infections and to avoid drinking alcohol until 24 hours after completing metronidazole therapy and 72 hours (3 days) after completing tinidazole therapy. Combining these medications with alcohol ingestion may produce a reaction characterized by flushing, nausea, vomiting, headache, and abdominal cramps (CDC, 2012b; Marrazzo & Cates, 2011; Vallerand & Sanoski, 2013).

⑤ Now Can You— Discuss Chlamydia, gonorrhea, and trichomoniasis?

1. Explain why infection with _Chlamydia trachomatis_ poses such a danger to young women?
2. Identify the U.S. population that is at highest risk for infection with gonorrhea?
3. Describe patient education that should accompany metronidazole therapy?

Pelvic Inflammatory Disease (PID)

Pelvic inflammatory disease (PID) is an acute infection of the uterus and fallopian tubes, which, if left untreated or unresolved, results in scarring, adhesions, or blockage of the fallopian tubes. A number of different organisms (e.g., *Escherichia coli, Mycoplasma hominis, Mycoplasma genitalium*) are usually involved, but the most common causative agents are *Chlamydia trachomatis* (more than 50%) and *Neisseria gonorrhoeae*. In the United States, PID accounts for nearly 180,000 hospitalizations every year, and one in seven reproductive-aged American women reports having received treatment for PID. Because PID may be caused by many organisms and encompasses a wide spectrum of pathological processes, the infection may be acute, subacute, or chronic. The two greatest reproductive consequences of acute PID are infertility and tubal pregnancy resulting from scarring of the fallopian tubes (Marrazzo & Cates, 2011; Soper, 2010).

> ### Nursing Insight— *Recognizing risk factors for pelvic inflammatory disease*
>
> When taking a sexual history, nurses should be aware of certain factors—such as a history of multiple sexual partners, a new partner in the past 6 months, lower age at first intercourse, lower economic status, vaginal douching, and cigarette smoking—that place women at increased risk for PID. Cigarette smoking may alter the cervical mucus by decreasing estrogen activity, thereby increasing the risk for bacterial ascent. Age constitutes another risk factor: Adolescents have the highest incidence of PID of any age group, and 70% of all cases of PID occur in women under age 25. Women who use intrauterine devices (IUDs) are also at increased risk if they have more than one sexual partner or if their partner has other sexual partners, because they are at higher risk for an STD (Marrazzo & Cates, 2011; Turner, 2012).

Symptoms of PID can range from none to severe abdominal, uterine, and ovarian pain and tenderness; abnormal bleeding or discharge; low back pain; nausea; and vomiting. The infected individual may also experience extreme tenderness when the cervix is moved on examination ("cervical motion tenderness"; the "chandelier sign"). Fever, chills, and an elevated white blood cell (WBC) count and erythrocyte sedimentation rate (ESR) may also be present, and women with more severe disease may demonstrate "peritoneal signs" such as shuffling gait associated with painful ambulation (Holland-Hall, 2012; Soper, 2010).

PID can be treated on an outpatient basis, but hospitalization may be necessary, depending on the individual case. For patients treated on an outpatient basis, reexamination within 48 to 72 hours is a crucial part of therapy. Combined drug therapy is advised, especially at the initiation of treatment, because the full spectrum of all organisms involved is often unknown. The CDC provides specific guidelines for PID treatment (http://www.cdc.gov/std/treatment/2010/pid.htm). Also, a PID Teaching Module for physicians, advanced practice nurses, and physician assistants is available at http://www2a.cdc.gov/STDTraining/Ready-To-Use/Manuals/PID/pid-notes-2009.pdf.

Human Papillomavirus (HPV)

Human papillomavirus (HPV), which causes genital warts (also called *condylomata acuminata*), is a DNA virus transmitted by skin-to-skin contact. There are more than 100 viral types currently identified, and of these, more than 30 types can infect the genital area. According to the CDC (2013a), HPV accounts for the majority of newly acquired STDs. Although more than 90% of HPV infections are cleared by the body's immune system within 2 years and cause no harm, some of the infections persist and can potentially lead to serious disease, including cervical cancer. (See Chapter 6 for further discussion.) Approximately one-half of all HPV genital infections occur in young women and men between the ages of 15 and 24 years. The majority of HPV infections are asymptomatic, unrecognized, or subclinical. Genital HPV infection can cause warty growths in the vagina or on the vulva, perineum, or anal area. The growths can be single or multiple, and they are soft and fleshy and usually painless. Diagnosis is usually made by visual confirmation of the lesions; confirmatory biopsy is rarely needed. Other strains of HPV infect the cervix and remain unnoticed until findings from a routine Pap test reveal the presence of the virus. Certain viral types are associated with the growth of abnormal cervical cells, which can lead to cancer of the cervix (CDC, 2011; Cox, Huh, Mayeaux, Randell, & Taylor, 2011).

> ### Optimizing Outcomes— **HPV prevention and testing**
>
> Strategies for prevention of HPV include sexual abstinence, confining sexual intimacy to a long-term monogamous relationship, and prophylactic vaccination. A vaccine against HPV types 6, 11, 16, and 18 (Gardasil) first became available in 2006 and is recommended for all females aged 9 to 26 years and for boys aged 11 or 12 years to age 21 years. In late 2014, the FDA approved a 9-valent recombinant HPV vaccine (Gardasil 9) that also covers HPV types 31, 33, 45, 52, and 58. These latter five are responsible for roughly one in five cases of cervical cancer. Gardasil 9, also administered as three intramuscular injections given over 6 months, is approved for use in females aged 9 through 26 and in males aged 9 through 15. Another immunogen, Cervarix, is a bivalent vaccine that protects against HPV 16 and 18. Available since 2009, Cervarix is licensed for use in females aged 10 to 25 years. All HPV vaccines are most effective if given before potential exposure to HPV through sexual contact. Although testing is available based on HPV-DNA in cervical cells, routine screening is not recommended except in specific circumstances following an abnormal Pap test (ACOG, 2010b; CDC, 2011; Marrazzo & Cates, 2011).

Several topical chemical agents are available for the treatment of external genital warts. These include trichloroacetic acid (TCA) or bichloroacetic acid (BCA) and podophyllin resin (provider administered) and podofilox gel or solution 0.5% (Condylox), sinecatechins ointment 15% (Veregen) (green tea extract), and imiquimod cream 5% (Aldara, Zyclara), which are patient administered. Cryotherapy (freezing), CO_2 laser surgery, electrosurgery, and surgical removal are other treatment options, depending on the severity of the lesions and resistance to treatment (Blereau, 2013; CDC, 2011; Fantasia, 2012; Marrazzo & Cates, 2011; Nelson, 2011).

When clinician-administered agents are used, the nurse should stress the importance of returning for regular treatment until the lesions have resolved. Once the warts have responded to therapy, no special follow-up is necessary. Owing to the risk of sequelae from cervical cancer, regular Pap tests are crucial for all women with documented HPV infection. Nurses should also encourage tobacco cessation to reduce the risk of HPV and neoplasia (Marrazzo & Cates, 2011).

Herpes Simplex Virus (HSV) 1 and 2

Herpes simplex virus 1 and 2 (HSV-1 and HSV-2), also known as human herpes virus 1 and 2 (HHV-1 and HHV-2), are members of the herpes virus family Herpesviridae that infect humans. Both HSV-1 and HSV-2 are transmitted horizontally during close contact with an infected person who is shedding virus from the skin, often in saliva or in genital secretions. Although transmission occurs most often when lesions are present, viral shedding and transmission can also occur in the absence of visible sores. HSV-1 is usually transmitted during childhood via nonsexual contacts. It is most commonly associated with cold sores or fever blisters on the mouth or face. Genital HSV-1 may result from oral–genital sexual contact with a person infected with oral HSV-1. Genital HSV-1 is unlikely to recur, and treatment may only be needed in persons with initial symptoms (Xu, Sternberg, Gottlieb, Berman, & Markowitz, 2010).

HSV-2 is primarily a sexually transmitted disease. HSV-2 is associated with genital lesions, although, depending on sexual practices, HSV-1 and HSV-2 are not exclusively associated with the respective sites. HSV-2 occurs more frequently in women than in men, which most likely results from the greater incidence of male-to-female transmission. HSV-infection rates are significantly higher among African Americans (46%) than among Caucasians (18%). Although HSV infection is not a reportable disease, it is estimated that 50 million Americans are infected with genital herpes (CDC, 2012b).

Most infected persons have no or only minimal signs or symptoms from HSV-1 or HSV-2 infection. As a result, the majority of genital herpes infections are transmitted by persons unaware that they have the infection or who are asymptomatic when transmission occurs. If symptoms develop during the first HSV-2 outbreak, they usually appear within 2 weeks after exposure and can be very pronounced. Owing to the fact that the body has not had an opportunity to develop antibodies, symptoms that result from a primary HSV infection are usually much more severe than with subsequent outbreaks (CDC, 2012b).

✦ *Nursing Insight— Recognizing signs and symptoms of HSV infection*

Symptoms of HSV-2 infection are similar to those that occur with the flu—malaise, muscle aches, and headache. Other symptoms include dysuria and the development of multiple fluid-filled, blister-like lesions, which can be extremely tender and persist for 2 to 3 weeks (Fig. 5-3). Before the appearance of the lesions, the patient may experience a period of prodromal symptoms characterized by skin sensitivity and nerve pain in the area where the lesions will appear. Reddening of the skin frequently follows these symptoms. The lesions form pustules and ulcers that dry up, crust over, and then heal without scarring. The woman may also experience itching, inguinal tenderness, vulvar edema, and a heavy watery or purulent vaginal discharge. In some instances, women with "chronic yeast infections" are actually experiencing herpes outbreaks that go undiagnosed because the typical herpetic lesions are not present (CDC, 2012b).

Typically, recurrent outbreaks are less severe than the primary infection and usually involve localized symptoms with less severe lesions that last 5 to 7 days. The prodromal characteristic genital tingling sensation is common with recurrence. The virus then enters a latent stage in the nerves at the base of the spine, only to reactivate when the patient's immune system is weakened. The lesions may occur along any skin surface supplied by that particular distribution (e.g., vulva, vagina, cervix, urethral meatus, buttocks). Because transmission of the virus is most likely during an active outbreak, patients should abstain from sexual contact during this time. However, viral transmission may occur at any time when the infected individual is producing and releasing ("shedding") the virus, and some individuals shed virus between active outbreaks (CDC, 2012b).

In most situations, a diagnosis of HSV is suspected based on the patient history and physical examination. Cell culture and polymerase chain reaction (PCR) are the preferred HSV tests for individuals who seek medical treatment for genital lesions. The sensitivity of viral culture testing is low, especially for recurrent lesions (blisters), and declines rapidly as the lesions begin to heal. Testing for the presence of HSV-2 antibodies in capillary blood or serum (i.e., HSV glycoprotein G-specific antibodies, IgG by immunoblot [HerpeSelect]) is also available for clinical use. However, screening of the general population is not indicated (CDC, 2012b).

The goal of treatment for herpes is to hasten healing and reduce symptoms. Several oral antiviral medications (e.g., acyclovir [Zovirax], valacyclovir [Valtrex], famciclovir [Famvir]) are available and may be used for primary or

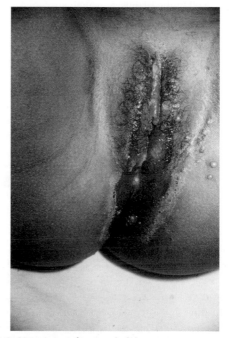

Figure 5-3 Herpes vulvovaginitis.

recurrent episodes or as daily suppressive therapy. The medications do not eradicate the infection, nor do they alter subsequent risk, frequency, or recurrences once the medication has been stopped. When indicated, acyclovir may be administered intravenously for 2 to 7 days (followed by oral antiviral therapy to complete at least 10 days of total therapy) for severe symptoms (CDC, 2011).

Optimizing Outcomes— Teaching women about HSV infection

Providing counseling and education forms an essential component of holistic care for women with herpes infections. Nurses should offer information about the etiology, signs, symptoms, modes of transmission, treatment options, and the possibility of suppression therapy to prevent partner transmission. It is important to advise women about the times when transmission is most likely and the need to avoid sexual contact beginning with the onset of prodromal symptoms until all lesions have healed. Some experts recommend the consistent use of condoms for all individuals with genital herpes. Nurses can help women explore potential precipitating factors in the reactivation of the latent herpes virus. Triggers may include stress, menstruation, febrile illnesses, chronic illnesses, and ultraviolet light. Some patients find that keeping a personal diary provides insights about precipitating events for their herpetic outbreaks.

Complementary Care: Measures to reduce HSV discomforts and outbreaks

For many women, certain comfort measures and dietary changes are useful in decreasing HSV symptoms and the frequency and severity of HSV outbreaks. Comfort measures may include taking warm sitz baths with baking soda or oatmeal; wearing cotton underwear; using a hair dryer (on the cool setting) to enhance drying of the lesions; applying compresses containing peppermint oil and clove oil to the lesions; and applying cool, wet, black tea bags or tea tree oil to the lesions. Oral analgesics including aspirin or ibuprofen may help relieve pain. Dietary strategies center on consumption of a diet rich in vitamin C, B-complex vitamins, zinc, and calcium and the daily use of kelp powder and sunflower seed oil as well as the amino acid l-lysine, which is thought to suppress the herpes simplex virus. Strategies to help reduce the emotional symptoms associated with herpes include support groups, relaxation techniques, self-hypnosis, biofeedback, and individual therapy (e.g., psychologist, social worker) (University of Maryland Medical Center, 2011).

? Global Health Case Study Efinanya T.

Painful Vaginal Vesicles

Efinanya T. is a 22-year-old Nigerian graduate student who visits the local health department because of her concerns over several vaginal "bumps" that she noticed a few days ago. During the interview, she tells the nurse that she first noticed a slight soreness in the area, but it had become increasingly more painful. She has never "had anything like this before." Efinanya denies vaginal discharge but has experienced dysuria over the past 2 days. She also has felt tired and achy. Efinanya is sexually active and uses oral contraceptives

for birth control. She and her boyfriend engage in oral and vaginal sex; upon questioning, Efinanya remembers that he recently has had a fever blister on his lip. Her physical examination reveals a temperature of 100.0°F, positive inguinal nodes, vulvar edema, and the presence of several vesicles surrounding the vaginal introitus.

critical thinking questions

1. What is the likely diagnosis?
2. What treatment may be prescribed for Efinanya?
3. What should the nurse teach Efinanya about this medication?
4. What else should the nurse teach Efinanya about herpes simplex virus?

Syphilis

One of the oldest known sexually transmitted diseases, syphilis is caused by the spirochetal bacterium *Treponema pallidum*. It is believed that the organism is transmitted through microscopic abrasions that can occur during sexual intercourse. Kissing, biting, and oral–genital sex may also be modes of transmission. Congenital syphilis occurs via maternal–fetal transmission. Syphilis cannot be contracted through toilet seats, daily activities, hot tubs, or sharing eating utensils or clothing. Left untreated, syphilis can cause severe systemic disease and death. According to the CDC (2013a), each year, approximately 55,400 people in the United States acquire new syphilis infections. There were 46,042 reported new cases of syphilis in 2011; of these, 13,970 cases were of primary and secondary (P & S) syphilis, the earliest and most infectious stages of the disease. In 2011, 72% of P & S syphilis occurred among men who have sex with men, and there were 360 reports of children with congenital syphilis in 2011. Although the rate of primary and secondary syphilis in the United States declined during 1990 to 2000, the rate increased annually from 2001 to 2009 before decreasing in 2010. The 2011 rate remained unchanged (CDC, 2013a).

Although the majority of reported syphilis cases in the United States occur among men who have sex with men, rates among women increased from 0.8 cases per 100,000 population in 2004 to 1.5 cases per 100,000 in 2008. The syphilis rate among women then declined to 1.1 cases per 100,000 population in 2010 and 1 case per 100,000 population in 2011. Rates of primary and secondary syphilis among women in 2011 were highest among non-Hispanic black women (5 cases/100,000 population), followed by Hispanic (0.6 cases/100,000 population), American Indian/Alaska Native (0.5 cases/100,000 population), non-Hispanic white (0.3 cases/100,000 population), and Asian/Pacific Islander (0.1/100,000 population) (CDC, 2012b).

Optimizing Outcomes— Through targeted syphilis screening efforts

The CDC (2013a) and the USPSTF (2009b) recommend that persons at increased risk for syphilis infection (i.e., all men who have sex with men) be tested at least annually for syphilis and that all pregnant women be screened for syphilis at the first prenatal visit to avoid transmission to their infants.

Syphilis is a complex disease with several stages. Different manifestations occur depending on the stage of the disease. In the primary stage, approximately 10 to 90 days after the initial exposure, a painless ulcer (chancre) appears at the point of contact, which is usually the genitalia. Lymphadenopathy may also be present. The lesion may persist for 4 to 6 weeks and usually resolves on its own without treatment (CDC, 2012b).

Secondary syphilis occurs 6 weeks to 6 months after the appearance of the chancre. During this stage, patients may have fever, a sore throat, weight loss, skin rash on the trunk and extremities (Fig. 5-4), headache, generalized malaise, mucous patches on the genitals or in the mouth, lymphadenopathy, alopecia, and the appearance of moist, flat warts in the genital and anal areas (condylomata lata). If left untreated, the symptoms resolve within 2 to 10 weeks. Approximately one-third of infected individuals will then develop tertiary syphilis (CDC, 2012b; Marrazzo & Cates, 2011).

Tertiary syphilis usually occurs 1 to 10 years after the initial infection, although in some cases systemic symptoms may not appear until 30 to 50 years later. This stage is characterized by the formation of gummas (soft, tumor-like balls of inflammation). Other manifestations of tertiary syphilis include neuropathic joint disease (degeneration of joint surfaces), neurosyphilis, and cardiovascular syphilis. It is estimated that approximately 20% to 30% of untreated individuals with syphilis develop tertiary syphilis (CDC, 2012b).

🌸 *Nursing Insight—* *Understanding the entity termed "latent syphilis"*

Latent syphilis is defined as having serological proof of infection without signs or symptoms of the disease. Latent syphilis may be "early" or "late." By definition, early latent syphilis is having the infection for greater than 2 years but without clinical evidence of the disease. This stage is treated with a single intramuscular injection of a long-acting penicillin. Late latent syphilis requires three weekly intramuscular injections of a long-acting penicillin (CDC, 2012b).

Effective tests and treatments for syphilis were developed during the 20th century. Microscopy of fluid from the primary or secondary lesion using darkfield illumination is highly accurate in detecting *T. pallidum*. Screening tests include the Rapid Plasma Reagin (RPR), the Venereal Disease Research Laboratory (VDRL), and the Syphilis Health Check, a 10-minute test that detects syphilis antibodies in human whole blood, serum, and plasma. When positive, the screening tests should be followed up by a more specific treponemal test. Tests based on monoclonal

antibodies and immunofluorescence, including treponema pallidum hemagglutination assay (TPHA) and fluorescent treponemal antibody absorption (FTA-ABS), are more specific tests. Tests based on ELISAs are also used to confirm results of the simpler screening tests for syphilis. Neurosyphilis is diagnosed via analysis of the cerebrospinal fluid. Because there is some evidence that the incidence of neurosyphilis is higher in HIV patients, some experts recommend that all HIV-positive individuals have a lumbar puncture to assess for asymptomatic neurosyphilis (CDC, 2011).

Penicillin, in the form of penicillin G, is the treatment of choice for syphilis, and the specific regimen and duration depends on the length of infection. Doxycycline and tetracycline may be used as alternative treatments for individuals who are allergic to penicillin (CDC, 2011). For the most current treatment guidelines, health professionals may visit the CDC Web site at http://www.cdc.gov/std/treatment/2010/default.htm.

⚠️ **clinical alert**

Teach patients about the possibility of a Jarisch-Herxheimer reaction

The Jarisch-Herxheimer reaction occurs when large quantities of toxins are released into the body as bacteria, typically spirochetal bacteria, and die during treatment with antibiotics. Death of the bacteria and the associated release of endotoxins occur more quickly than the liver and kidneys can remove the toxins. Fever, chills, headache, myalgia, and exacerbation of skin lesions are the hallmarks of this acute reaction. In syphilis, the duration is usually only a few hours but can persist for much longer with other diseases. Treatment, aimed at reducing symptoms, centers on the use of analgesics and antipyretics.

🔄 **Now Can You—** **Discuss PID, HPV, HSV, and syphilis?**

1. Identify six risk factors for PID?
2. Describe strategies for HPV prevention?
3. Discuss the nurse's role in teaching women about HSV infection?
4. Differentiate among the primary, secondary, and tertiary stages of syphilis?

Hepatitis

Hepatitis is the leading cause of liver cancer and the most common reason for liver transplantation. In the United

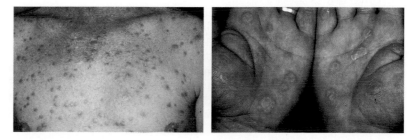

Figure 5-4 Secondary syphilitic rash on chest and palms.

States, an estimated 1.4 million individuals are living with chronic hepatitis B virus (HBV) and 3.2 million persons are living with chronic hepatitis C virus (HCV). Many are unaware that they are infected. Each year, an estimated 21,000 persons become infected with the hepatitis A virus (HAV), 38,000 with hepatitis B, and 17,000 with hepatitis C (CDC, 2012a).

✾ *Nursing Insight*— *Hepatitis A virus*

Formerly known as "infectious hepatitis," hepatitis A is an acute infectious disease of the liver caused by HAV. Every year, approximately 10 million people worldwide are infected with the virus, and the incidence of infection is highest in developing countries and in regions with poor hygiene standards. HAV causes no clinical signs and symptoms in over 90% of infected children, and because the infection confers lifelong immunity, the disease is of no special significance to the indigenous population. When present, symptoms may include fever, fatigue, loss of appetite, nausea, vomiting, abdominal pain, dark urine, clay-colored bowel movements, joint pain, and jaundice; symptoms typically last less than 2 months. In the United States, HAV is primarily contracted by susceptible young adults, the majority of whom are infected with the virus during trips to countries with a high incidence of the disease. There is no specific treatment for HAV. Hepatitis A can be prevented by vaccination (full two-dose series), good hygiene, and sanitation (CDC, 2012a).

HEPATITIS B VIRUS (HBV)

In 2009, an estimated 38,000 persons in the United States were newly infected with HBV. The highest incidence of HBV occurs in persons aged 20 to 49 years, and the virus is 50 to 100 times more contagious than HIV. It causes liver disease and can be fatal. Each year, approximately 2,000 to 4,000 Americans die of complications resulting from HBV infection. The rate of new HBV infections has declined by approximately 82% since 1991, when a national strategy was initiated to eliminate HBV infection in the United States; the decline has been greatest among children born since 1991, when routine vaccination of children was first implemented (CDC, 2012a).

Hepatitis B virus is a species of the genus *Orthohepadnavirus,* which is a part of the Hepadnaviridae family of viruses. This virus causes the disease hepatitis B. The incubation period from the time of exposure to the onset of symptoms is 6 weeks to 6 months. HBV is found in highest concentrations in blood and in lower concentrations in other body fluids such as semen, vaginal secretions, and wound exudates. Although heterosexual intercourse is the predominant mode of transmission, HBV may also be spread through blood-to-blood contact. Blood-to-blood contact can occur through the sharing of razors, toothbrushes, and manicure tools, as well as through contaminated instruments used for dental procedures, tattooing, and body piercing. Vertical transmission occurs when a pregnant woman passes the virus to her fetus. HBV is not spread through food or water, sharing eating utensils, breastfeeding, hugging, kissing, hand holding, coughing, or sneezing (Apuzzio et al., 2012; CDC, 2012a).

⬡ Optimizing Outcomes— **Identifying populations at increased risk for HBV**

Nurses should be aware of certain factors that place men, women, children, and intimate partners at increased risk for HBV. Taking a detailed patient history can help nurses to identify these individuals, who include (CDC 2012a):

- Infants born to infected mothers
- Sex partners of infected persons
- Sexually active persons who are not in a long-term (greater than 6 months) mutually monogamous relationship
- Men who have sex with men
- Injection drug users
- Household contacts of persons with chronic HBV infection
- Health-care and public safety workers at risk for occupational exposure to blood or blood-contaminated body fluids
- Hemodialysis patients
- Residents and staff of facilities for developmentally disabled persons
- Travelers to countries with intermediate or high prevalence of HBV infection

Signs and symptoms of infection with HBV are often absent, especially in children under age 5 years and in newly infected immunosuppressed adults. However, it is estimated that up to 50% of persons older than 5 years have initial signs and symptoms of the infection, such as fever, fatigue, a loss of appetite, nausea, vomiting, abdominal pain, dark-colored urine, clay-colored stools, joint pain, and jaundice. On average, symptoms appear from 60 to 150 days after exposure to HBV and last for several weeks (CDC, 2012a).

✾ *Nursing Insight*— *Acute and chronic HBV infection*

Acute HBV infection ranges from asymptomatic or mild disease to fulminate hepatitis (rare). The disease is more severe among older adults (older than 60 years). The risk for chronic infection varies according to the age at infection and is greatest among young children: Approximately 90% of infants and 25% to 50% of children (aged 1–5 years) will remain chronically infected with HBV. The vast majority (more than 95%) of adults with HBV infection recover completely and do not become chronically infected. Approximately 25% of those who become chronically infected during childhood and 15% of those who become chronically infected after childhood die prematurely from cirrhosis or liver cancer, and the majority remain asymptomatic until the onset of cirrhosis or end-stage liver disease. In the United States, chronic HBV infection results in an estimated 2,000 to 4,000 deaths each year (CDC, 2012a). Nearly 90% of individuals living in the United States with chronic HBV infection are immigrants born in areas (e.g., Africa, Asia, Caribbean [Haiti, Jamaica, Dominica, St. Lucia], South America) where the virus prevalence is greater than 2% (Tarrant, Block, & McMahon, 2013).

Individuals at high risk for contracting HBV should be screened on a regular basis. The USPSTF (2009a) recommends that all women should be screened for HBV at the first prenatal visit, regardless of whether they have been tested previously, and screening should be repeated later in the pregnancy for women with high-risk behaviors. No routine screening is recommended for the general population. Testing for HBV is complex. There are a number of different markers identified in a blood test, some of which indicate active infection, chronic carrier state, or past infection (ACOG, 2011b; CDC, 2012a; USPSTF, 2012).

❋ Collaboration in Caring— *Providing vaccines for hepatitis B prevention*

Two single-antigen vaccines (Engerix-B and Recombivax HB) and three combination vaccines are licensed in the United States. The combination vaccines include the following: Comvax (combined hepatitis *B-Haemophilus influenzae* type b [Hib])—cannot be administered at birth, before age 6 weeks, or after age 71 months); Pediarix (combined hepatitis B, diphtheria, tetanus, acellular pertussis [DtaP], and inactivated poliovirus [IPV] vaccine)—cannot be administered at birth, before age 6 weeks, or after age 7 years; and Twinrix (combined hepatitis A and hepatitis B vaccine—recommended for persons aged 18+ years who are at increased risk for both HAV and HBV). The vaccination schedule most often used for children and adults is three intramuscular injections; the second and third doses administered 1 and 6 months after the first dose. After a person has been exposed to HBV, appropriate prophylaxis (i.e., hepatitis B vaccine), given as soon as possible but preferably within 24 hours, can effectively prevent infection. Although persons who have already been infected with HBV will receive no benefit from vaccination, there is no risk to a previously infected person who receives the vaccination (CDC, 2012a).

The CDC (2012a) Advisory Committee on Immunization Practices has published recommendations for hepatitis B vaccination. At-risk individuals who should receive HBV vaccination are presented in Box 5-2. The CDC Advisory Committee has also determined that adults who receive care in health-care, evaluation, and treatment settings should also receive HBV vaccination. Specific settings are presented in Box 5-3.

There is no specific therapy for acute hepatitis B infection; treatment is supportive. Several antiviral drugs (adefovir dipivoxil [Preveon, Hepsera], interferon alfa-2b [PEG-Intron], pegylated interferon alfa 2a [Pegasys], lamivudine [Epivir], entecavir [Baraclude], telbivudine [Tyzeka]) are used for treatment of chronic infection. Individuals with chronic HBV infection require medical evaluation and regular monitoring to determine whether the disease is progressing and to identify liver damage or hepatocellular carcinoma (cancer of the liver) (CDC, 2012a; Rustgi, Carriero, Bachtold, & Zeldin, 2010).

⑤ Optimizing Outcomes— **Patient education and counseling after HBV diagnosis**

Once a person has received a diagnosis of HBV, the nurse should stress the importance of HBV screening for close family members, household contacts, and sexual partners. Uninfected close family members, household contacts, and sexual partners should then be vaccinated, and the infected individual provided with disease-management information and referral to a specialist (Tarrant et al., 2013).

Box 5-2 Individuals Who Should Be Vaccinated Against Hepatitis B

- All infants, beginning at birth
- All children aged less than 19 years who have not been vaccinated previously
- Susceptible sex partners of hepatitis B surface antigen (HbsAg)–positive persons
- Sexually active persons who are not in a long-term, mutually monogamous relationship (e.g., more than one sex partner during the previous 6 months)
- Persons seeking evaluation or treatment for an STD
- Men who have sex with men
- Injection drug users
- Susceptible household contacts of HbsAg-positive persons
- Health-care and public safety workers at risk for exposure to blood or blood-contaminated body fluids
- Persons with end-stage renal disease, including predialysis, hemodialysis, peritoneal dialysis, and home dialysis patients
- Residents and staff of facilities for developmentally disabled persons
- Travelers to regions with intermediate or high rates of endemic HBV infection
- Persons with chronic liver disease

PERSONS WITH HIV INFECTION

- Unvaccinated adults with diabetes mellitus who are aged 19 through 59 years (discretion of clinicians for unvaccinated adults with diabetes mellitus who are aged older than 60 years)
- All other persons seeking protection from HBV infection—acknowledgment of a specific risk factor is not a requirement for vaccination

Source: CDC (2012a).

Box 5-3 Settings Where Hepatitis B Vaccination Should Be Administered to All Adults Who Receive Care

- STD treatment facilities
- HIV testing and treatment facilities
- Facilities providing drug-abuse treatment and prevention services
- Health-care settings targeting services to injection drug users
- Correctional facilities
- Health-care settings targeting services to men who have sex with men
- Chronic hemodialysis facilities and end-stage renal disease programs
- Institutions and nonresidential day-care facilities for developmentally disabled persons

Source: CDC (2012a).

HEPATITIS C VIRUS (HCV)

Hepatitis C (*Flaviviridae hepacivirus*) is a small, enveloped, single-stranded RNA virus. Largely unknown to the American public, hepatitis C virus (HCV) infection is the most common chronic bloodborne infection in the United States. According to the CDC (2012b), approximately 3.2 million persons are chronically infected. Previously known as "non-A, non-B hepatitis," up to 85% of individuals infected with HCV will progress to chronic viral hepatitis. There are six genotypes of the virus; genotype 1, the most difficult to treat, makes up approximately 75% of the HCV population in the United States (Page, 2012; Rapsilber, 2012).

HCV is primarily spread through blood-to-blood contact and less efficiently through semen, saliva, or urine. As with HBV, transmission of HCV can potentially occur through blood contact with shared needles, razors, and toothbrushes. Persons at risk for HCV include those with STDs such as hepatitis B and HIV and those with multiple sex partners, a history of blood transfusions, or a history of IV drug use. Currently, no vaccine for HCV infection is available (CDC, 2012a).

Newly acquired HCV infection is often asymptomatic. When symptoms occur, however, they may include fever, fatigue, dark-colored urine, clay-colored stools, abdominal pain, anorexia, nausea, vomiting, joint pain, and jaundice. Approximately 20% to 30% of individuals newly infected with HCV experience fatigue, abdominal pain, poor appetite, or jaundice. The average time period from exposure to symptom onset (if any) is 4 to 12 weeks (CDC, 2012a).

Nursing Insight— *Progression of acute HCV infection to chronic HCV infection to death*

Hepatitis C causes tissue inflammation, which results in hepatic fibrosis, which leads to scarring. The scarring adversely affects liver function, leading to the development of cirrhosis, which eventually leads to liver failure and transplant. Of every 100 persons infected with HCV, approximately 75 to 85 will develop chronic infection; 60 to 70 will develop chronic liver disease; 5 to 20 will develop cirrhosis over a period of 20 to 30 years; and 1 to 5 will die of the consequences of chronic infection (e.g., liver cancer [hepatocellular carcinoma] or cirrhosis). Chronic HCV infection, the leading indication for liver transplantation in this country, accounts for more than 15,000 deaths in the United States each year (CDC, 2012a; Page, 2012; Rapsilber, 2012).

According to the CDC (2012a), certain individuals and populations should be tested for HCV infection (Box 5-4). Blood tests that may be performed to test for HCV infection include screening tests for antibody to HCV (e.g., EIA, enhanced chemiluminescence immunoassay

---

Box 5-4 Testing for HCV Infection

The CDC (2012a) recommends that the following individuals are at increased risk for HCV infection and should undergo testing:

- Persons born from 1945 through 1965
- Persons who have ever injected illegal drugs, including those who injected only once many years ago
- Recipients of clotting factor concentrates made before 1987
- Recipients of blood transfusions or solid organ transplants before July 1992
- Patients who have ever received long-term hemodialysis treatment
- Persons with known exposures to HCV (e.g., health-care workers after needle sticks involving HCV-positive blood, recipients of blood or organs from a donor who later tested HCV positive)
- All persons with HIV infection
- Patients with signs or symptoms of liver disease (e.g., abnormal liver enzyme tests)
- Children born to HCV-positive mothers (to avoid detecting maternal antibody, testing should not be performed prior to 18 months of age)

[CIA]), recombinant immunoblot assay [RIBA]), qualitative tests to detect the presence or absence of the virus, and quantitative tests to detect the amount of virus. The CDC provides a table on interpretation of HCV test results for health professionals, available at http://www.cdc.gov/hepatitis/HCV/PDFs/hcv_graph.pdf.

Following diagnosis, HCV-infected patients should be evaluated for the presence of chronic liver disease and determination of the need for hepatitis B vaccination. Combination therapy with pegylated interferon and ribavirin is the treatment of choice for individuals with chronic hepatitis C. According to the CDC (2012), success rates are improved with the addition of polymerase and protease inhibitors to standard pegylated interferon/ribavirin combination therapy. The goal of therapy is to halt the progression of fibrosis and to prevent the development of cirrhosis by eradicating the virus (Casey, 2014; Mayhew, 2011; Page, 2012).

Optimizing Outcomes— With holistic nursing care for women with chronic hepatitis

Nurses can empower women with chronic hepatitis infection by providing education and counseling about strategies to optimize health, reduce the transmission of infection, and communicate concerns with intimate sexual partners. Referrals to local resources such as professional counselors and peer support groups may also be of benefit. Nurses can teach women about the importance of maintaining a high level of personal hygiene with measures such as performing strict hand washing after toileting and ensuring the careful disposal of all tampons, sanitary pads, and bandages. Patients can also be taught to avoid sharing razor blades, toothbrushes, needles, and manicure implements and to promptly clean blood spills with soap and water. Non-HBV-vaccinated male sexual partners should consistently use latex condoms. Nutritional strategies may include the consumption of a low-protein, low-fat diet; avoidance of protein or amino acid supplements; the use of an antioxidant formula vitamin supplement; and the avoidance of alcohol and tobacco. Patients are also taught about medication side effects (e.g., fatigue, headache, gastrointestinal symptoms, rash, and hematological symptoms [anemia, neutropenia, thrombocytopenia]) and strategies for coping with them (e.g., hydration, energy-conservation, skin moisturizers, antiemetics, NSAIDs) and advised to avoid medications that are hepatotoxic (e.g., Tylenol) (Page, 2012; Rapsilber, 2012; Rustgi et al., 2010; Tarrant et al., 2013).

HEPATITIS D VIRUS (HDV)

Hepatitis D virus (HDV), also known as "delta hepatitis," is a single-stranded circular RNA molecule with some double-stranded attachments. HDV infection can only occur in a person already infected with HBV; a person can be infected by HBV and HDV simultaneously or by HBV first. Infection with HDV is clinically indistinguishable from other forms of hepatitis. After exposure, the incubation period is 21 to 45 days. Up to 90% of cases of HDV are asymptomatic, but when present, symptoms include jaundice, fatigue, abdominal pain, confusion, pruritus, anorexia, nausea, vomiting, and joint pain. Chronic hepatitis D, a long-term liver infection, is possible (Hepatitis Foundation International, 2013).

Serum testing is complex and includes assays for serum HDAg, serum HDV RNA, anti-HDV antibody, and tissue markers for HDV infection. Transmission of HDV occurs through body fluids, including blood, semen, vaginal fluids, and saliva. Perinatal transmission is rare. Nurses can teach women to reduce their risk of contracting HDV through the avoidance of exposure to infected blood, contaminated needles, and an infected person's personal items such as toothbrushes, razors, and nail clippers, and the consistent practice of safer-sex strategies (e.g., latex condoms during vaginal, anal, and oral sex). Women may also wish to consider vaccination against hepatitis B. Interferon alfa-2b treatments may be of benefit to a small proportion of infected individuals (Hepatitis Foundation International, 2013).

Now Can You—Discuss aspects of viral hepatitis?

1. Identify populations at greatest risk for infection with HBV?
2. Identify seven settings where hepatitis B vaccination should be administered to adults who receive care?
3. Explain how the hepatitis virus may be transmitted?

Chancroid, Lymphogranuloma Venereum, Granuloma Inguinale, Pediculosis Pubis, and Scabies

Although they occur less commonly, STDs including chancroid, lymphogranuloma venereum, granuloma inguinale, pediculosis pubis, and scabies may be identified in the clinical setting.

CHANCROID

Caused by the gram-negative streptobacillus *Haemophilus ducreyi*, infection with chancroid begins with a small bump (usually on the labia majora) that quickly develops into a painful ulcer with a base that is covered with a gray or yellow-gray material. Symptoms include dysuria and dyspareunia. Inguinal adenopathy is present in approximately one-third of infected individuals. The diagnosis is made via special culture media. Treatment consists of a single oral dose (1 g) of azithromycin (Zithromax) *or* a single intramuscular dose (250 mg) of ceftriaxone (Rocephin) *or* oral ciprofloxacin (Cipro) (500 mg bid) for 3 days *or* oral erythromycin base (E-Mycin, E.E.S.) (500 mg tid) for 7 days (CDC, 2011).

LYMPHOGRANULOMA VENEREUM

Lymphogranuloma venereum (LGV) is caused by three different types of the bacterium *Chlamydia trachomatis*. The infection is not caused by the same bacteria that cause genital Chlamydia. Primarily an infection of the lymphatics and lymph nodes, LGV gains entrance through breaks in the skin or via the mucous membranes. The primary infection produces a self-limited, painless genital ulcer at the contact site approximately 3 to 12 days after exposure. Owing to its hidden location, women frequently are unaware of its presence. The second stage, which usually occurs from 10 to 30 days later, involves the lymph nodes and lymphatic drainage pathways. Localized symptoms include cervicitis, perimetritis, salpingitis, and lymphadenitis; systemic symptoms include fever, decreased appetite, and malaise. The diagnosis is based on clinical suspicion, epidemiological information, and the exclusion of other causes, along with *C. trachomatis* testing. Serological testing is also available. LGV is treated with doxycycline (Doxycin, Vibramycin) 100 mg orally bid for 21 days *or* erythromycin base (E-Mycin, Robimycin) 500 mg orally qid for 21 days (CDC, 2011).

GRANULOMA INGUINALE

Granuloma inguinale (also known as "donovanosis") is a genital ulcerative disease caused by the intracellular gram-negative bacterium *Klebsiella granulomatis*. The disease commonly produces painless, progressive, beefy-red ulcerative lesions; regional lymphadenopathy is absent. The lesions most commonly occur on the labia or perineum. The diagnosis is made based on the patient's sexual history, absence of inguinal lymphadenopathy, and identification of the lesions. Tissue biopsy may be used to aid in the diagnosis. Granuloma inguinale is treated with doxycycline (Adoxa) 100 mg orally bid for at least 3 weeks and until all lesions have completely healed. Alternative regimens include azithromycin (Zithromax) (1 g orally once per week for at least 3 weeks) *or* ciprofloxacin (Cipro) (750 mg orally bid for at least 3 weeks) *or* erythromycin base (E-Mycin) (500 mg orally qid for at least 3 weeks) *or* trimethoprim-sulfamethoxazole (Bactrim) (one double-strength [160 mg/800 mg] tablet orally bid for at least 3 weeks) (CDC, 2011).

PEDICULOSIS PUBIS

Pediculosis pubis is a disease caused by the pubic louse *Pthirus pubis*. Lice are parasitic insects that can be found on the head and body, including the pubic area. Human lice survive by feeding on human blood. Lice infestations are primarily spread by close person-to-person contact. Lice move by crawling—they are unable to hop or fly. The *Pthirus pubis* (pubic louse, "crab" louse) is very short (1.1 to 1.8 mm in length) and crablike in appearance (Fig. 5-5). Pubic lice are typically found attached to hair in the pubic area but can sometimes be found on coarse hair in the eyebrows, eyelashes, beard, mustache, chest, or armpits. Pubic lice are usually spread through sexual contact and are most common in adults. Although they do not transmit disease, secondary bacterial infection can occur from scratching of the skin. Pubic lice and nits (eggs) may be large enough to be seen with the naked eye, although a magnifying lens may be necessary to find them. Patients with pediculosis pubis should be screened for other STDs, as coinfections are common (CDC, 2012b).

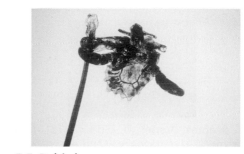

Figure 5-5 Pubic louse.

> **⊚ Optimizing Outcomes—** **Through prevention and control of pubic lice**
>
> The nurse counsels infected women about strategies to help prevent and control the spread of pubic lice. Patients are taught to (CDC, 2012b):
>
> * Ensure that all sexual contacts are examined and all infested persons are treated.
> * Avoid sexual contact until treatment and reevaluation have been completed.
> * Machine wash all clothing and bedding in hot (at least 130°F) water and machine dry on the high-heat drying cycle. Clothing and items that are not washable can be dry-cleaned or sealed in a plastic bag and stored for 2 weeks.
> * Avoid the sharing of clothing, bedding, and towels.
> * Avoid the use of fumigant sprays or fogs—these products can be toxic if inhaled or absorbed through the skin.

A lice-killing lotion containing 1% permethrin or a mousse containing pyrethrins and piperonyl butoxide can be used to treat pubic lice. These products are readily available over the counter without a prescription at a local drugstore. When used exactly according to the instructions listed on the package, these medications are safe and effective (CDC, 2012b).

SCABIES

Human scabies is caused by an infestation of the skin by the human itch mite *Sarcoptes scabiei* var. *hominis*. The microscopic scabies mite infects the epidermis by burrowing into the upper layer of the skin where it lives and lays its eggs. Scabies is usually spread by direct, prolonged, skin-to-skin contact with an infected person. The infected individual typically experiences intense itching, especially at night, and a pimplelike skin rash. Upon examination, scaly papules and insect burrows may be observed in the interdigital spaces of the hands and flexor areas of the wrist; in the axillae; and on the waist, feet, ankles, and buttocks (Fig. 5-6). Secondary bacterial skin infections may result from itching and scratching. The diagnosis is made by history, physical examination, and observation of the insect burrows; confirmation can be made by visualization of the scabies mite, eggs, or feces under low-power microscopy (CDC, 2011; Fantasia et al., 2011).

Scabicides, prescription-only products that kill scabies mites, are used to treat infestations. Scabicide lotion or cream (e.g., permethrin cream 5%) should be applied to all areas of the body from the neck down to the feet

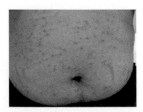

Figure 5-6 Scabies. (Venes, D. [Ed.]. [2013]. *Taber's cyclopedic medical dictionary* [22nd ed., p. 2082]. Philadelphia, PA: F.A. Davis.)

and toes, left on for the recommended amount of time, and then washed off. Because scabies may be present in bedding, clothing, and towels, patients should be counseled to wash all items in hot water and dry them in a hot dryer. Alternately, items may be sealed in a plastic bag for at least 72 hours. Owing to the high rate of infectivity, all household and sexual partners should be treated regardless of symptoms (CDC, 2011; Fantasia et al., 2011).

The Nurse's Role in Fostering Reproductive Health Through STD Education and Counseling

When educating women about STDs, nurses should include basic information along with sexual decision-making skills. When dealing with adolescents, it is often helpful to discuss basic communication skills needed to negotiate in a relationship and how to operate from an internal value system rather than submit to peer pressure. Educating women about the workings of their bodies and encouraging them to be active participants in their own health care enhance their personal control over their reproductive health. Nurses can empower women of all ages by providing them with specific strategies for making safe choices in their intimate relationships. When appropriate, teaching about strategies for "safer sex" provides guidance and serves to foster wellness and promote reproductive health (Box 5-5). During STD counseling, the nurse can emphasize that condoms offer the best protection against the transmission of disease and stress that intimate sexual contact should be avoided if the person or partner has any sore areas or visible lesions (Marrazzo & Cates, 2011; Matkins, 2013).

During private counseling sessions, it is important to inquire about substance use and other high-risk behaviors that may increase the likelihood of exposure to an STD. A woman who drinks heavily or who practices binge drinking may not remember the details of sexual encounters that took place while intoxicated. A history of injected drug use increases the risk for infection with hepatitis and HIV; women who smoke have a higher rate of cervical cancer (Marrazzo & Cates, 2011).

⊚ Where Research and Practice Meet:
STD Social Networking Site for Adolescents

Yager and O'Keefe (2012) developed and implemented "Teen Sexual Health Information," a social networking (Facebook) site designed to provide adolescents with STD information, testing, and treatment sites. Intended to help adolescents make informed decisions about their sexual health, the Web site included videos, photographs, fact sheets about STDs, free and reduced-cost clinic locations for STD testing and treatment, and links to other STD information Web sites. Project evaluation data revealed increased connections between adolescents and health-care professionals and demonstrated the ease with which information on a social networking site can be accessed. The researchers concluded that the social networking site Facebook could serve as a viable option for circulating sexual health information to the technology-savvy adolescent population.

Box 5-5 Safer Sex Strategies for Sexual Intimacy and HIV and STD Prevention

STRATEGIES CONSIDERED TO BE SAFE

- Sexual fantasies
- Massage
- Hugging
- Body rubbing
- Dry kissing
- Masturbation without contact with the partner's semen or vaginal secretions
- Erotic conversation, books, movies, videos, or DVDs
- Eroticizing feet, fingers, buttocks, abdomen, ears, or other body parts
- All sexual activities when both partners are monogamous and known by testing to be free of HIV and other STDs

STRATEGIES WITH A LOW RISK, CONSIDERED TO BE POSSIBLY SAFE

- Wet kissing with no broken skin, cracked lips, or damaged mouth tissue
- Hand-to-genital touching or mutual masturbation
- Vaginal or anal intercourse using latex or plastic condom
- Oral sex on a woman using a latex or plastic barrier, such as a female condom, dental dam, or modified male condom (especially if the woman does not have a vaginal infection with discharge and is not menstruating)
- Oral sex on a man using a latex or plastic condom
- All sexual activities, when both partners agree to a monogamous relationship and trust each other

STRATEGIES CONSIDERED UNSAFE IN THE ABSENCE OF HIV TESTING AND TRUST AND MONOGAMY

- Blood contact of any kind, including menstrual blood
- Any vaginal or anal intercourse without a latex or plastic condom
- Oral sex on a woman without a latex or plastic barrier, such as a female condom, dental dam, or modified male condom, especially if she has a vaginal infection with discharge or is menstruating
- Semen in the mouth
- Oral–anal contact
- Sharing sex toys or douching equipment
- Any sex that causes tissue damage or bleeding (e.g., rough vaginal or anal intercourse, rape, fisting)

Source: Marrazzo & Cates (2011).

✿ *Nursing Insight*— *Contraceptive choice and safer sex*

Nurses should recognize that women who use nonbarrier contraceptive methods (e.g., oral contraceptive pills [OCPs], IUDs, subdermal hormonal implants) usually choose these methods for the freedom involved. Thus, it is important to inform oral contraceptive users that the "pill" may cause changes in the cervix and in the immune system that increase susceptibility to HIV infection. Women who are in new or nonmonogamous relationships should be encouraged to use a barrier method along with the OCP, IUD, or subdermal hormonal implant.

The nurse should approach the counseling sessions with sensitivity and awareness that the individual may feel uncomfortable with sharing personal information about the sexual history or STD infection in the past. When possible, partners should be included in discussions concerning reproductive health issues.

⑤ **Optimizing Outcomes**— **Reducing the likelihood of STD transmission and progression of disease**

To promote health maintenance and safety and reduce the likelihood of STD transmission, nurses can teach women:

- How to use condoms (male and female, if appropriate) properly
- How to perform a genital self-examination
- To limit the number of sexual partners
- To avoid the sharing of personal care items, such as toothbrushes and razors
- To promptly report signs and symptoms of infection (e.g., vaginal discharge, pelvic pain, dysuria, irregular bleeding, dyspareunia, bleeding with intercourse)
- To take all prescribed antibiotics, even if symptoms resolve
- To abstain from sexual intercourse until both partners have completed treatment (to prevent reinfection)
- To return for evaluation, as indicated, after treatment has been completed

All women are potentially at risk for STDs and should be screened appropriately. Women who are sexually active in same-sex relationships, particularly adolescents, young women, and women with both male and female partners, might be at increased risk for STDs and HIV as a result of certain risk behaviors. Women who have sex with women (WSW) are at risk for acquiring bacterial, viral, and protozoal infections from current and prior partners, both male and female. Although the efficiency of STD transmission is greater with penile-vaginal intercourse, infection is also spread via other practices such as oral–genital sex, oral–digital sex, skin-to-skin contact, and through the sharing of sex toys. As with any population, effective STD communication should include honest, open discussion about sexual and behavioral risks (ACOG, 2013; CDC, 2011; Delk & Wiczyk, 2010; Fantasia et al., 2011; Hrivnak, 2013; Shafii, Burstein, & Blythe, 2011).

Nurses should also inquire about vaginal douching, a common practice among women in the United States. Findings from a 2001 survey (Sutton, Bruce, & Sternberg, 2006) showed that approximately 22% of women douche, with the prevalence highest among black women (50%). More recently, DiClemente and colleagues (2012) found that in a group (N = 701) of young (aged 14 to 20) African American females, prominent risk factors for douching behavior included older age, lower socioeconomic status, and older sex partners. To date, no study has shown that douching is in any way beneficial to a woman's reproductive health or that it decreases the risk for contracting an STD. In fact, women who douche are at increased risk for STDs, especially if they are less educated, are economically disadvantaged, have more sexual partners, have higher-risk sexual partners, or have a past history of pelvic inflammatory disease. Owing to their biological and behavioral vulnerability to STDs, at-risk adolescents may experience even greater risks associated with douching (Vermund & Allen, 2009; Womenshealth.gov, 2012).

🌸 *Nursing Insight*— *Douching and STDs*

Douching increases the risk for STDs by washing away the resident lactobacilli, which increase vaginal acidity, thereby creating an inhospitable environment for pathogens. The lactobacilli also adhere to epithelial cells that prevent pathogen adherence. Without a preponderance of beneficial lactobacilli, the vaginal acidity decreases and pathogens can more readily adhere to the vagina (Schwebke, 2012). Younger women who douche and are more sexually active may be at an especially high risk for contracting an STD; the risk with douching may not be as great for older women (Vermund & Allen, 2009).

Nurses who work with women of all ages can provide counseling about the harmful effects of douching. The information should be presented in a patient-centered, nonjudgmental manner that is appropriately attuned to the patient's age, culture, sexual orientation, and developmental level. When appropriate, engaging the support of influential family members (e.g., mothers, sisters, mothers-in-law) may also be of benefit in effecting the desired behavioral change (Vermund & Allen, 2009).

Nursing diagnoses for women with STDs are developed after careful consideration of all patient assessment data, the plan of treatment, and specific directives from the health-care provider. One appropriate diagnosis, for example, may focus on the threat to physiological functioning: "Acute Pain/Impaired Tissue Integrity related to effects of the infection process/excoriation of pruritic areas/hygiene practices." Another may address the emotional dimensions of the diagnosis: "Anxiety/Situational Low Self-Esteem/Disturbed Body Image related to perceived effects on intimate relationships and long-term sequelae of infection," or "Social Isolation and Impaired Social Interaction related to perceived effects on relationships with others if the STD status is not known." A nursing diagnosis that addresses educational needs is "Deficient Knowledge related to transmission/prevention/reinfection/management of infection or safer sex behaviors."

Nursing interventions center on the use of therapeutic communication to foster nonjudgmental, culturally appropriate discussion to facilitate learning and understanding. Providing emotional support is an essential component of care. The nurse assesses the patient's (and partner's, if appropriate) level of knowledge about the infection and uses this information to develop an individualized teaching plan. Emphasis is placed on the use and importance of safe sexual practices and, depending on the treatment regimen, the need to complete all prescribed medication and return for further evaluation. Referral to support groups may be appropriate.

In some situations, the patient may confide that she is too embarrassed to reveal information about the STD to her intimate partner and ask for guidance. The nurse can assist her by offering strategies, such as role-playing, for approaching the partner and sharing the information. It is important to emphasize that although this is a difficult topic for discussion, most individuals would rather know about the possibility that they are infected rather than not know. Exploring ways of communicating sensitive information is an important nursing intervention that can strengthen the therapeutic relationship, enhance adherence with the treatment plan, and improve STD case finding.

❝What to say❞ — *Exploring strategies for communicating STD infection information*

When counseling the patient about how she may approach her intimate partner about her STD, the nurse may suggest that she use statements such as "I care about you and I want you to know that I am concerned about your health. I want you to know that I am undergoing treatment for an STD—and you need to be evaluated as well."

Ⓢ Now Can You— Describe the nurse's role in promoting reproductive health?

1. Identify eight "safer sex" strategies?
2. Explain patient teaching about the practice of douching?
3. Formulate three potential nursing diagnoses for a woman with an STD?
4. Discuss aspects of patient education and counseling about STDs?

Summary Points

◆ STDs encompass more than 25 infectious organisms that cause reproductive tract infections.

◆ Potential complications of STDs include infertility, ectopic pregnancy, chronic pelvic pain, liver disease, liver cancer, and death.

◆ Chlamydia, the most commonly reported infectious disease in the United States, is the leading cause of preventable infertility and ectopic pregnancy.

◆ Once on the verge of elimination, syphilis has reemerged as a common STD.

◆ In the United States, women represent one of the fastest growing segments of the HIV epidemic.

◆ Gonorrhea and Chlamydia are prevalent in the adolescent population and disproportionately prevalent in minority groups.

◆ Infection with *Trichomonas vaginalis* increases the risk of HIV transmission.

◆ Pelvic inflammatory disease is most often caused by the organisms *Chlamydia trachomatis* and *Neisseria gonorrhoeae*.

◆ Hepatitis is the leading cause of liver cancer and the most common reason for liver transplantation.

◆ In the area of reproductive health promotion, an important nursing role centers on education about STDs, safer sex strategies, and actions to reduce the likelihood of STD transmission.

Review Questions

Multiple Choice

1. Self-care measures that reduce the transmission of STDs include:
A. Withdrawal of the penis before ejaculation
B. Douching immediately after sexual intercourse
C. Use of barrier methods of contraception
D. Mutual masturbation

2. Strategies for safer sex that avoid contact with bodily fluids include:
  A. Erotic massage
  B. Oral–genital stimulation
  C. Careful anal intercourse
  D. Consensual sharing of sex toys

3. Factors that place women at increased risk for HIV infection include:
  A. History of premenstrual syndrome
  B. History of prostitution
  C. History of a seizure disorder
  D. History of an ectopic pregnancy

4. The most common STD that frequently produces no signs or symptoms in women is:
  A. Chancroid
  B. Herpes
  C. Chlamydia
  D. Syphilis

5. The first sign of syphilis is a sore that is:
  A. Painful
  B. Filled with clear fluid
  C. Itchy and scaly
  D. Painless

REFERENCES

American College of Obstetricians and Gynecologists (ACOG). (2008). Prenatal and perinatal human immunodeficiency virus testing: Expanded recommendations. Committee Opinion No. 418 (Reaffirmed 2011). *Obstetrics & Gynecology, 112*(9), 739–742.

American College of Obstetricians and Gynecologists (ACOG). (2010a). Gynecologic care for women with human immunodeficiency virus. Practice Bulletin No. 117. (Reaffirmed 2012). *Obstetrics & Gynecology, 116*(11), 1492–1509.

American College of Obstetricians and Gynecologists (ACOG). (2010b). Human papillomavirus vaccination. Committee Opinion No. 467. *Obstetrics and Gynecology, 116*(9), 800–803.

American College of Obstetricians and Gynecologists (ACOG). (2011a). Expedited partner therapy in the management of gonorrhea and chlamydia by obstetrician-gynecologists. Committee Opinion No. 506. *Obstetrics & Gynecology, 118*(3), 761–766.

American College of Obstetricians and Gynecologists (ACOG). (2011b). Hepatitis B, hepatitis C, and human immunodeficiency virus infections in obstetricians-gynecologists. Committee Opinion No. 489. *Obstetrics & Gynecology, 117*(5), 1242–1246.

American College of Obstetricians and Gynecologists (ACOG). (2012). Human immunodeficiency virus and acquired immunodeficiency syndrome and women of color. Committee Opinion No. 536. *Obstetrics & Gynecology, 120*(3), 735–739.

American College of Obstetricians and Gynecologists (ACOG). (2013). Addressing health risks of noncoital sexual activity. Committee Opinion No. 582. *Obstetrics & Gynecology, 122*(6), 1378–1383.

Apuzzio, J., Block, J., Cullison, S., Cohen, C., Leong, S., London, W., . . . McMahon, B. (2012). Chronic hepatitis B in pregnancy: A workshop consensus statement on screening, evaluation, and management. *The Female Patient, 37*(4), 22–27.

Barry, P.M., Kent, C.K., Philip, S.S., & Klausner, J.D. (2010). Results of a program to test women for rectal Chlamydia and gonorrhea. *Obstetrics and Gynecology, 115*(4), 753–759.

Blerau, R.P. (2013). Genital lesions in women. *Consultant, 53*(6), 406.

Bulechek, G.M., Butcher, H.K., Dochterman, J.M., & Wagner, C. (2013). *Nursing interventions classification (NIC)* (6th ed.). St. Louis, MO: Elsevier Mosby.

Casey, T. (2014). Hepatitis C treatment guidelines and cost concerns of new drugs. *Consultant, 54*(4), 292.

Centers for Disease Control and Prevention (CDC). (2006). Revised recommendations for HIV testing of adults, adolescents, and pregnant women in health-care settings. *MMWR Recommendations and Reports, 55*(RR14), 1–17.

Centers for Disease Control and Prevention (CDC). (2011). Sexually transmitted diseases treatment guidelines, 2010. *Morbidity and Mortality Weekly Report, 59*(RR-12), 1–110.

Centers for Disease Control and Prevention (CDC). (2012a). *Hepatitis information for health professionals.* Retrieved from http://www.cdc.gov/hepatitis/HBV/index.htm

Centers for Disease Control and Prevention (CDC). (2012b). *2011 sexually transmitted diseases surveillance.* Retrieved from http://www.cdc.gov/std/stats11/toc.htm

Centers for Disease Control and Prevention (CDC). (2013a). *CDC fact sheet. Incidence, prevention, and cost of sexually transmitted infections in the United States.* Retrieved from http://www.cdc.gov/std/stats/STI-Estimates-Fact-Sheet-Feb-2013.pdf

Centers for Disease Control and Prevention (CDC). (2013b). *HIV in the United States.* Retrieved from http://www.cdc.gov/hiv/statistics/basics/ataglance.html

Centers for Disease Control and Prevention (CDC). (2013c). *Sexually transmitted diseases fact sheets.* Retrieved from http://www.cdc.gov/std/syphilis/STDFact-Syphilis.htm

Centers for Disease Control and Prevention (CDC). (2014). Recommendations for the laboratory-based detection of *Chlamydia trachomatis* and *Neisseria gonorrhoeae*—2014. Retrieved from http://www.cdc.gov/std/laboratory/2014LabRec/recommendations.htm

Chapin, K. (2013). Diagnosis of trichomoniasis: Comparison of wet mount with nucleic acid amplification assays. *OBG Management, 25*(Suppl. 2), 51–52.

Cox, J.T., Huh, W., Mayeaux, E.J., Randell, M., & Taylor, M. (2011). Management of external genital and perianal warts: Proceedings of an expert panel meeting. *The Female Patient, 36*(11), S1–S13.

Delk, C., & Wiczyk, H. (2010). Approach to health care for lesbian and bisexual women. *The Female Patient, 35*(1), 26–29.

DiClemente, R., Young, A., Painter, J., Wingood, G., Rose, E., & Sales, J. (2012). Prevalence and correlates of recent vaginal douching among African American adolescent females. *Journal of Pediatric & Adolescent Gynecology, 25*(1), 48–53. doi:10.1016/j.jpag.2011.07.017

Fantasia, H.C. (2012). Sinecatechins ointment 15% for the treatment of external genital warts. *Nursing for Women's Health, 16*(5), 418–422. doi:10.1111/j.1751-486X.2012.01765.x

Fantasia, H.C., Fontenot, H.B., Sutherland, M., & Harris, A.L. (2011). Sexually transmitted infections in women. *Nursing for Women's Health, 15*(1), 47–57. doi:10.1111/j.1751-486X.2011.017610.x

Graseck, A.S., Secura, G.M., Allsworth, J.E., Madden, T., & Peipert, J.F. (2010). Home screening compared with clinic-based screening for sexually transmitted infections. *Obstetrics and Gynecology, 115*(4), 745–752.

Hepatitis Foundation International. (2013). Hepatitis D (HDV). Retrieved from http://www.hepatitisfoundation.org/HEPATITIS/Hepatitis-D.html

Holland-Hall, C. (2012). Pelvic inflammatory disease. *The Female Patient, 37*(5), 23–28.

Hrivnak, J. (2013). Health issues in lesbian patients. *Advance for NPs & PAs, 4*(10), 17–20.

Kahn, J.O., & Walker, B.D. (1998). Acute human immunodeficiency virus type 1 infection. *New England Journal of Medicine, 339*(1), 33–39.

Kapur, R., & Effron, D. (2011). Young woman with atypical presentation of Fitz-Hugh-Curtis syndrome. *Consultant, 51*(2), 94–96.

Kettinger, L.D. (2012). A practice improvement intervention increases Chlamydia screening among young women at a women's health practice. *Journal of Obstetric, Gynecologic & Neonatal Nursing, 42*(1), 81–90. doi:10.1111/j.1552-6909.2012.01427.x

Kurtyka, D. (2012). HIV/AIDS in 2012. *Advance for NPs & PAs, 3*(7), 19–24.

McNulty, C.A., Freeman, E., Howell-Jones, R., Hogan, A., Randall, S., Ford-Young, W., . . . Oliver, I. (2010). Overcoming the barriers to Chlamydia screening in general practice—a qualitative study. *Family Practice, 27*(3), 291–302. doi:10.1093/fampra/cmq004

McNulty, C.A., Hogan, A., Ricketts, E., Wallace, L., Oliver, I., Campbell, R., Kalwij, S., . . . Charlett, A. (2013). Increasing Chlamydia screening tests in general practice: A modified Zelen prospective cluster randomised controlled trial evaluating a complex intervention based on the theory of planned behaviour. *Sexually Transmitted Infections, 90*(3), 171–177. doi:10.1136/sextrans-2013-051029

Maes, C.A., & Louis, M. (2011). Nurse practitioners' sexual history-taking practices with adults 50 and older. *The Journal for Nurse Practitioners—JNP, 7*(3), 216–222.

Marrazzo, J.M., & Cates, W., Jr. (2011). Reproductive tract infections, including HIV and other sexually transmitted infections. In R.A Hatcher, J.

Trussell, A.L Nelson, W. Cates, D. Kowal, & M.S. Policar (Eds.), *Contraceptive technology* (20th ed., pp. 571–620). Decatur, GA: Bridging the Gap Communications.

Matkins, P.P. (2013). Sexually transmitted infections in adolescents. *North Carolina Medical Journal, 74*(1), 48–51.

Mayhew, M.S. (2011). Hepatitis C treatment. *The Journal for Nurse Practitioners—JNP, 7*(10), 875–876.

Moorhead, S., Johnson, M., Maas, M.L., & Swanson, E. (2013). *Nursing outcomes classification (NOC)* (5th ed.). St. Louis, MO: Elsevier Mosby.

Nelson, A.L. (2011). Current and emerging options for treating external genital warts. *The Female Patient, 36*(Suppl. 7), S1–S8.

Page, J. (2013). Recent developments in the treatment of chronic hepatitis C. *The Journal for Nurse Practitioners—JNP, 8*(3), 225–230.

Rapsilber, L. (2012). What to do with a positive hep C test. *The Clinical Advisor, 15*(10), 16–26.

Roberts, S.W., Sheffield, J.S., McIntire, D.D., & Alexander, J.M. (2011). Urine screening for *Chlamydia trachomatis* during pregnancy. *Obstetrics & Gynecology, 117*(4), 883–885. doi:10.1097/AOG.0b013e3182107d47

Royer, H.R., & Cerf, C. (2009). Young women's beliefs about the terms sexually transmitted disease and sexually transmitted infection. *Journal of Obstetric, Gynecologic, & Neonatal Nursing, 38*(6), 686–692.

Rustgi, V., Carriero, D., Bachtold, M., & Zeldin, G. (2010). Update on chronic hepatitis B. *The Journal for Nurse Practitioners—JNP, 6*(8), 631–639.

Schwebke, J. (2012). Trichomonas: Clinical analysis of a highly prevalent and misdiagnosed infection. *The Female Patient, 37*(Suppl. 8), 1–4.

Schwebke, J. (2013). New approaches to the diagnosis of vaginitis. *OBG Management, 23*(Suppl. 10), 1–10.

Shafii, T., Burstein, G.R., & Blythe, M.J. (2011). Sexually transmitted infections. *The Female Patient, 36*(11), 30–37.

Soper, D.E. (2010). Pelvic inflammatory disease. *Obstetrics & Gynecology, 116*(2), 419–428.

Stewart, A., & Graham, S. (2013). Sexual risk behavior among older adults. *Clinical Advisor, 16*(4), 28–38.

Sutton, M.Y., Bruce, C., & Sternberg, M.R. (2006, May). *Prevalence and correlates of vaginal douching among women in the United States, 2001–2002.* Paper presented at the National STD Prevention conference, Jacksonville, FL.

Tarrant, D., Block, J., & McMahon, B. (2013). Screening for hepatitis B. *The Journal for Nurse Practitioners—JNP, 9*(4), 233–237.

Taylor, A., & Gosney, M.A. (2011). Sexuality in older age: Essential considerations for healthcare professionals. *Age Ageing, 40*(5), 538–543. doi:10.1093/ageing/afr049

Taylor, D., & James, E.A. (2012). Risks of being sexual in midlife: What we don't know can hurt us. *The Female Patient, 37*(5), 17–20.

Turner, D. (2012). Pelvic inflammatory disease: A continuing challenge. *The American Journal for Nurse Practitioners, 16*(1/2), 20–23.

University of Maryland Medical Center. (2011). *Herpes simplex virus.* Retrieved from http://www.umm.edu/altmed/articles/herpes-simplex-000079.htm

U.S. Department of Health and Human Services (USDHHS). (2013). *Healthy People 2020: Topics & objectives: Sexually transmitted disease.* Retrieved from http://www.healthypeople.gov/2020/topicsobjectives2020/objectiveslist.aspx?topicId=37

U.S. Department of Health and Human Services (USDHHS) Panel on Antiretroviral Guidelines for Adults and Adolescents. (2011). *Guidelines for the use of antiretroviral agents in HIV-1—infected adults and adolescents.* Retrieved from http://aidsinfo.nih.gov/contentfiles/lvguidelines/adultandadolescentgl.pdf

U.S. Food and Drug Administration (FDA). (2014). *FDA approves Gardasil 9 for prevention of certain cancers caused by five additional types of HPV.* Retrieved from http://www.fda.gov/NewsEvents/Newsroom/PressAnnouncements/ucm426485.htm

U.S. Preventive Services Task Force (USPSTF). (2008). USPSTF recommendations for STI screening. Retrieved from http://www.uspreventiveservicestaskforce.org/uspstf08/methods/stinfections.htm

U.S. Preventive Services Task Force (USPSTF). (2009a). *Screening for hepatitis B virus infection in pregnancy.* Retrieved from http://www.uspreventiveservicestaskforce.org/uspstf/uspshepbpg.htm

U.S. Preventive Services Task Force (USPSTF). (2009b). U.S. Preventive Services Task Force Reaffirmation of recommendation statement: Screening for syphilis infection in pregnancy. *Annals of Family Medicine, 150*(5), 705–709.

U.S. Preventive Services Task Force (USPSTF). (2013). Recommendation statement: Screening for HIV. Retrieved from http://www.uspreventiveservicestaskforce.org/uspstf/uspshivi.htm

Vallerand, A.H., & Sanoski, C.A. (2013). *Davis's drug guide for nurses* (13th ed.). Philadelphia, PA: F.A. Davis.

Vermund, S.H., & Allen, K.L. (2009). Douching is a remediable risk factor for sexually transmitted infections. *Female Patient, 34*(7), 37–39.

Womenshealth.gov. (2012). *Douching fact sheet.* Retrieved from http://www.womenshealth.gov/publications/our-publications/fact-sheet/douching.html

Wysocki, S., & Woodward, J.A. (2010). Expedited partner therapy for Chlamydia. *Women's Health Care: A Practical Journal for Nurse Practitioners, 9*(5), 21–25.

Xu, F., Sternberg, M., Gottlieb, S., Berman, S., & Markowitz, L. (2010). Seroprevalence of herpes simplex virus type 2 among persons aged 14–49 years—United States, 2005–2008. *Morbidity and Mortality Weekly Report, 59*(15), 456–459.

Xu, F., Stoner, B., Taylor, S., Mena, L., Tian, L., Papp, J., . . . Markowitz, L. (2011). Use of home-obtained vaginal swabs to facilitate rescreening for *Chlamydia trachomatis* infections. *Obstetrics & Gynecology, 118*(2), 231–239. doi:10.1097/AOG.0b013e3182246a83

Yager, A.M., & O'Keefe, C. (2012). Adolescent use of social networking to gain sexual health information. *The Journal for Nurse Practitioners—JNP, 8*(4), 294–298. doi:10.1016/j.nurpra.2012.01.016

DavisPlus | For more information, go to **http://www.davisplus.fadavis.com/**.

CONCEPT MAP

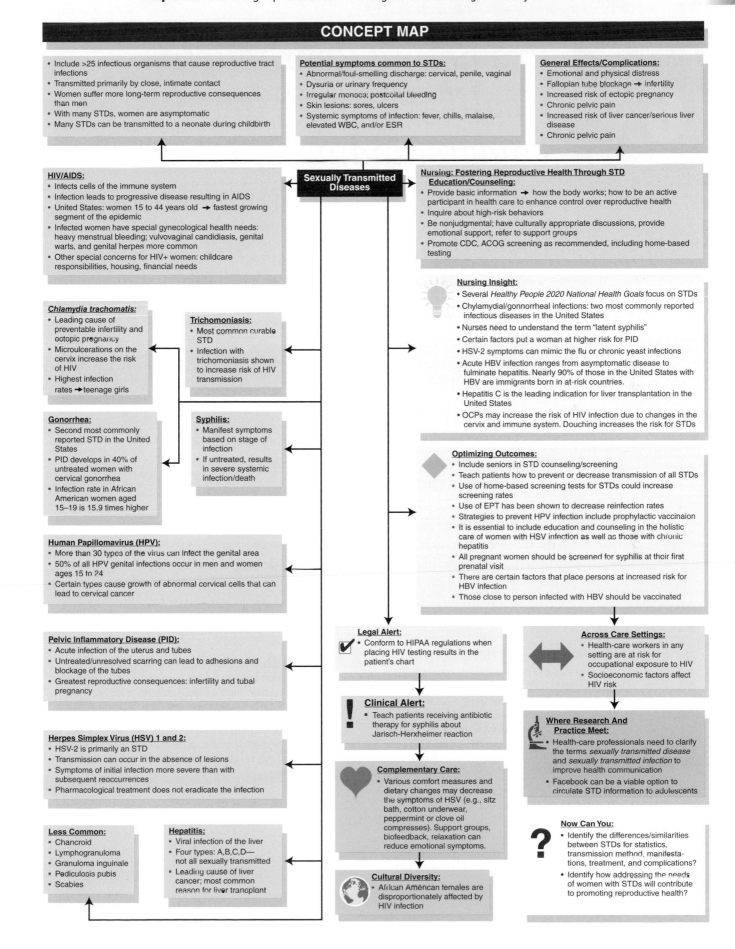

Sexually Transmitted Diseases

- Include >25 infectious organisms that cause reproductive tract infections
- Transmitted primarily by close, intimate contact
- Women suffer more long-term reproductive consequences than men
- With many STDs, women are asymptomatic
- Many STDs can be transmitted to a neonate during childbirth

Potential symptoms common to STDs:
- Abnormal/foul-smelling discharge: cervical, penile, vaginal
- Dysuria or urinary frequency
- Irregular menses; postcoital bleeding
- Skin lesions: sores, ulcers
- Systemic symptoms of infection: fever, chills, malaise, elevated WBC, and/or ESR

General Effects/Complications:
- Emotional and physical distress
- Fallopian tube blockage → infertility
- Increased risk of ectopic pregnancy
- Chronic pelvic pain
- Increased risk of liver cancer/serious liver disease
- Chronic pelvic pain

HIV/AIDS:
- Infects cells of the immune system
- Infection leads to progressive disease resulting in AIDS
- United States: women 15 to 44 years old → fastest growing segment of the epidemic
- Infected women have special gynecological health needs: heavy menstrual bleeding; vulvovaginal candidiasis; genital warts, and genital herpes more common
- Other special concerns for HIV+ women: childcare responsibilities, housing, financial needs

Nursing: Fostering Reproductive Health Through STD Education/Counseling:
- Provide basic information → how the body works; how to be an active participant in health care to enhance control over reproductive health
- Inquire about high-risk behaviors
- Be nonjudgmental; have culturally appropriate discussions, provide emotional support, refer to support groups
- Promote CDC, ACOG screening as recommended, including home-based testing

Nursing Insight:
- Several *Healthy People 2020 National Health Goals* focus on STDs
- Chylamydial/gonorrheal infections: two most commonly reported infectious diseases in the United States
- Nurses need to understand the term "latent syphilis"
- Certain factors put a woman at higher risk for PID
- HSV-2 symptoms can mimic the flu or chronic yeast infections
- Acute HBV infection ranges from asymptomatic disease to fulminate hepatitis. Nearly 90% of those in the United States with HBV are immigrants born in at-risk countries.
- Hepatitis C is the leading indication for liver transplantation in the United States
- OCPs may increase the risk of HIV infection due to changes in the cervix and immune system. Douching increases the risk for STDs

Chlamydia trachomatis:
- Leading cause of preventable infertility and ectopic pregnancy
- Microulcerations on the cervix increase the risk of HIV
- Highest infection rates → teenage girls

Trichomoniasis:
- Most common curable STD
- Infection with trichomoniasis shown to increase risk of HIV transmission

Gonorrhea:
- Second most commonly reported STD in the United States
- PID develops in 40% of untreated women with cervical gonorrhea
- Infection rate in African American women aged 15–19 is 15.9 times higher

Syphilis:
- Manifest symptoms based on stage of infection
- If untreated, results in severe systemic infection/death

Optimizing Outcomes:
- Include seniors in STD counseling/screening
- Teach patients how to prevent or decrease transmission of all STDs
- Use of home-based screening tests for STDs could increase screening rates
- Use of EPT has been shown to decrease reinfection rates
- Strategies to prevent HPV infection include prophylactic vaccinaion
- It is essential to include education and counseling in the holistic care of women with HSV infection as well as those with chronic hepatitis
- All pregnant women should be screened for syphilis at their first prenatal visit
- There are certain factors that place persons at increased risk for HBV infection
- Those close to person infected with HBV should be vaccinated

Human Papillomavirus (HPV):
- More than 30 types of the virus can infect the genital area
- 50% of all HPV genital infections occur in men and women ages 15 to 24
- Certain types cause growth of abnormal cervical cells that can lead to cervical cancer

Pelvic Inflammatory Disease (PID):
- Acute infection of the uterus and tubes
- Untreated/unresolved scarring can lead to adhesions and blockage of the tubes
- Greatest reproductive consequences: infertility and tubal pregnancy

Legal Alert:
- Conform to HIPAA regulations when placing HIV testing results in the patient's chart

Across Care Settings:
- Health-care workers in any setting are at risk for occupational exposure to HIV
- Socioeconomic factors affect HIV risk

Clinical Alert:
- Teach patients receiving antibiotic therapy for syphilis about Jarisch-Herxheimer reaction

Herpes Simplex Virus (HSV) 1 and 2:
- HSV-2 is primarily an STD
- Transmission can occur in the absence of lesions
- Symptoms of initial infection more severe than with subsequent reoccurrences
- Pharmacological treatment does not eradicate the infection

Where Research And Practice Meet:
- Health-care professionals need to clarify the terms *sexually transmitted disease* and *sexually transmitted infection* to improve health communication
- Facebook can be a viable option to circulate STD information to adolescents

Complementary Care:
- Various comfort measures and dietary changes may decrease the symptoms of HSV (e.g., sitz bath, cotton underwear, peppermint or clove oil compresses). Support groups, biofeedback, relaxation can reduce emotional symptoms.

Now Can You:
- Identify the differences/similarities between STDs for statistics, transmission method, manifestations, treatment, and complications?
- Identify how addressing the needs of women with STDs will contribute to promoting reproductive health?

Less Common:
- Chancroid
- Lymphogranuloma
- Granuloma inguinale
- Pediculosis pubis
- Scabies

Hepatitis:
- Viral infection of the liver
- Four types: A,B,C,D— not all sexually transmitted
- Leading cause of liver cancer; most common reason for liver transplant

Cultural Diversity:
- African American females are disproportionately affected by HIV infection

Promoting Reproductive Health Through an Understanding of Cervical Cytology Screening, Human Papillomavirus, and Cervical Cancer

 Life is what happens to you when you're making other plans

—Betty Talmadge

LEARNING TARGETS *At the completion of this chapter, the student will be able to:*

- ◆ Describe the cervical epithelium and the process of metaplasia.
- ◆ Discuss methods of cervical cytology screening.
- ◆ Identify treatment options for various preinvasive conditions of the cervix.
- ◆ Identify risk factors for human papillomavirus (HPV).
- ◆ Discuss the HPV–cervical cancer link and identify risk factors for cervical cancer.
- ◆ Develop materials for patient education and counseling regarding cervical cytology screening, human papillomavirus, and cervical cancer.

PICO(T) Questions

The intent of Evidence-Based Practice (EBP) is to provide nursing care that integrates the best available evidence. An initial step in EBP is to write a PICO(T) question that effectively guides the research. A PICO(T) question is an acronym that stands for population (P), intervention or issue (I), comparison of interest (C), outcome (O), and time frame (T). Depending on the question, all or some of the question components are used in the research process. Use these PICO(T) questions to spark your thinking as you read the chapter.

1. Does (I) health education regarding HPV awareness and prevention lead to (O) higher condom use among (P) sexually active high school students compared with (C) students who do not receive HPV health education?

2. What (O) nursing interventions are shown to provide support to (P) women who undergo a follow-up procedure for (I) abnormal cervical cytology findings?

Evidence-Based Practice

Wilson, R.T., Giroux, J., Kasicky, K.R., Fatupaito, B.H., Wood, E.C., Crichlow, R., . . . Cobb, N. (2011). Breast and cervical cancer screening patterns among American Indian women at IHS clinics in Montana and Wyoming. *Public Health Reports, 126*(6), 806–815.

The purpose of this study was to examine factors associated with primary and secondary breast and cervical cancer screening among American Indian/Alaska Native (AI/AN) women receiving care from the Indian Health Service (IHS) in Montana and Wyoming. Previous research has shown that the incidence of breast and cervical cancers among American Indian women varies significantly in relation to U.S. region of residence. For example, AI women living in the Northern Plains region (includes the states of Illinois, Indiana, Iowa, Michigan, Minnesota, Montana, Nebraska, South Dakota, Wisconsin, and Wyoming) have the second highest incidence of both cancers (breast cancer = 115.9/100,000 population; cervical cancer = 12.5/100,000 population). Compared with non-Hispanic white women throughout the United States, AI/AN women have a lower incidence of breast cancer but a higher incidence of cervical cancer, and a risk of death that is 50% to 80% higher once the diagnosis is made. For both cancer sites, AI/AN women are more likely than non-Hispanic white women to be diagnosed with late-stage cancer. In the Northern Plains, the incidence of metastatic cervical cancer among AI women is six times higher than for non-Hispanic white women in the same region.

Study participants included AI women aged 18 years and older who received care at IHS facilities on five reservations in Montana and one reservation in Wyoming. The populations served by these clinics include approximately 6,554 women 45 years of age and older and 9,980 women between 18 and 44 years of age. Inclusion criteria were as follows: women aged 18 years of age or older with at least two clinic visits (excluding emergency room visits) to the same clinic during a 78-month period. Those having had a mastectomy and/or hysterectomy prior to the initiation of the study were excluded.

Data, gathered through chart reviews, included the following: age, percentage AI blood quantum (total percentage of blood that is considered tribal native owing to bloodlines), ZIP code of residence, facility type (hospital or clinic), date and purpose of last visit, total number of visits during the study period, and dates of all mammograms and Pap tests during the study period and reason for those exams (e.g., screening, diagnosis of symptoms).

One thousand ninety-four women aged 18 and older met the inclusion criteria for the Cervical Cancer Screening Study (CCSS) sample; 700 women aged 45 years and older met the inclusion criteria for the Breast Cancer Screening Study sample (BCSS). The mean age of the CCSS group was 45 years; the mean age of the BCSS group was 60.5 years. Other data were as follows:

Blood quantum percentage:
- CCSS sample: ≥50% for 34.5% of the participants; <50% for 20.5% of the participants; none was recorded for 45.1% of the participants.
- BCSS sample: ≥50% for 31.6% of the participants; <50% for 23.3% of the participants; none was recorded for 45.1% of the participants.

Mean distance in miles to the nearest IHS clinic:
- CCSS sample: 12.7 miles
- BCSS sample: 13.1 miles

Mean distance in miles to the nearest mammography facility:
- CCSS sample: 15.8 miles
- BCSS sample: 16.1 miles

Purposes of the last visit and percentage of participants:
- CCSS sample: preventive—32.1%; chronic disease management—24.2%; inpatient—10%; emergency room—35.6%; unknown reason—7.1%
- BCSS sample: preventive—30.1%; chronic disease management—31.9%; inpatient—5%; emergency room—31.4%; unknown reason—5.9%

During the study period, 37.7% of the participants in the BCSS sample had a mammogram; of these, 8% were abnormal. The reasons noted for deciding to have a mammogram were 82.2% for screening, 5.3% for a previously abnormal mammogram, and 3.4% for a baseline mammogram. The prevalence of Pap test screening was 37.8%; of these, 6.3% had an abnormal result. The main reason for obtaining a Pap test was for screening, as noted by 91.5% of the participants.

Further analysis revealed that the prevalence of obtaining a mammogram was higher among women with blood quantum levels of >50%. Prevalence for screening was also greater (40%) for women living in a town with a mammography facility and lowest for those living 1 to 14 miles from a facility. Among women aged ≥65, 19.3% received a Pap test during the study period, as compared with 41.2% of women aged 18 to 44. Screening was also positively associated with the distance to the nearest facility—more than 30% of those living in the same town or less than 30 miles away received screening during the study period, as compared with 21.4% of those living ≥30 miles from the facility. Among those with prior abnormal Pap tests, 45% of women ≥65 years received a Pap test during the study, compared with 52.8% of those aged 18 to 44 years. Distance from the screening facility was not determined to be significant, although it may influence decisions about seeking screening services as well as needed follow-up.

The study findings were consistent with previous reports that found that AI women have among the lowest breast and cervical cancer screening rates in the United States. The researchers also noted that the *Healthy People 2010* (now *Healthy People 2020*) goals for breast cancer screening of at least 90% (now 93%) and cervical cancer screening of at least 70% (now 81%) have not been met for AI women.

---

1. How is this information useful to clinical nursing practice?

2. Based on these findings, what are implications for further research?

See Suggested Responses for Evidence-Based Practice on Davis*Plus.*

Introduction

This chapter describes cervical cytology and Pap test screening, and concludes with a discussion of human papillomavirus (HPV) and its association with premalignant and malignant cervical disease. According to the Centers for Disease Control and Prevention (CDC) (2013b), approximately 79 million Americans are currently infected with HPV, and another 14 million people become newly infected each year. HPV is so common that nearly all sexually active men and women get it at some point in their lives. Around 360,000 sexually active adults in the United States acquire (HPV-related) genital warts each year, and approximately 12,000 American women get cervical cancer each year. HPV infection is known to be the primary cause of cervical cancer. Other cancers that may be caused by HPV include pharyngeal, vulvar, vaginal, penile, and anal (CDC, 2014).

Although HPV has been recognized since 1907, it has only been within the past three decades that an understanding of the virus has evolved and its link to cervical and other cancers has been clearly established. The past 10 years have brought major advances in cervical screening technologies with the advent of liquid-based Pap tests and HPV DNA testing. Most recently, three HPV vaccines have become available. The vaccines are indicated for the prevention of cervical cancer, genital warts, and dysplastic or precancerous cervical lesions caused by several of the HPV virus types (American Cancer Society [ACS], 2014; CDC, 2014).

The Cervix and the Cervical Transformation Zone

To enhance understanding about the uterine cervix and the cervical Pap test to screen for cancer, it is important for the nurse to be knowledgeable about cervical cytology and the normal cellular changes that occur throughout a woman's life. The surface of the cervix and the canal that leads into the uterus—termed the "endocervical canal"—is composed of two types of cells: squamous epithelium and columnar epithelium.

A & P review Cervical Cell Types, the Squamocolumnar Junction, and the Transformation Zone

The cervix, which is typically 2.5 cm long, communicates with the endometrial cavity of the corpus uteri (uterine body) through the internal os and with the vagina through the external os. The vaginal portion (also called the exocervix, ectocervix, or portio vaginalis) is covered by stratified *squamous epithelium*. The squamous epithelium is smooth and light pink in appearance. The cervical canal is covered by *columnar epithelium*, which also forms endocervical glands, more correctly called "clefts." In young women, columnar epithelium can also be noted on the outer surface of the cervix around the external cervical os. The glandular tissue has a rough texture and is dark pink in color.

The area in which the squamous epithelium and the columnar epithelium come together on the cervix is called the *squamocolumnar junction (SCJ)*. The SCJ is located where the more delicate, darker pink columnar cells that line the uterus meet the sturdier, lighter pink squamous epithelium of the vagina. Throughout the reproductive years, some columnar cells at the SCJ are replaced by squamous epithelium through a process termed *squamous metaplasia*. The area between the old and new SCJ is called the *transformation zone* (Fig. 6-1). The size of the transformation zone varies from 2 to 15 mm. In most adult women, the squamocolumnar junction is not an abrupt meeting point but a zone containing irregular areas of glandular and squamous epithelium. This site undergoes continuous cell growth and replacement. The squamous type of cell replaces the columnar type of cell in a constant cycle of cell turnover, which is influenced by the female hormones. Metaplasia, which is a normal process of cell turnover, occurs most rapidly during adolescence and pregnancy. Cervical cancer usually develops in this area of rapid cell division. The immature cells undergoing the transformation from columnar to squamous tissue are especially vulnerable to events that can change the genetic material of the cells. These changes, or mutations, may result in the development of premalignant or malignant cells (Schiffman & Wentzensen, 2010). ◆

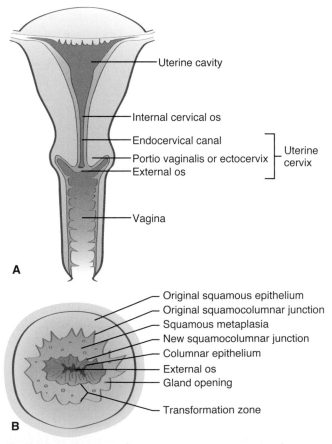

Figure 6-1 The transformation zone. *A,* Sagittal section of uterine corpus, uterine cervix, and vagina. *B,* Cross section of cervix at level of external os.

🌸 *Nursing Insight*— *Natural migration of the transformation zone*

In infants and postmenopausal women, the transformation zone is located deep within the endocervical canal. In women of childbearing age, beginning at puberty, the transformation zone moves out of the endocervical canal and lies primarily on the ectocervix; this movement is termed *cervical ectopy.* Elevated hormone states that occur, for example, during pregnancy and with the use of hormonal contraception may cause the transformation zone to become enlarged or more greatly exposed (Woodson, 2010).

Cervical Cancer Screening

DEVELOPMENT OF THE PAPANICOLAOU (PAP) TEST

Prior to the 1940s when the Papanicolaou (Pap) test for cervical cytological screening became widely available, cervical cancer was the most common cause of cancer death in women in the United States. Over the past 30 years, the incidence of invasive cervical cancer has decreased by 70%. This dramatic improvement in cervical cancer–related morbidity and mortality has largely been attributed to screening with the Pap test.

🌸 *Nursing Insight*— *Origins of the Pap test*

The Pap test is named for Dr. George Papanicolaou, the physician who, along with Dr. Herbert Traut, developed the procedure in the 1930s. The Pap test is a cytological study used to detect cancer in cells that an organ has shed. Although used most often in the diagnosis and prevention of cervical cancers, the Pap test is also of value in detecting pleural or peritoneal malignancies and in the evaluation of cellular changes caused by radiation, infection, or atrophy. In women's health, the Pap test is a screening technique used to detect cervical cancer or cervical abnormalities that may progress to cancer. The test can detect 95% of all cervical cancers and precancerous abnormalities. In the years since World War II, the Pap test has become the most widely used cancer screening method in the world, and it is the most successful cancer screening technique in medical history. Pap screening reduced cervical cancer death rates by almost 70% between 1955 and 1992, and the rate continues to decline by about 2% each year (Venes, 2013).

🌸 *Nursing Insight*— *Screening and early detection for cervical cancer*

The goal of screening for cervical cancer is to detect cervical cell changes and early cervical cancers before any symptoms develop. *Screening* refers to the use of tests (e.g., the Pap test) and exams to find a disease, such as cancer, in individuals who have no symptoms. *Early detection* means applying a strategy that results in an earlier diagnosis of cervical cancer than otherwise might have occurred. Screening tests offer the best chance to detect cervical cancer at an early stage when successful treatment is likely. Screening for cervical cancer is especially beneficial because it affords an opportunity to detect abnormal cell changes (precancers) so that they can be treated before they progress to cervical cancer (ACS, 2014).

PAP TEST TECHNIQUES

The Pap test may be included in a pelvic examination. A sample of cervical epithelium is gathered from the squamocolumnar junction, which can often be visualized on the cervix. An adequate Pap test should contain both columnar cells and squamous cells, which indicates that the squamocolumnar junction was sampled. The Pap test is obtained before any digital examination of the vagina is performed and before any endocervical bacteriological specimens are collected. Prior to insertion, the vaginal speculum may be moistened with warm water, saline, or an aqueous gel; level I evidence indicates that modest lubrication of the external surface of the speculum does not impair cytological and infectious evaluation of the cervix. The examiner may use a large cotton-tipped applicator to remove excess cervical discharge before the cytological specimen is obtained (Harmanli & Jones, 2010; Hill & Lamvu, 2012).

Various sampling devices (e.g., spatula [paddle], cervix brush, plastic "broom") may be used (Fig. 6-2). When conventional Pap tests are performed, a single microscope slide, combining both the endocervical and ectocervical samples, or two separate glass slides can be used. The exocervix (outer area) is first sampled with the spatula (Fig. 6-3). This is done first to minimize the possibility of obscuring the

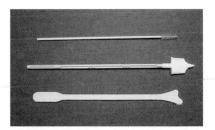

Figure 6-2 Tools for the Pap test *(top to bottom):* Cytobrush, cervical cytobroom, and wooden spatula. (Venes, D. [2009]. *Taber's cyclopedic medical dictionary* [21st ed., p. 1697]. Philadelphia, PA: F.A. Davis.)

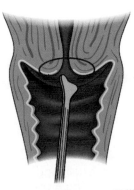

Figure 6-3 Taking a cervical smear. (Dillon, P.M. [2007]. *Nursing health assessment: A critical thinking, case studies approach* [2nd ed., p. 637]. Philadelphia, PA: F.A. Davis.)

cells with blood. The endocervix (inner area) is then sampled with the brush placed into the cervical os. The plastic "broomlike" brush is designed to simultaneously sample the endocervix and the exocervix. This device is inserted and rotated 360 degrees for a total of three to five times. If the patient has had a hysterectomy, the vaginal cuff (the portion of the vagina that remains open to the peritoneum following removal of the uterus) is sampled. The vaginal wall is usually not sampled unless the woman is approaching menopause, and in that case, a second sample may be obtained to evaluate the hormonal effects on vaginal tissue (American College of Obstetricians and Gynecologists [ACOG], 2012a; Policar, 2011).

The cytology sample is promptly transferred onto one or two thin glass slides and the sampling device is discarded. With this method of Pap testing, the most important consideration is rapid fixation. The slide should be sprayed with a preservative within 5 seconds to prevent drying of the specimen (Fig. 6-4). Drawbacks of the conventional "slide method" of Pap test collection include the possibility of inadequate cellular sampling, the presence of artifacts (e.g., blood, discharge, lubricant) that obscure the cervical cells, the clinician's failure to properly "fix" the specimen in a timely manner, and inaccurate interpretation by the laboratory cytologist (ACOG, 2012a).

Today, the majority of cervical cytology screening performed in the United States uses a liquid-based process (e.g., ThinPrep Pap Test, BD SurePath Pap Test). With the liquid-based technique, exfoliated cells are collected from the transformation zone of the cervix and transferred to a vial of liquid alcohol-based preservative. The sample is then processed in the laboratory and a slide is produced for interpretation. With this method, almost all of the sample

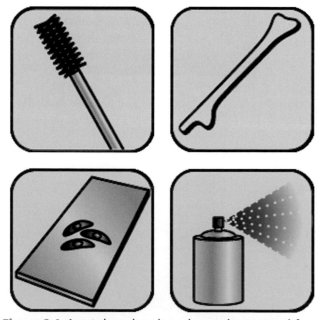

Figure 6-4 A cytology brush and spatula are used for specimens obtained during a conventional Pap test. The specimen is placed onto a thin glass side and immediately sprayed with a preservative (fixative). (Dillon, P.M. [2007]. *Nursing health assessment: A critical thinking, case studies approach* [2nd ed., p. 65]. Philadelphia, PA: F.A. Davis.)

cells are transferred to the liquid preservative, and most of the contaminating blood, inflammatory cells, and debris are filtered out. However, heavy menstrual blood may limit the number of squamous cells available for interpretation. Prompt suspension of the cells in the liquid preservative eliminates the problem of air-drying artifact, a factor that can limit the interpretation of conventional cervical cytology (ACOG, 2012a).

> ### ❀ *Nursing Insight*— *Comparing the conventional Pap test with the liquid-based Pap test*
>
> In the conventional Pap test, cell samples are obtained from the vagina, cervix, and cervical canal and spread on a glass slide. In liquid-based Pap testing, cell samples are collected using a special brush that is immediately washed in an alcohol-based fluid. In the laboratory, a special machine filters out the cells from the solution and deposits them in a thin, uniform monolayer (a single layer of cells) on a glass slide. Analysis usually includes initial computer screening followed by slide review by a cytotechnologist. The liquid-based Pap test method removes contaminants such as blood and mucus, which frequently obscure cells in the conventional Pap test. The monolayer of cells is also easier to examine under the microscope, resulting in an increased rate of detection of abnormal cells. The disadvantage of the liquid-based method primarily centers on the increased cost incurred by the collection fluid and the continuing operation of the laboratory-filtering machine.

With the liquid-based technology, between 50,000 and 70,000 diagnostic cells are available for screening; with the conventional process, approximately 4,000 to 300,000 cells are "smeared" onto a slide, where they often overlap or are obscured by noncervical material. In addition, according to the laboratory-based cytotechnologists, the liquid-based tests are easier to read. Although the liquid-based cytology is more expensive than conventional cytology, it provides the added ability to test for HPV, *Neisseria gonorrhoeae*, and *Chlamydia trachomatis* from the same sample (ACOG, 2012a).

❝What to say❞ — *Informing patients of Pap test limitations*

Counseling patients about Pap test limitations constitutes a central role for nurses in women's health care. Nurses can advise about the limits of Pap test accuracy while reassuring them that the Pap test is one of the most reliable methods for detecting preinvasive cancer of the cervix. However, there is no guarantee that any single Pap test will identify abnormal cells that may be present. Rescreening, when necessary, carries the burden of an additional expense, which may or may not be covered by insurance, whether funded by private, state, or federal sources (ACOG, 2012a).

> 🌀 **Now Can You**— **Describe normal cervical epithelium and the cervical Pap test?**
>
> 1. Identify the types of cells normally found in the cervix?
> 2. Define the terms *squamous metaplasia, squamocolumnar junction,* and *transformation zone*?

3. Describe the proper technique for obtaining a Pap test, and compare the liquid-based method with the conventional slide method?

INITIATION AND RECOMMENDED FREQUENCY OF CERVICAL CANCER SCREENING

Cancer of the cervix is usually a slow-growing neoplasm that is almost always caused by infection with the sexually transmitted disease human papillomavirus (HPV). (See later discussion of HPV in this chapter.) Speculum examination for cervical cytology screening should begin at age 21 years, regardless of the patient's history of sexual activity (ACOG, 2012b). Cervical neoplasia develops in susceptible individuals in response to infection with a high-risk type of HPV (i.e., types 16 and 18, which cause about 70% of all cervical cancers). HPV causes carcinogenesis in the transformation zone of the cervix, where the process of squamous metaplasia replaces columnar epithelium with squamous epithelium. Squamous metaplasia is particularly active in the cervix during adolescence and early adulthood. HPV is commonly acquired by young women shortly after the initiation of vaginal intercourse, but in most situations, the HPV is cleared by the immune system within 1 to 2 years without producing neoplastic changes. The risk of neoplastic transformation increases in women whose HPV infections persist. The recommendation to initiate cervical cancer screening at age 21 years regardless of the age of onset of sexual intercourse is based in part on the very low incidence of cancer in younger women. It is also based on the potential for adverse effects associated with follow-up of young women with abnormal cytology screening results (ACOG, 2012a; Somerall, 2013; U.S. Preventive Services Task Force [USPSTF], 2012).

🌸 Nursing Insight—*Potential adverse effects associated with cervical cancer screening in adolescents*

Initiating cervical cancer screening in the adolescent population may result in increased anxiety, morbidity, and expense from the testing and overuse of follow-up procedures. The emotional impact of labeling an adolescent with both a sexually transmitted disease (i.e., HPV) and a potential precancer must be considered in light of the fact that the adolescent period is characterized by emerging sexuality and a heightened concern for self-image. Sexually active adolescents (i.e., females younger than 21 years) should be counseled and tested for STDs and educated about safer sex and contraception. These measures may be carried out without cervical cytology screening and, in the asymptomatic patient, without the use of a speculum (ACOG, 2012a; Burkman, 2010; Einstein & Cox, 2013; USPSTF, 2012).

Cervical cytology screening is recommended every 3 years for women aged 21 to 29 years, with either conventional or liquid-based cytology. For women aged 30 to 65 years, current recommendations call for a combination of cytology and human papillomavirus (HPV) testing (cotesting) every 5 years, or cytology alone every 3 years. HPV testing should not be used alone for cervical cancer screening. No screening is necessary for women older than 65 years, provided that they have had adequate negative prior screening results; also, no screening is necessary for women who have undergone total hysterectomy for indications other than a high-grade precancerous lesion or cervical cancer. Women with any of the following risk factors may require more frequent cervical cytological screening (ACOG, 2012a; USPSTF, 2012):

- Women who are infected with HIV
- Women who are immunosuppressed (e.g., those who have received solid organ transplants)
- Women who were exposed to diethylstilbestrol (DES) in utero
- Women previously treated for cervical intraepithelial neoplasia (CIN) 2, CIN 3, or cancer

🌀 Optimizing Outcomes— **Educate patients about strategies to optimize cervical cancer screening**

Nurses can teach patients about strategies to optimize cervical cancer screening. In the ideal situation, the Pap test should be collected at midcycle. Patients should avoid intercourse, douching, or the use of vaginal medications for 24 to 48 hours prior to the test. The presence of infection (e.g., yeast) can cause vaginal inflammation and interfere with the test results. Over-the-counter vaginal creams, gels, foams, or suppositories used within 24 to 48 hours before the Pap test is obtained may interfere with the collection of an adequate cytological specimen.

🌸 *Cultural Diversity: Cervical Cancer Screening*

Hispanic women with limited English proficiency (i.e., difficulty reading, speaking, writing, or understanding English) who live in the United States tend to have low rates of cervical cancer screening, owing to factors such as language and cultural barriers. Nurses can help to overcome the barriers and, it is hoped, improve cervical cancer screening in this population by facilitating effective communication (e.g., same-language care provider, use of professional translators, careful attention to word choice to avoid implying patient responsibility for abnormal Pap test results), delivering health-promotion messages within a familial context, and when possible, scheduling patients with same-sex practitioners (Warren & Thomas, 2011).

CERVICAL CANCER SCREENING IN THE OLDER WOMAN

Cervical cancer tends to occur in midlife. It rarely develops in women younger than age 50, and most cases of cervical cancer and related deaths occur in women older than age 50. Interestingly, women 65 and older have 19.5% of the new cases of cervical cancer but only represent 14.1% of the U.S. female population. However, as is true with younger women, most cases of cervical cancer occur in unscreened or inadequately screened women. Unfortunately, many older women do not realize that the risk of developing cervical cancer is still present as they age. Sadly, up to two-thirds of older women with cervical cancer have not received adequate Pap screening prior to their cancer diagnosis. Thus, all women with a cervix should continue to receive Pap test screening according to standard guidelines and their care provider's recommendations (ACS, 2014).

Where Research and Practice Meet:
HPV and Cervical Cancer Knowledge in Older
Women

Montgomery, Bloch, Bhattacharya, and Montgomery (2010) distributed a self-administered survey to 149 women aged 40 to 70 years to assess their HPV and cervical cancer knowledge, health beliefs, and preventive practices. The participants demonstrated low-level knowledge of HPV and cervical cancer; more than one-half of them responded incorrectly to 50% of the questions regarding knowledge of cervical cancer/HPV. Moreover, one-third of the questions about the relationship of HPV and risks for cervical cancer were answered incorrectly by more than 75% of the women. Although most women were aware that HPV is a sexually transmitted disease that can potentially cause genital warts, they were unaware of the HPV–cervical cancer relationship. Study findings underscore the need for HPV and cervical cancer awareness and education for women older than age 40; nurses are uniquely situated to address these needs.

Joint recommendations of the American Cancer Society, the American College of Obstetricians and Gynecologists, the American Society for Colposcopy and Cervical Pathology, and the American Society for Clinical Pathology (2012) for cervical cancer screening methods are summarized in Box 6-1. The U.S. Preventive Services Task Force (USPSTF) (2012) also recommends screening cessation in women older than 65 years with negative test results who have had adequate prior screening and are not otherwise considered to be high risk for cancer. All expert groups are in agreement that cervical cancer screening can be discontinued in women who have had a hysterectomy if the surgery was performed for benign reasons and there is no past history of high-grade cervical lesions.

 legal alert— Document all communications concerning Pap tests

When Pap test results are received, it is essential that patients be promptly notified of abnormal results. Neglect to do so may result from a breakdown in communication between the care provider and the office staff or from poor follow-up efforts to contact patients. Documentation of test results and patient follow-up efforts is equally important. It is essential that information regarding efforts to report results, make treatment recommendations, and order appropriate follow-up, as well as efforts to obtain patient history and informed consent or informed refusal, be documented in the chart (U.S. Department of Health and Human Services, Health Resources and Services Administration, 2013).

 Where Research and Practice Meet:
Cervical Cancer Screening Trends

In the January 2013 issue of the CDC *Morbidity and Mortality Weekly Report,* two studies reflect how well cervical cancer screening aligns with current national recommendations. Investigators used Pap test survey data from CDC's Behavior Risk Factor Surveillance System 2000 to 2010 to discover that screening has become more consistent with current cervical cancer screening recommendations. For example, the percentage of women aged 18 to 21 years who reported never being screened increased from 23.6% in 2000 to 47.5% in 2010. Also, among women aged 30 years and older who had a hysterectomy, Pap testing declined from 73.3% in 2000 to 58.7% in 2010 (CDC, 2013b).

Box 6-1 Cervical Cancer Screening Methods: 2012 Joint Recommendations of the American Cancer Society, the American College of Obstetricians and Gynecologists, the American Society for Colposcopy and Cervical Pathology, and the American Society for Clinical Pathology

- No screening for women younger than 21 years.
- Women aged 21–29 years: Cervical cytology alone every 3 years.
- Women aged 30–65 years: Human papillomavirus and cervical cytology cotesting every 5 years or cytology alone every 3 years.
- Women older than 65 years: No screening is necessary after adequate negative prior screening results. Women with a history of CIN 2, CIN 3, or adenocarcinoma in situ should continue routine age-based screening for at least 20 years.
- Women who have had a total hysterectomy for benign indications (i.e., women without a cervix and with no prior history of high-grade CIN [CIN 2, CIN 3]), adenocarcinoma in situ, or cancer in the past 20 years: No screening is necessary.
- Women vaccinated against HPV: Follow age-specific recommendations (same as unvaccinated women).

Sources: ACOG (2012a, 2013); Saslow et al. (2012).

Across Care Settings: **Ensuring cervical cancer screening for medically underserved women**

In this country, all states are making cervical cancer screening more available to medically underserved women through the National Breast and Cervical Cancer Early Detection Program (NBCCEDP). The program provides free or low-cost breast and cervical cancer screenings to women with no health insurance. The goal of NBCCEDP is to reach as many women in medically underserved communities as possible, including older women, women without health insurance, and women who are members of racial and ethnic minorities. Nurses can contact the Department of Health in their practice state for specific information regarding program location and eligibility requirements, or they may contact the CDC at 1-800-CDC-INFO, or visit the CDC Web site at www.cdc.gov/cancer/nbccedp.

INTERPRETING CERVICAL CYTOLOGY FINDINGS: THE BETHESDA SYSTEM TERMINOLOGY

The Bethesda System is the classification for abnormal cervical cytology and histology that is most commonly used today. First developed in 1988 under sponsorship of the National Institutes of Health (NIH), the updated 2001 Bethesda System terminology is used to describe the categories of epithelial cell abnormalities, including atypical squamous cells (ASC), low-grade or high-grade squamous intraepithelial lesions (LSIL or HSIL), and glandular cell abnormalities, including atypical glandular cells (AGC) and adenocarcinoma in situ (AIS). Histology diagnoses of abnormalities are reported as CIN 1–3 (ACOG, 2013; Solomon et al., 2002). The 2001 Bethesda System terminology is presented in Box 6-2.

Box 6-2 The 2001 Bethesda System Terminology

SQUAMOUS CELL
- Atypical squamous cells (ASC)
- Of undetermined significance (ASC-US) (the most minor form of cytological abnormality detected on the Pap test)
- Cannot exclude high-grade squamous intraepithelial lesions (SIL)*
- Low-grade squamous intraepithelial lesions (LSIL—encompasses HPV, mild dysplasia, and cervical intraepithelial neoplasia [CIN] 1)**
- High-grade squamous intraepithelial lesions (HSIL—encompasses HPV, moderate and severe dysplasia, carcinoma in situ [CIS], and CIN 2 and CIN 3)
- Squamous cell carcinoma

GLANDULAR CELL
- Atypical glandular cells (AGC)—a cytological abnormality of the glandular cells that line the endocervix or uterus
- Atypical glandular cells, favors neoplasia
- Endocervical adenocarcinoma in situ
- Adenocarcinoma

---

* SIL: cytological abnormalities identified on the Pap test, classified as low-grade (LSIL) or high-grade (HSIL).
** CIN: cervical cancer precursor (confirmed by biopsy), divided into low-grade (CIN 1) and high-grade (CIN 2/3) (ACOG, 2013; Frey & Gupta, 2011; Solomon et al., 2002).

Optimizing Outcomes— With the Bethesda System: a standardized approach for cytology/histology findings and interpretation to guide patient care

Over the years, the Bethesda System has undergone a number of major changes in approach and terminology in attempts to standardize reporting systems worldwide and provide more information about what was actually identified in the cellular sample. Developed by major medical groups including the ACOG, the ACS, the Association of Reproductive Health Professionals (ARHP), and the American Society for Colposcopy and Cervical Pathology (ASCCP), the original guidelines have undergone review several times in past years in response to emerging data on the role of HPV in cervical cancer. The latest (2012) ASCCP consensus guidelines reflect evidence-based advances in the understanding of the natural history of HPV, its influence on the development of cervical dysplasia (precancerous changes) and cancer, and the role of Pap tests with a liquid-based sample (ACOG, 2013; Massad et al., 2013).

Optimizing Outcomes— With new terminology designed to unify all lower genital tract HPV intraepithelial neoplasia

In 2012, the Lower Anogenital Squamous Terminology (LAST) Standardization Project created new histology terminology for HPV-related lesions of the lower genital tract. With the new terminology, the low-grade squamous intraepithelial lesion (LSIL) finding was designated as the all-encompassing term for cervical intraepithelial neoplasia (CIN) 1, vaginal intraepithelial neoplasia 1 (VaIN 1), vulvar intraepithelial neoplasia 1 (VIN 1), penile intraepithelial neoplasia 1 (PeIN 1), perianal intraepithelial neoplasia 1 (PAIN 1), and anal intraepithelial neoplasia 1 (AIN 1). The new terminology is intended to reflect current knowledge of HPV biology and pathogenesis, facilitate clear communication across different medical specialities, and ultimately optimize patient care (Darragh et al., 2012; Waxman, Chelmow, Darragh, Lawson, & Moscicki, 2012).

 Now Can You— Discuss cervical cytology screening?

1. Identify the appropriate time for initiation and recommended frequency for cervical cancer screening according to guidelines established by ACOG and other professional organizations?
2. Explain why cervical cancer screening in the adolescent population is discouraged?
3. Teach a patient how to prepare for her Pap test and include three strategies intended to optimize the test results?

FOLLOW-UP FOR UNSATISFACTORY PAP TEST RESULTS AND ABNORMAL CERVICAL CYTOLOGY SCREENING RESULTS

In April 2013, the American Society for Colposcopy and Cervical Pathology (ASCCP) updated guidelines for the management of abnormal cervical cytology and cervical cancer precursors. The guidelines, which apply only to women who are found to have abnormalities during routine screening, are stratified by risk, according to the woman's age, cytological diagnosis, and HPV status (Einstein & Cox, 2013). The guideline algorithms are available at www .jlgtd.com and www.greenjournal.org. Updated guidelines for the management of women with unsatisfactory Pap test results are presented in Box 6-3.

Depending on the woman's age and the Pap test result, further evaluation or treatment or both may be indicated. Young women aged 21 to 24 are at high risk for HPV infection but are at very low risk for cancer. Owing to the fact that aggressive management usually involves more

---

Box 6-3 Updated Guidelines for the Management of Unsatisfactory Pap Test Results—American Society for Colposcopy and Cervical Pathology, 2013

If unsatisfactory Pap test results
- Repeat cytology in 2–4 months
  If the unsatisfactory Pap test is part of a cotest, the following strategies are appropriate:
- If the HPV test is positive, repeat the Pap test or perform colposcopy
- If HPV genotyping was reported and is positive for type 16 or 18, perform colposcopy
  Perform colposcopy when two consecutive Pap tests are unsatisfactory. If normal cytology but no/insufficient endocervical cells present:
- Ages 21–29 years: routine screening with cytology in 3 years
- Ages 30+ years:
  - If cotesting done: HPV negative—routine screening with cotesting in 5 years; if HPV-positive—either cotest in 1 year, or perform immediate genotyping
  - If HPV testing not done: HPV testing recommended; management guided by results

---

Source: Massad et al., (2013).

harm than benefit, observation without HPV testing is recommended for this population. For women 30 years and older, reflex HPV DNA testing is performed to determine whether HPV is present and whether referral for colposcopy is indicated. The liquid-based Pap samples can be immediately tested for HPV if there is an ASC-US (atypical squamous cells of undetermined significance) result. Women with an ASC-US Pap test result who test positive for HPV should have a repeat cotest in 1 year; those who are HPV positive with low-grade squamous intraepithelial lesions (LSIL) should be referred for colposcopy with directed biopsy and endocervical sampling (ACOG, 2012a, 2013; Einstein & Cox, 2013; Massad et al., 2013).

Colposcopy

Colposcopy is a medical diagnostic procedure that uses a colposcope to provide an illuminated, magnified view of the cervix and the tissues of the vagina and vulva. The colposcope is a low-powered binocular microscope with a powerful light source mounted to allow visualization of the vagina and cervix during a pelvic examination. This instrument allows for a close-up view of the cervix and surrounding tissue for evaluation. The main goal of colposcopy is to prevent cervical cancer by the early detection and treatment of precancerous lesions.

"What to say" — *Preparing the patient for colposcopy*

The nurse can do much to allay a patient's anxiety about colposcopy. The nurse may offer the following description of the procedure to help the patient understand what to expect:

"Once you have emptied your bladder, I will assist you into position (dorsal lithotomy) for a pelvic examination. The clinician (colposcopist) will insert a vaginal speculum and most likely use cotton swabs to apply an acetic acid (vinegar) solution to the cervix. Abnormal areas turn white (acetowhite) and become more prominent in response to the acetic acid, allowing for improved visualization. Areas that turn white after the application of acetic acid or have an abnormal vascular pattern are often considered for biopsy. If no lesions are visible, an iodine solution (Schiller's or Lugol's solution) may be applied to the cervix and vagina to help highlight areas of abnormality. The colposcopist determines the areas with the highest degree of visible abnormality and may obtain biopsies from these areas. A numbing medication (lidocaine) is used to diminish discomfort, especially if many biopsy samples are taken. Although not common, potential complications include bleeding and infection. To minimize the risk of infection, you should use a panty liner or sanitary napkin and avoid sexual intercourse until all vaginal bleeding or discharge has stopped. Your health-care provider may advise you to take a mild pain reliever such as ibuprofen approximately 30 minutes to 1 hour before the procedure and afterward as needed for cramping and discomfort. Be sure to promptly notify your health-care provider if you develop any signs of infection, such as fever, continued pain, bleeding, foul-smelling vaginal discharge, or painful urination (dysuria), or have any concerns. Also, it is a good idea to bring a support person with you."

Endocervical Sampling

Endocervical sampling is performed if the colposcopy is unsatisfactory (e.g., no lesions are identified, or the endocervical canal cannot be fully visualized) and in women who have follow-up colposcopy after treatment for CIN 2 or 3 with a positive endocervical margin. Endocervical sampling may be conducted either with vigorous endocervical brushing or by the traditional endocervical curettage (ECC), a procedure that uses a sharp, spoon-shaped instrument (curette). A small tissue sample is obtained and sent to a pathology laboratory for evaluation. Examination of the tissue allows for determination of whether abnormal lesions are located inside the endocervical canal; this information is an important determinant in the treatment plan (ACOG, 2012a, 2013).

During the endocervical sampling procedure, which usually takes only a few minutes, the patient will most likely experience abdominal pain and menstrual-like uterine cramps. Endocervical sampling is not indicated in the pregnant patient. Monsel's solution (basic ferric sulfate solution, a hemostatic agent) is applied with large cotton swabs to the surface of the cervix to control bleeding. This solution, which is mustard colored, turns black when exposed to blood. After the procedure, the Monsel's solution is expelled naturally. The nurse can explain to the patient that she may experience a thin, coffee ground–like vaginal discharge for several days after the procedure (ACOG, 2013).

Optimizing Outcomes— Addressing abnormal Pap test results during pregnancy

The management of abnormal Pap test results during pregnancy takes into consideration the duration of the pregnancy, the woman's desire to maintain the pregnancy, and the degree of cellular abnormality. Colposcopy is used for diagnosis, and the primary goal of both cytology and colposcopy is to identify invasive cancer that requires treatment before or at the time of delivery. Cervical biopsies are safe and should be performed for suspected high-grade disease or cancer. Biopsy during pregnancy has not been linked to fetal loss or preterm birth. Endocervical sampling should not be performed. Unless invasive cancer is identified, treatment is postponed until after the pregnancy has ended (ACOG, 2013).

MANAGEMENT OF ABNORMAL CERVICAL CYTOLOGY/COLPOSCOPY FINDINGS

There are several ways to treat the lesions identified in a colposcopic examination; the treatment depends on the location and severity of the lesions. Four types of interventional techniques are available: cryosurgery, laser ablation, conization, and the loop electrosurgical excision procedure.

Cryosurgery

Cryosurgery (cryotherapy), a gynecological treatment that involves the freezing of cervical tissue, is performed in the office setting. The patient is assisted into a dorsal lithotomy position and a vaginal speculum is inserted. Cryo probes are placed over the abnormal areas on the cervix. Liquid nitrogen flows through the cryo probes at a temperature of approximately −50°C, making the metal cold enough to freeze and destroy the tissue. Cryosurgery is relatively painless and produces very little scarring. An "ice ball" forms on the cervix, killing the superficial abnormal cells. The most effective treatment result is obtained by a process of freezing for 3 minutes, allowing the area to thaw, and then refreezing for 3 more minutes. Throughout the procedure, the patient may experience slight cramping and/or a sensation of cold or heat. Cryosurgery effectively destroys all of the abnormal cervical tissue in more than 85% of cases (ACOG, 2013).

"What to say" — *Teaching patients about aftercare following cryosurgery*

Offering explanations about what to expect following cryosurgery and alerting patients to danger signs constitutes an important nursing role. The nurse can counsel the patient that she:

- May return to most normal activities the day following the cryosurgery
- Will experience a foul-smelling, watery vaginal discharge, caused by sloughing of the necrotic cervical tissue, for a few weeks
- Should avoid inserting anything (tampons, douches) into the vagina and refrain from intercourse for at least 2 to 3 weeks
- Should promptly call her health-care provider if she experiences any symptoms of infection (fever, vaginal bleeding heavier than a normal menstrual cycle, severe or increasing pelvic pain, foul-smelling or yellow-green vaginal discharge)
- Should be sure to return for her follow-up appointment and comply with her health-care provider's recommendations for repeat Pap testing

A long-term complication of cryosurgery concerns the migration of the squamocolumnar junction (the transformation zone—the area on the cervix where the outer squamous cells meet the inner glandular columnar cells). Following the procedure, the squamocolumnar junction migrates upward into the cervical canal. The relocation of the transformation zone may create the need for a more invasive procedure in the future if abnormal lesions occur that are not visible with the colposcope (i.e., the abnormal cells are located inside the endocervical canal). Although rare, cryosurgery may cause scarring of the cervix and lead to stenosis (narrowing) of the cervical opening, making future cervical cytology screening (Pap testing) and evaluation (colposcopy) difficult (ACOG, 2013).

Laser Ablation

Laser ablation (destruction) involves the use of a thin, high-energy beam of light precisely directed at the abnormal tissue to cause cell destruction through vaporization. Depending on the circumstances, the procedure may be performed in the office or outpatient setting of the clinic or hospital. The technique uses a laser (mounted on a colposcope) to vaporize the transformation zone, where the abnormal cells are located. Advantages of laser ablation include rapid healing (3–4 weeks), minimal scarring, and no retraction of the transformation zone. Following laser ablation, patients may experience less vaginal discharge than with cryosurgery, but they may experience more discomfort immediately after the procedure. Vaginal spotting or bleeding may occur for several days after the surgery.

"What to say" — *Preparing the patient for cervical laser ablation*

Prior to the procedure, the nurse provides information, answers questions, and asks the patient to empty her bladder. The nurse may offer the following description of the procedure to help the patient understand what to expect:

- Medication will be given to decrease cramping and to numb the area to be treated.
- Everyone in the room will wear special glasses and surgical masks.
- Because laser burns or vaporizes cells, there will be a small amount of smoke present, and a smoke evacuator is used to remove the smoke from the air.
- The entire procedure (when done in the office or clinic) will take approximately 5 to 20 minutes, depending on the size of the abnormal area.
- Recovery time is minimal; most women leave within 20 minutes following the procedure.
- Some vaginal discharge is normal, but immediately report bleeding heavier than a menstrual period or yellow-green, foul-smelling discharge.
- A mild analgesic such as acetaminophen or ibuprofen may be taken as needed for pain, but severe abdominal pain should be reported immediately.
- Intercourse, douching, or the use of tampons should be avoided for 3 weeks.
- A fever above 100°F (38°C) should be reported immediately.
- Tub baths and showers may be taken, and you may return to work the day after the treatment.
- It is a good idea to ask a support person to accompany you to the appointment.
- Be sure to keep your follow-up appointment and follow your health-care provider's recommendations for repeat Pap testing.

Conization: Cold Knife Conization; Laser Conization; Loop Electrosurgical Excision Procedure (LEEP)

Conization of the cervix is defined as excision of a cone-shaped or cylindrical wedge from the uterine cervix that includes the transformation zone and all or a portion of the endocervical canal (Fig. 6-5). This procedure may be done when the lesion found on colposcopy extends into the endocervical canal and cannot be fully seen. Cold knife conization (CKC; also known as "cone biopsy") involves the use of a scalpel without electrosurgical current; laser conization employs use of a laser for the excision of tissue. Cold knife and laser conization, which are usually performed in the hospital outpatient surgical center, may be done for diagnostic purposes, or for therapeutic purposes, to remove precancerous cells. Techniques for diagnostic and therapeutic conization are virtually identical. Depending on the circumstances and setting, patients may receive a local anesthetic with IV sedation, regional anesthesia, or general anesthesia. Potential complications of cervical conization include infection, bleeding, and cervical scarring

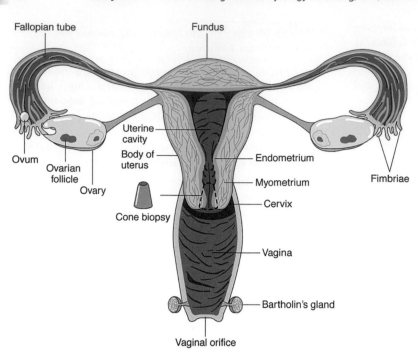

Fallopian tube

Fundus

Uterine cavity

Ovum

Ovarian follicle

Ovary

Body of uterus

Endometrium

Myometrium

Cervix

Cone biopsy

Fimbriae

Vagina

Bartholin's gland

Vaginal orifice

Figure 6-5 Cervical conization. (Williams, L.S., & Hopper, P.D. [Eds.]. [2007]. *Understanding medical-surgical nursing* [3rd ed. p. 928]. Philadelphia, PA: F.A. Davis.)

or stenosis (narrowing); the procedure may also increase the risk of cervical incompetence and preterm birth (ACOG, 2013; Burkman, 2010).

Conization performed with electrosurgical loop is called the loop electrosurgical excision procedure (LEEP), or large loop excision of the transformation zone (LLETZ). LEEP uses a low-voltage electrical current to remove abnormal cervical tissue. With this procedure, the cervix is anesthetized with a local anesthetic, and a fine wire loop electrode is used to simultaneously remove and cauterize a portion of the cervix. The advantage of the electrosurgical loop procedure and other excisional techniques (e.g., CKC) over the ablative therapies (e.g., cryosurgery, laser vaporization) is that the tissue is removed, not destroyed. Thus, the tissue is available for evaluation by a pathologist. Also, the LEEP procedure is fast (20–30 minutes), virtually bloodless, and may be performed in the office. Following the procedure, healing is rapid, and there is only a mild vaginal discharge afterward. Patients may experience mild pain and cramping for the first few hours after the LEEP; the discomfort can be relieved by oral medications. Possible short- and long-term complications include bleeding, cervical stenosis, preterm birth, infertility, and loss of cervical mucus (ACOG, 2013; Burkman, 2010).

"What to say" — *Preparing the patient for cervical conization*

An important nursing role in caring for the patient who will undergo cervical conization centers on education and support. Prior to the conization, the nurse answers questions and addresses concerns. The nurse may offer the following description of the procedure to help the patient understand what to expect:

- The procedure will take less than 1 hour.
- Some form of anesthesia will be used to control pain.
- Depending on the type of anesthesia to be used, nothing should be taken by mouth for 8 hours prior to

the procedure (when IV sedation or general anesthesia is planned).

- The physician will first insert a vaginal speculum and then use a knife (CKC), laser, or heated loop (LEEP) to remove a cone-shaped section of tissue (containing any abnormal cells) from the cervix.
- Self-absorbable sutures may be placed in the cervix to control bleeding.
- Analgesics may be taken as needed for pain control after the conization.
- If the conization is performed in an outpatient surgery center, and depending on the type of anesthesia used, you may leave after you are fully awake, but someone must be with you to drive you home.
- If the conization is planned as an office procedure (LEEP), an electrosurgical dispersive pad (a gel-covered adhesive electrode that provides a safe return path for the electrosurgical current) will be placed on your thigh and removed after the procedure.
- Vaginal bleeding or discharge may be present for several days after the conization; a panty liner or sanitary napkin should be worn to protect clothing.
- Tampons, douches, and sexual intercourse should be avoided for 4 to 6 weeks.
- You should avoid lifting items heavier than 25 pounds for at least 1 week.
- Tub baths and showers may be taken as desired.
- Any signs of infection or other complications (e.g., fever, chills, foul-smelling discharge from the vagina, worsening abdominal pain, heavy vaginal bleeding [may not occur until about 1 week after the procedure, when the healing scar is shed from the cervix]) should be promptly reported to your health-care provider.
- It is important to return for the postoperative examination and to follow your health-care provider's recommendations for repeat Pap testing.

Now Can You— Discuss diagnostic/treatment modalities for abnormal cervical cytological screening results?

1. Describe colposcopy, and explain how to prepare a patient for a colposcopic examination?
2. Discuss the importance of endocervical sampling?
3. Compare and contrast cervical cryosurgery, laser ablation, and conization, and provide patient teaching for each of these treatment modalities?

Human Papillomavirus

The human papillomavirus (HPV), a double-stranded DNA tumor virus, is the most common sexually transmitted disease in the United States. More than 40 HPV types can infect cutaneous and mucosal surfaces, including the anogenital epithelium and the mouth and throat. Although anogenital and cutaneous HPV infections are very common, only a small fraction of genital infections actually progress to cancer. Cervical cancer, rarely found among women in celibate religious orders, has long been associated with intimate sexual activity. Owing to the rising epidemic of the sexually transmitted HPV infection, the average age of women with abnormal Pap test findings is declining steadily. HPV is most prevalent among the younger population of women, although it does occur with the same frequency in older women as well (Lemieux, 2010; Pruitt, 2012).

Nursing Insight— *The papillomavirus–cancer link*

Many of the papilloma viruses cause papillomas. Papillomas are not cancers and are more commonly called warts. The most important risk factor in the development of cervical cancer is infection with a high-risk strain of HPV. The virus–cancer connection occurs as a result of alterations in the cervical cells that can lead to the development of CIN, which can then lead to cancer. HPV is passed from one individual to another during skin-to-skin contact. Although the virus is frequently transmitted during vaginal intercourse, anal intercourse, or oral sex, intercourse does not have to take place for HPV to be spread from one person to another. Skin-to-skin contact with an area of the body infected with HPV is the only requirement for transmission (ACS, 2014).

Nursing Insight— *The National Health Initiative addresses HPV*

An important Healthy People 2020 National Health Goal specifically focuses on HPV:

• Reduce the proportion of females with human papillomavirus (HPV) infection
• Reduce the proportion of females with human papillomavirus (HPV) types 6 and 11
• Reduce the proportion of females with human papillomavirus (HPV) types 16 and 18
• Reduce the proportion of females with other human papillomavirus (HPV) types

(U.S. Department of Health and Human Services [USDHHS], 2013).

Nurses can help the nation to meet this goal and objectives by providing education about methods of preventing HPV and information about how to recognize the signs and symptoms of HPV-related infection. Nurses can design studies and engage in research to provide evidence-based practice strategies for issues such as teaching women about safer sex practices, teaching youth about the methods of transmission of HPV infection and the long-term consequences of the disease, fostering HPV prevention through vaccination and exploring the use of alternative sites for vaccination delivery, and ways that health professionals can increase HPV awareness in their practice settings.

HPVs are a family of more than 100 virus types with a multitude of manifestations that include common warts, plantar warts, skin cancers, anal and genital warts, recurrent respiratory papillomatosis (a rare, benign infection of type HPV 6 or 11—it passes from mothers to neonates during vaginal childbirth), head and neck cancers, genital cancers, and cervical cancer. Young men and women between the ages of 15 and 24 account for approximately half of all new HPV infections (CDC, 2013a, 2013c; Whyte, 2012).

Nursing Insight— *Maternal HPV and neonatal laryngeal papillomatosis*

Vertical transmission of oncogenic HPV from the mother to her fetus via the placenta is possible but not fully understood; additional research in this area is indicated. Transmission to the infant of HPV type 6 or 11 is known to be possible during vaginal childbirth, but it is rare. Most experts believe that the risk of cesarean birth to both the mother and her infant exceeds the risk of neonatal genital warts or laryngeal papillomatosis (the presence of HPV 6– or 11–induced warts in the larynx or upper airway). However, cesarean birth may be indicated for women with genital warts if the pelvic outlet is obstructed or if vaginal birth would result in excessive bleeding. Once the maternal warts are no longer present, especially if the woman has had no detectable HPV lesions for 6 months or more, transmission of HPV to the infant during a vaginal birth becomes increasingly unlikely (CDC, 2014; D'Souza & Dempsey, 2011; Porterfield, 2011).

Where Research and Practice Meet:
Incidence of HPV Infection in New Sexual Relationships

According to a study conducted by Burchell, Tellier, Hanley, Coutlee, and Franco, more than half (56%) of young adults who reported that they were involved in a new sexual relationship were infected with HPV; of those, nearly half (44%) were infected with an HPV type that causes cancer. The results also indicated a high probability of HPV transmission between partners. When one partner had HPV, the researchers observed that in 42% of couples, the other partner also had the infection. If one partner was infected with HPV, the other partner's chance of also being infected with the same HPV type increased more than 50 times. According to the researchers, study findings support the belief that HPV infection is very common among young adults and underscore the importance of prevention programs for HPV-associated diseases such as cervical cancer screening and HPV vaccination (Burchell et al., 2010).

Approximately 40 HPV strains are believed to be capable of infecting the genital tract. HPV types 6 and 11 have been identified as "low risk," or nononcogenic (not capable of causing cancer). These are the types most likely to be associated with condylomata acuminata (genital warts), benign cervical changes, and low-grade cervical intraepithelial lesions. HPV types 42, 43, 44, 54, 61, 70, and 72 are also considered nononcogenic. Important associations have been identified between HPV type 16 and squamous cell carcinoma, and between type 18 and cervical adenocarcinoma. Many other HPV types (i.e., types 31, 33, 35, 39, 45, 51, 52, 56, 58, 59, 68, 73, 82) are also considered to be "high risk," or oncogenic (they carry the potential to cause cervical cancer), and one or more of these particular types is detected in nearly every patient diagnosed with cervical cancer. Oncogenic types have been identified in cervical, vaginal, vulvar, anal, penile, and oropharyngeal cancers, and HPV types 16,18, 31, and 45 cause the greatest number of cancers. High-risk HPV produces no visible symptoms; instead, it is detected by DNA testing for the virus, or on the basis of abnormal Pap test results (ACS, 2014; Chelmow, Waxman, Cain, & Lawrence, 2012; Gattoc, Flowers, & Ault, 2012; Gisvold, 2013; Schwartz, 2011).

HPV DNA TESTING

Most HPV infections produce no symptoms, and frequently a woman learns that she has been exposed to the virus only after undergoing a routine Pap test. Reflex HPV DNA testing, performed on a sample of vaginal or cervical cells collected during a pelvic examination, is most commonly performed on cells collected from residual preservative when liquid-based cytology is used. The HPV DNA test can often be performed on the same sample collected for the Pap test. HPV DNA testing assesses exfoliated cervical cells for the presence of one or more of 13 or 14 of the 15 to 18 potentially cancer-causing HPV types (ACOG, 2012a).

> ⊜ **Optimizing Outcomes**— **Through cotesting: a combination of cytology + HPV DNA testing**
>
> Although the Pap test can detect cellular changes caused by high-risk types of HPV, it is not as sensitive as is the HPV test, which specifically detects the viral DNA. DNA testing for HPV has gained widespread acceptance as an additional cervical cancer–screening tool and as follow-up to abnormal changes detected with a Pap test. Today, there are several DNA HPV tests that can detect either the majority of the high-risk types of HPV or specific subtypes, such as HPV 16 and HPV 18. The tests are performed on cervical or vaginal cells collected through self-sampling or obtained by a health-care provider during a pelvic examination. In 2014, the Food and Drug Administration (FDA) recommended that the cobas HPV test (manufactured by Roche Pharmaceuticals) be used as a first-line primary screening tool in women aged 25 years and older to assess their risk of cervical cancer based on the presence of clinically relevant high-risk HPV DNA. The cobas HPV test detects DNA from 14 high-risk HPV types including HPV 16 and 18 and 12 others. Presently, ACOG recommends that women 30 years or older be offered an HPV DNA test in addition to their Pap test and pelvic exam, and this recommendation is supported by various organizations, including the ACS, the National Institutes of Health (NIH), the ASCCP, the NPWH, and the

American Medical Women's Association (AMWA). The HPV DNA test is not recommended for screening adolescents because infections with HPV are relatively common in this age group and often resolve without treatment or complications (ACOG, 2013; FDA, 2014; Massad et al., 2013).

POTENTIAL MANIFESTATIONS OF HPV INFECTION

In women with HPV infection, abnormal findings on Pap screening are common. Of persons infected with HPV, only about 1% develop external genital warts, while approximately 10% develop cervical lesions. When present, HPV lesions most often occur on the posterior part of the vaginal introitus. Other locations include the buttocks, vulva, vagina, urethra, anus, and cervix. Four different types of genital warts have been identified (Box 6-4). It is possible to be infected with several different genotypes of HPV; some may be associated with a low risk, whereas others are associated with a high risk for the development of cervical cancer (ACS, 2014; ACOG, 2013).

"What to say" — *Counseling patients about abnormal Pap test results and HPV*

It is incumbent upon the nurse to listen carefully and fully to patient concerns about HPV and cervical cancer and offer support in coping with abnormal or positive results. Nurses should be sensitive to the fact that sharing the results of an abnormal Pap test with a patient can evoke feelings of anxiety, fear, and difficulty assimilating the implications of the results. In this situation, the nurse may wish to include the following information:

"Your abnormal Pap test result is not a diagnosis of a disease; it merely alerts us to the fact that there is a need for closer surveillance (e.g., more frequent testing) or further evaluation (e.g., colposcopy). Because it takes so long for cervical changes caused by HPV to develop into cancer, women who obtain Pap tests regularly are very unlikely ever to develop cervical cancer because there is plenty of opportunity to identify and treat the problem at an early stage" (Woodson, 2010).

HPV is an elusive virus with a clinical course that is characterized by spontaneous regressions and recurrences. Once a woman contracts genital HPV, she may develop a

---

> **Box 6-4** **Types of Genital Warts**
>
> *Condyloma acuminata* are soft, moist, pink, red, or gray lesions that may occur singularly or in multiples. The warts occur on moist surfaces and often cluster to form a cauliflower shape.
>
> *Smooth papular warts* are small, dome-shaped papules that are usually skin colored. They occur on hair-bearing or non-hair-bearing skin and do not occur on mucosal tissue.
>
> *Keratotic genital warts* have a thick layer and often look like "common" warts. They develop on hair-bearing or on non-hair-bearing skin and other nonskin tissues.
>
> *Flat warts* are generally flat or slightly raised with flat tops. These lesions can occur on moist or on dry tissue (Cox et al., 2011).

latent HPV infection, a subclinical HPV infection, a clinical HPV infection (manifested by the appearance of warts and/or cervical changes), or regression of the HPV lesions (Box 6-5). For most women, HPV infection resolves without intervention. It is estimated that up to 70% of HPV infections clear in 1 year and 91% of infected women do not have detectable levels of cervical HPV infection after 2 years. It is unknown whether the virus is truly absent or is simply reduced to undetectable levels. For the remaining 10% of women, persistent infection with certain types of HPV constitutes the major risk factor for cervical cancer (ACOG, 2012a; Kahn, Feemster, & Hillard, 2011).

Box 6-5 Potential Manifestations of HPV Infection

Following exposure to HPV, one or more of the following may occur:

Latent HPV infection: No detectable warts are present (i.e., undetectable by visual inspection, cytology, or HPV testing) and the person is noncontagious. However, because the virus can move from latency to "expressed" HPV disease (e.g., warts, cervical cell changes), there is no guarantee that the person will remain noncontagious indefinitely.

Subclinical HPV infection: Applies to changes in the skin cells of the lower genital tract that cannot be seen with the naked eye. The most common subclinical change is intraepithelial neoplasia of the cervix (cervical "precancerous change"; dysplasia; CIN 1, 2, or 3) that can be seen following the application of vinegar (acetic acid) to the skin, followed by close examination (e.g., colposcopy magnification) of areas that turn white (acetowhitening). Although subclinical HPV may appear anywhere in the lower genital tract, acetowhitening is very nonspecific and often unrelated to HPV. Tissue biopsy must be used to confirm the diagnosis of HPV infection.

Clinical HPV: The presence of warts and precancerous changes on the external genitalia (vulvar and perianal intraepithelial neoplasia; cervical and other lower genital tract cancers) that can be seen with the naked eye. Common clinical manifestations of HPV are:

- *Condyloma acuminata:* Raised, cauliflower-appearing (papillary) warts. Most are caused by the low-risk HPV 6 or 11 and are generally found on the external vulva, although they may also appear in the vagina, cervix, and anus.
- *Condyloma planum:* "Flat" warts; although most are caused by HPV 16 or other high-risk types, they should be treated as genital warts and not as a true precancerous condition.
- *High-grade intraepithelial neoplasia:* "Precancerous" flat HPV lesions that may appear on the vulva and the perianal and anal canal area. They can be very white (due to thick layers of keratin) or red (due to an increased blood supply) or various shades of brown to dark gray (due to increased pigment).
- *Cancer:* HPV is the cause of virtually all cancers of the cervix, as well as about 80% of vaginal cancers and 90% of anal cancers. In any of these areas, the cancer may appear as a nodule, erosion, ulcer, or thickening.

IMMUNE MEDIATED REGRESSION

- Most HPV lesions eventually resolve because of a host immune response to the virus. This is especially true for genital warts and CIN 1 because neither is truly precancer. Approximately 40%–50% of CIN 2 will resolve spontaneously; CIN 3 is considered a true cancer precursor, although some CIN 3 may resolve spontaneously to an immune-mediated regression.
- It is not known whether an immune-mediated regression clears that particular HPV type from the body completely or just suppresses it to the point where it is not likely to be contagious or cause HPV-induced disease in the future.

Sources: ACS (2014); Gravitt (2011).

Nursing Insight— *HPV and chronological age; STD screening*

HPV infections are most common in teenagers and women in their early 20s, with prevalence decreasing as women age. Most women will come in contact with HPV shortly after they become sexually active. Couples who are contemplating a sexual relationship should always be encouraged to undergo STD testing prior to initiating intercourse. However, because HPV is so very common and most often undetectable, neither the CDC nor the American Medical Association recommends clinical examinations for HPV as a component of STD screening. By age 50, more than 80% of women will have had HPV at some time in their lives. In adolescents and young women, HPV infections and dysplasia are likely to resolve spontaneously. This finding suggests that HPV infections detected in older women are more likely to reflect persistent infections acquired in the past (ACOG, 2010, 2012).

Now Can You— Discuss certain aspects of HPV?

1. Identify the population at highest risk for contracting HPV?
2. Briefly discuss the link between HPV and cervical cancer?
3. Explain the process of "cotesting" and identify patients for whom this procedure is most appropriate?

THE NURSING ROLE IN REDUCING PATIENT RISK FOR CERVICAL CANCER

Currently, researchers continue to investigate factors that may promote the development of cervical cancer. The role and the progression of HPV-induced lesions into cancer have recently become clearer. Research has demonstrated that cigarette smoking interferes with women's ability to clear an HPV infection and is associated with an increased risk of new HPV infection, persistent HPV infection, and cervical cancer. Also, a dose–response relationship with the amount of tobacco consumed has been noted. Cessation of smoking can lead to a decrease in cervical lesion size, whereas continuing to smoke can negatively affect the treatment outcome once cervical changes have become apparent (Fonseca-Moutinho, 2011). Other potential factors that link HPV with cervical cancer include long-term oral contraceptive use, young age, nutritional deficiency, presence of other genital tract infections, and immunodeficiency, such as occurs with HIV infection. For women with a healthy immune system, it may take decades for cervical cancer to develop from an initial exposure to high-risk viral types (ACOG, 2012a).

Optimizing Outcomes— Identifying risk factors associated with HPV infection and HPV-related cervical disease

To guide clinical HPV screening and educational efforts, nurses who work with women of all ages should be aware of certain risk factors that are associated with HPV infection and/or HPV-related cervical disease, including the following:

- A sex partner more than 2 years older
- More than three lifetime sex partners
- A new sex partner in the past 12 months

- Illegal drug use in the past 12 months
- Engaging in intercourse while impaired by alcohol
- Never having been married
- Having a male partner who is not circumcised

Sources: ACS (2013); Mayo Clinic (2014); National Cancer Institute (NCI) (2012).

A recent review of the literature revealed that several studies have linked HPV and cervical cancer to intimate partner violence in women, likely because women victims are less able to successfully negotiate strategies for safer sex, such as condom usage and monogamy, with an abusive partner. Also, female victims of violence are more likely to smoke, which increases the risk for cervical cancer. Women who have sex with women (WSW) are also at risk of contracting HPV. Although less common than heterosexual transmission, woman-to-woman HPV transmission is possible. Many WSW report a history of sexual encounters with men and may have engaged in intercourse without condoms. WSW may be less likely to seek regular pelvic examinations and Pap tests, although these health-promoting practices are recommended for women regardless of their sexual partners' gender (Crane, 2010; Hrivnak, 2013; Institute of Medicine, 2011; McCormish, 2012; Pruitt, 2012).

 Optimizing Outcomes— Educating lesbians about strategies to reduce HPV transmission

Women who have sex with women should be made aware that they are at risk for HPV infection and therefore require Pap screening. Nurses must educate all women about the contagiousness of HPV and emphasize that it is not exclusive to women who have heterosexual intercourse. It is also essential that patients understand that HPV risk increases with the number of sexual partners, regardless of gender, and that certain sexual practices (e.g., engaging in oral-genital and genital-genital contact without barrier devices; not cleaning sex toys between use; engaging in digital penetration without gloves, condoms, or finger cots) are associated with infection risk. Vaccination against HPV should be offered to all women who meet the prescribing criteria (i.e., younger than age 26) (Crane, 2010).

An important role for nurses in reproductive health promotion centers on counseling and education about strategies to enhance the immune system and reduce the risk for contracting HPV and other STDs. For example, the nurse can teach patients that refraining from smoking; limiting the use of alcohol; consuming a healthy, nutritious diet; maintaining a healthy weight; and avoiding exposure to chemical and environmental hazards are health practices that enhance the strength of the immune system. Observing sexual abstinence or, if sexually active, consistently using condoms or receiving prophylactic HPV vaccination are other preventive strategies to reduce the risk for infection. The nurse can counsel women that they can lower their chance of getting HPV by remaining in a faithful relationship with one partner, by limiting the number of sex partners, and by choosing a partner who has had no or few prior sex partners (CDC, 2013a; Linton, 2013).

The patient with genital warts may benefit from HPV counseling sessions that include her intimate partner.

Where Research and Practice Meet:
Young Women's Beliefs About HPV

Royer and Falk (2011) conducted a survey with 302 women aged 18 to 24 to assess their perceptions of HPV and to examine whether the perceptions differed based on a personal history of HPV diagnosis or STD testing. Study findings suggested that young women tend to have misconceptions about the cause, symptoms, and chronicity of HPV and considerable concerns about the psychosocial consequences of HPV diagnosis. Understanding women's beliefs about HPV can help guide development of patient-centered interventions to reduce HPV prevalence and improve management of those diagnosed with HPV.

Meeting with both partners provides an opportunity for the couple to learn that HPV infection is common and probably shared between partners and affords the possibility for other STD evaluation and screening along with Pap screening. The nurse can again emphasize the importance of routine cytological screening for cervical cancer.

Optimizing Outcomes— With condoms to reduce the risk of contracting HPV

Latex condoms offer some protection against HPV, and consistent condom use appears to reduce the risk of HPV transmission by about 70%. However, condoms protect only those areas of skin that they cover—and many infected individuals have HPV in noncovered areas of their skin that come into contact with their partner's skin. Secretions may also be a source of HPV-infected skin cells that could come into contact with a partner's uncovered skin areas. Spermicides and condoms coated with spermicide are not effective in preventing HPV and may cause microscopic abrasions that facilitate transmission of HPV and other STDs. Because female condoms cover more of the female introital epithelium at risk for HPV, they may provide a more protective barrier for both partners. However, the female condom may also be more easily dislodged during intercourse (CDC, 2014; Schiffman & Wentzensen, 2010).

"What to say" — *When discussing HPV with patients*

When discussing HPV, the nurse can be instrumental in dispelling various myths and misconceptions about genital HPV. Providing current, evidence-based information empowers the woman to make informed choices and decisions about her reproductive health. Depending on the situation, sharing the following information may be appropriate:

"Genital HPV is very common. It is primarily transmitted through sexual contact involving genital skin, and penetrative intercourse is not required. The only way to entirely eliminate the possibility of being exposed to HPV is abstinence from any form of genital-genital or oral-genital contact. The lifetime likelihood of getting genital HPV is estimated at 75% to 90%, and the risk of exposure to HPV is estimated to be approximately 15% to 25% per partner. That is, for every sexual partner one has, there is up to a 25% chance of being exposed to some type of HPV.

Because HPV rarely causes symptoms, most people who get HPV never know they have it—they do not develop genital warts, receive an abnormal Pap test result, or develop any other manifestations of HPV that they can identify. An HPV diagnosis does not necessarily mean that your partner has not been monogamous; it means only that the infection was contracted at some point in that person's life. HPV testing is not indicated for partners of persons with genital warts. An abnormal Pap test result does not necessarily mean that a woman is at high risk for cervical cancer. The abnormal result can be related to infection, local irritation, a low-risk HPV type, or a higher risk HPV type. Depending on your age and the degree of abnormality, further evaluation or cotesting for HPV DNA may be recommended. Only one in four cases of cervical lesions, if left untreated, will progress to cancer, and treatment is almost always successful in preventing cancer if the cells are discovered early. Undergoing routine Pap testing according to the recommendations of your healthcare provider is an important preventive strategy" (ACOG, 2010, 2012a; CDC, 2014).

HPV VACCINES

A vaccine (Gardasil) against HPV types 6, 11, 16, and 18 became available in 2006. Gardasil is the first HPV vaccine in the United States. The quadrivalent recombinant (non-live virus) vaccine is recommended for females aged 9 to 26 years. (The quadrivalent HPV vaccine may also be given to males aged 9 through 26 years to reduce their likelihood of acquiring genital warts; ideally, the vaccine should be administered before potential exposure to HPV through sexual contact.) Vaccination consists of three intramuscular injections given over 6 months, with the second dose to be given 2 months after the first dose and the third dose given 6 months after the first dose. If the HPV vaccine schedule is interrupted, the vaccine series does not need to be restarted (ACOG, 2014; CDC, 2014; Linton, 2013).

The HPV vaccine is supplied in prefilled syringes for single use only and in single-use vials; the vials must be stored under refrigeration and protected from light. The vaccine is highly protective, especially when the vaccination occurs before sexual activity. Although the vaccine does not prevent infection with all types of HPV, it provides protection against the HPV types associated with 70% of cervical cancers (16, 18), and 90% of external genital warts (6, 11). It is also effective in the prevention of vaginal, vulvar, and anal dysplasia and cancer caused by HPV types 16 and 18. However, if a woman has already been infected with HPV 16, 18, 6, or 11, the vaccine offers no protection, and only limited or no protection against the other HPV types. Hence, the protection afforded by the vaccine is lower in women who have had sex prior to vaccination. The quadrivalent vaccine has also been demonstrated to protect against vulvar and vaginal cancers (CDC, 2014; Gattoc et al., 2012; Linton, 2013; McGuire, 2011).

In late 2014, the FDA approved a 9-valent recombinant HPV vaccine (Gardasil 9) that also covers HPV types 31, 33, 45, 52, and 58. These latter five are responsible for roughly one in five cases of cervical cancer. Gardasil 9, also administered as three intramuscular injections given over 6 months, is approved for use in females aged 9 through 26 and in males aged 9 through 15 (FDA, 2014).

Cervarix is a bivalent vaccine that protects against HPV 16 and 18. Approved by the FDA in 2009, Cervarix also consists of three intramuscular injections given over 6 months; the second dose is given 1 month after the first dose and the third dose is given 6 months after the first dose. Cervarix is approved for use in girls and women aged 10 through 25 to prevent cervical cancer (Carlos, Dempsey, Patel, & Dalton, 2010; CDC, 2014).

 legal alert— Offer HPV vaccines to appropriate patients

It is important that an HPV vaccine be administered before people become sexually active. The CDC's Advisory Committee on Immunization Practices (CDC, 2010) recommends that Gardasil and Cervarix be routinely given to girls when they are 11 or 12 years old. However, Gardasil can be started as early as age 9 and can also be given to women 13 to 26 years old. Cervarix is approved for use in females 9 through 25 years of age. Although the vaccine series should begin before the initiation of sexual intercourse, a "catch-up" series is recommended for young women in the older age group who are already sexually active. HPV testing should not be conducted before HPV vaccination. HPV vaccines are not recommended for use in pregnant women, but pregnancy testing is not needed before vaccination. Completion of the HPV vaccine series should occur before pregnancy or after a pregnancy is complete. The HPV vaccines are contraindicated for persons with a history of immediate hypersensitivity to any vaccine component. The quadrivalent HPV vaccine (Gardasil) is contraindicated for persons with a history of immediate hypersensitivity to yeast. The bivalent HPV vaccine (Cervarix) in prefilled syringes is contraindicated for persons with an anaphylactic latex allergy. Because the HPV vaccines are not live vaccines, they may be administered either simultaneously or at any time before or after an inactivated or live vaccine. Syncope may occur after vaccination; to avoid patient injury related to a syncopal episode, the nurse should observe the patient for 15 minutes after any vaccination, with the adolescent seated or lying down. The most commonly reported adverse reactions to the vaccinations include pain, redness, and swelling at the injection site and fever, fatigue, headache, muscle and joint aches, and gastrointestinal distress. Because the vaccines do not cover all of the HPV types that can cause cervical cancer, routine Pap test screening is still recommended for those who have been vaccinated against HPV (ACOG, 2010, 2014; CDC, 2014; Kahn et al., 2011; Linton, 2013).

Where Research and Practice Meet:
Confirming HPV Vaccine Safety and Efficacy

Klein and colleagues (2012) conducted a retrospective, observational study of nearly 200,000 young females to assess the safety of the quadrivalent HPV vaccine (HPV4) following routine administration. The investigators found that the HPV4 vaccine appeared to be associated with syncope on the day of vaccination and skin infections in the 2 weeks after the vaccination. The study did not detect any evidence of new safety concerns among females aged 9 to 26 years secondary to vaccination with HPV4. Nurses can share the findings from this study with parents and patients when educating them about the general safety of routine vaccination with HPV4 to prevent cancer.

Markowitz and colleagues (2013) analyzed HPV prevalence data from the vaccine era (2007–2010) and the prevaccine era (2003–2006) that were collected during the National Health and Nutrition Examination Surveys. Among females aged 14 to 19 years, the vaccine-type HPV prevalence (HPV 6, 11, 16, or 18) decreased from 11.5% in 2003 to 2006 to 5.1% in 2007 to 2010, a decline of 56%. The vaccine effectiveness of at least one dose was 82%. The researchers concluded that within 4 years of vaccine introduction, the vaccine-type HPV prevalence decreased among females aged 14 to 19 years despite low vaccine uptake; also, the findings suggest that the estimated vaccine effectiveness was high.

 legal alert— **Be knowledgeable about immunization laws in your practice state**

Federal law does not explicitly require parental consent for immunizations such as the HPV vaccine. However, it does require that prior to administration the parent or guardian receive federally mandated vaccine information statements on any immunizations their children will receive. State law is the authority on whether parental consent is required. Minor consent laws are based on status (e.g., emancipated, married, in armed services, "mature" minor, pregnant, incarcerated) and services they are seeking (e.g., pregnancy-related care, family planning, and sexual health services) (Center for Adolescent Health & the Law, 2014; CDC, 2012). It is essential that the health-care provider have an understanding of the laws in the particular practice state; this information is available at http://www.cahl.org./

🌸 *Nursing Insight— HPV vaccination no longer required for U.S. immigration*

In December 2009, the Centers for Disease Control and Prevention (CDC) removed the HPV vaccine from the list of required vaccines for immigrant applicants. According to the Advisory Committee on Immunization Practices (ACIP), HPV immunization was removed from the list of recommended vaccines because HPV is the most common sexually transmitted disease in the United States, it is not close to being eliminated at this time, and it is not known to cause outbreaks (CDC, 2009).

 Where Research and Practice Meet: **Identifying Disparities in Attitudes, Acceptability, and Beliefs About the HPV Vaccine; Disparities in Vaccine Completion Rates**

Several epidemiological and behavioral studies have identified disparities in attitudes, acceptability, and beliefs about the HPV vaccine (Burns et al, 2010). Watts and colleagues (2009) found that acceptance of the HPV vaccine was high among Latina women for themselves and their daughters, and this was primarily motivated by the concern for cancer prevention. An investigation by Cates and colleagues (2009) discovered racial differences between blacks

and whites in HPV knowledge in a rural southern U.S. sample; whites were significantly more informed about the HPV vaccine. Blacks were significantly less likely to perceive cervical cancer as a threat to their daughters' health and had lower intentions to vaccinate their daughters against HPV than did whites. Based on their research, Gottlieb and Brewer (2009) concluded that the demographic factors of race and educational level were found to influence the use of information sources to learn about the HPV vaccine; this finding may be used to guide communication-based interventions for future research and practice. Other investigators (Brewer & Fazekas, 2007; Dorell, Yankey, Santibanez, & Markowitz, 2011; Fazekas, Brewer, & Smith, 2008; Kahn et al., 2008; Marshall, Phillip, Don, & Peter, 2007; Mehta et al., 2012; Small & Patel, 2012; Teitelman et al., 2011) reported factors (e.g., lack of knowledge, lack of insurance or resources to pay for the vaccine, difficulties making appointments owing to embarrassment, long waits, and inconvenient appointment times, perception that the vaccine is unsafe, fear that receipt of the vaccine would encourage sexual behavior, fear of needles, lack of provider recommendation, and personal perception of being at low risk for HPV and cervical cancer) that may inhibit patients' intention to receive the HPV vaccine or parents' intention to have their child receive the HPV vaccine. These studies highlight the importance of the nurse's role in developing culturally appropriate health promotion programs that target vaccination education and outreach. To successfully accomplish this goal, nurses must seek the latest evidence-based information about vaccines, remain knowledgeable about current vaccination guidelines, and possess an awareness of various behavioral disparities that place some populations at greater risk than others (Burns et al., 2010; Pruitt, 2012).

In related research, Chou and colleagues (2011) explored disparities in HPV vaccine completion rates in more than 1,400 young women. Only one-third of patients in the study group who initiated the series received all three shots in the recommended 12 months. The investigators concluded that their results supported findings from other studies that cite various barriers to vaccination (e.g., cost, access to health care, cultural beliefs, lack of vaccine awareness, misperceptions about vaccination) and suggested that strategies to improve preventive HPV vaccination compliance should especially target inner-city young people. Thomas, Stehens, and Blanchard (2010) described an innovative strategy that infused hip hop music into cell phone technology to facilitate a health promotion message about the HPV vaccine for young African American women attending universities and colleges. Based on their findings, the researchers suggested that the use of hip hop as a vehicle for sending HPV vaccine reminders is valuable in promoting the health of all young women.

🌸 **Collaboration in Caring—** *Securing funding resources for HPV vaccination*

Most health insurance plans cover the recommended HPV vaccines, although some plans may not cover any or all vaccines. The Vaccines for Children (VFC) program helps families of eligible children who may not otherwise have access to vaccines. The program provides vaccines at no cost to physicians who serve eligible children. Children younger than 19 years of age are eligible for VFC vaccines if they are Medicaid eligible, American Indian, or Alaska Native, or have no health insurance. "Underinsured children" who have health insurance that does not cover vaccination can receive VFC vaccines through Federally Qualified Health Centers or Rural Health Centers (CDC,

2014). For more information about the program, nurses may visit the CDC Web site at http://www.cdc.gov/vaccines/programs/vfc/index.html.

The Association of Women's Health, Obstetric and Neonatal Nurses (AWHONN) supports HPV vaccination for the prevention of cervical cancer along with regular cervical cancer screening with Papanicolaou and HPV tests, as recommended. The organization also supports policies that ensure universal access to HPV vaccination and cervical cancer screening and treatment. In the revised and reaffirmed "HPV Vaccination for the Prevention of Cervical Cancer" Position Statement (November 2010), AWHONN endorsed the establishment of adolescent health visits (to include health counseling, physical assessment, and vaccinations) and called for the establishment of programs specifically designed to educate young women and men, parents, and providers about HPV and the importance of HPV vaccination (AWHONN, 2010).

In an effort to increase public awareness of the need for vaccination, Merck (manufacturer of Gardasil) launched a multimedia campaign about HPV and cervical cancer prevention using their vaccine. Other organizations including the CDC and the National Federation of Planned Parenthood have created consumer education Web sites. And recently, the Society for Adolescent Medicine, the National Basketball Association, the Women's National Basketball Association, and Sanofi Pasteur (a vaccine manufacturer) have collaborated in launching a national program designed to heighten public awareness of the importance of vaccinations for teens.

🌸 Collaboration in Caring— *A team approach to a teen-targeted immunization campaign*

The NBA and the WNBA have collaborated with the Society for Adolescent Medicine and Sanofi Pasteur (a vaccine manufacturer) to create Vaccines for Teens, a national program designed to educate parents and their teens about the need to get vaccinated. The campaign Web site (http://www.vaccinesforteens.net/) is one component of the larger effort to make parents and teens aware of the dangers of four serious diseases (meningococcal disease/meningococcal meningitis, pertussis, influenza, and HPV) that can easily be spread from person to person. The Web site, which includes a brief athlete-narrated video, describes each disease and provides links for additional resources.

🌸 Cultural Diversity: *Cervical Cancer Screening and Prevention in Muslim Women in the United States*

Muslim women, who represent a growing minority in the United States, have unique cultural and religious traditions that may create barriers to cervical cancer screening and prevention. Nurses who work with these women should be sensitive to the importance of protecting their patients' modesty by creating an environment that encourages preservation of privacy. Strategies to enhance patient comfort include seeking the woman's particular preferences at the initiation of care, avoiding pressuring for answers to intimate questions (e.g., social/sexual history), allowing extra time for disrobing, reassuring her that no man can enter the examination room, providing a female clinician, and asking permission to perform each component of the clinical examination (taking care to expose only the body part that is being examined). Discussion about HPV vaccination is an important component of preventive health care. Muslim women may be more open to discussions of reproductive issues in the company of their peers and should be encouraged to participate in opportunities for health-care screening and prevention offered in both community settings and in traditional health-care environments (Guimond & Salman, 2013).

HPV EDUCATION AND COUNSELING FOR TEENS AND THEIR PARENTS

An essential area for nurses in HPV awareness and prevention centers on education and counseling for adolescents and teens and their parents. Because both males and females may be at risk for acquiring HPV, educational efforts should target both genders. It is important that reproductive health counseling provide developmentally appropriate information. Preteens tend to be concrete thinkers, and teenagers are more likely to engage in risky health behaviors. Understanding the tasks associated with normal adolescent development is an essential element that guides the nurse in establishing and directing a therapeutic dialogue. Communicating with young patients about HPV, the HPV vaccine, and other health issues may be enhanced by listening attentively, using terms the adolescent understands, remaining focused, and avoiding lectures and writing during the course of the conversation (Buitrago, 2011; Fisher, Alderman, Kreipe, & Rosenfeld, 2011; Walter & Chung, 2013).

🌸 Nursing Insight— *Understanding normal adolescent development*

The period of adolescence is characterized by rapid physical, emotional, and intellectual changes and development. Developmental tasks of adolescence center on establishing autonomy and identity, integrating physical changes into a new body image, and operating within the peer group. Adolescents experience feelings of invulnerability that may lead to an increased willingness to expose themselves to risk. Adolescents often tend to underestimate the personal risk of health hazards and unhealthful behaviors (Fisher et al., 2011).

During the course of the conversation, it is helpful to focus on strategies to minimize HPV risk (e.g., minimizing sexual partners, using condoms, avoiding smoking) and discuss the HPV vaccination in terms of its value for the prevention of genital warts and cervical dysplasia. The nurse should emphasize the importance of completing the HPV vaccine series, once initiated. The nurse can encourage the teen to take responsibility for her health by discussing how a healthy lifestyle can contribute to disease prevention. Teens should also be reminded of the importance of cervical cancer screening beginning at age 21.

The North American Society for Pediatric and Adolescent Gynecology (NASPAG) is a nonprofit organization dedicated to educating health-care professionals in pediatric and adolescent gynecology. NASPAG's mission is to provide a forum for education, research, and communication among health professionals who provide gynecological care to children and adolescents. The Web address for NASPAG is http://www.naspag.org/.

Nurses can also teach parents about strategies to enhance effective HPV communication with their daughters. Some parents may believe that giving their daughters the HPV vaccine somehow implies that they are encouraging sexual activity. In this situation, it may be beneficial to use a seat belt analogy: Just as the seat belt does not give someone permission to drive recklessly, the HPV vaccination does not imply that it is okay to have sex (Woodson, 2010). Nurses should encourage frequent, age-appropriate dialogue between parents and their children. For younger girls, ongoing parent–adolescent communication about issues such as personal sexual risk and partner relationship dynamics is an important strategy in STD prevention. The nurse can model for parents how to have honest, open communications about HPV information and use discussion about HPV and the vaccine as a basis for future discussions about sexuality and reproductive health as their daughters grow older. Parent–daughter communication about partner sexual pressure has been associated with increased condom use (Woodson, 2010).

TREATMENT FOR HPV-RELATED GENITAL WARTS

The risk of developing genital warts after sexual intercourse with someone who has warts is greater than 65%. Once exposed to genital warts, most individuals will develop them within 4 weeks to 8 months. Genital warts are usually not painful, but they can interfere with normal bodily functions, such as urination and defecation, making these actions painful and uncomfortable. Although no treatment has been developed for latent HPV infection, several therapies are available to manage external genital warts and clearly identifiable subclinical HPV lesions on the vulva, cervix, and vagina. The goal of all therapies is to destroy the visible lesions and reduce patient symptoms. In the majority of patients, treatment produces wart-free periods. Treatment, however, does not eliminate HPV infection. Eradication of the virus is not considered to be conclusive even after there is no visible evidence of wart tissue because of the high incidence of recurrence (Woodson, 2010).

⑤ Optimizing Outcomes— **With treatment for genital warts (Condylomata acuminata)**

Treatment options for genital warts (Condylomata acuminata) include the provider-administered medications podophyllin resin, trichloroacetic acid (TCA), or bichloracetic acid (BCA) and podophyllin resin, which are carefully applied to each wart and allowed to air-dry. Patient-applied medications include podofilox solution or gel 0.5% (Condylox); imiquimod

cream 5% (Aldara, Zyclara); and sinecatechins ointment 15% (Veregen) (green tea extract).

Podofilox solution is applied with a cotton swab; the gel formulation is applied by finger twice daily for 3 consecutive days, followed by 4 days without treatment. The treatment cycle may be repeated for up to four cycles. The nurse should advise the patient that mild or moderate pain or local ulceration may develop after application and instruct her to wash off the treated areas with soap and water 6 to 8 hours after treatment.

Imiquimod 5% cream is applied to warts only once daily at bedtime, every other day, for a total of three doses in a 7-day period. The regimen may be repeated until the lesions clear, but not for longer than 16 weeks. Patients should be instructed to wash all treated areas with soap and water 6 to 10 hours after application of the medication. Also, because imiquimod is mixed in a petroleum-based formula, latex condoms and diaphragms should be avoided until the medication has been washed off. Local inflammatory reactions (e.g., erythema, irritation, induration, ulcerations, vesicles) may occur with treatment.

Sinecatechins ointment is applied with the finger three times a day until the wart clears, but not longer than 16 weeks. Patients should be instructed to wash their hands before and after application, but that it is not necessary to wash off the ointment from the treated area prior to the next application. The nurse should also advise them of the possibility of local skin reactions to the medication, and counsel them that sinecatechins ointment may damage latex condoms and diaphragms. Podophyllin, podofilox, and imiquimod should not be used during pregnancy. No one treatment is ideal for all warts.

Surgical therapies used to eliminate the lesions include cryosurgery, manual excision, electrosurgical excision, and laser vaporization. Injection of interferon is another treatment, but one that is usually reserved for recurrent lesions unresponsive to standard treatments such as cryosurgery with liquid nitrogen or cryoprobe, electrocautery, and laser vaporization. Interferon is a naturally occurring substance that boosts the immune system and interferes with the ability of viruses to reproduce (CDC, 2014; Cox, Huh, Mayeaux, Randell, & Taylor, 2011; Nelson, 2011).

One's degree of contagiousness following treatment depends on how successful the treatment was in destroying the HPV lesions (where potentially infectious HPV particles are known to be present) and how successful the individual's immunity is in suppressing any HPV that might still be present in apparently normal skin. Most people treated for external warts do not experience a complete resolution, even after several treatments. This is because most treatments destroy the HPV lesions but cannot eliminate any HPV in surrounding apparently normal skin. Until the individual's immune system responds and suppresses the remaining HPV, new lesions may appear (CDC, 2014).

Once no further HPV lesions are detectable by clinical examination, and no new lesions have appeared over several subsequent months, the chance of shedding enough HPV to be contagious dramatically falls. Although it is impossible to advise anyone exactly when they have little to no chance of passing HPV to a partner, as months pass with no new lesions found by a clinician, the possibility of being contagious becomes increasingly remote (CDC, 2014).

(?) Global Health Case Study Maya S.

Condylomata acuminata

Maya S. is a 26-year-old Honduran woman who has lived in the United States for the past 3 months. She visits the community health clinic to inquire about treatment for her "venereal warts." During the interview, Maya tells the nurse that she has had the warts for several years but is concerned that they have "spread" and look unsightly. Her cousin has used a preparation with green tea extract with good results, and Maya would like a prescription for the medication. Maya's menstrual history is normal. She is single and has never had a pregnancy. She is sexually active and uses oral contraceptives prescribed in her native country. She takes no other medications. Her medical history is unremarkable and she has no known allergies. She is a nonsmoker, uses alcohol socially, and denies other drug use. Her vital signs are within normal limits.

critical thinking questions

1. What type of evaluation does the nurse anticipate?

2. What testing should be performed during the pelvic examination?

3. What instructions does the nurse offer about this medication?

4. What other counseling should the nurse provide?

(S) Now Can You— **Discuss HPV education, vaccination, and treatment?**

1. Develop HPV educational programs specifically suited for adolescents, parents of adolescents, reproductive-age women, and older women?

2. Identify six risk factors associated with HPV infection and HPV-related cervical disease?

3. Discuss HPV vaccination: identify who should receive the vaccines, how and when the vaccines should be given, nursing implications for administration, and patient education concerning vaccination?

4. Identify medical and surgical treatment modalities for HPV-related genital warts?

Cervical Cancer

Cervical cancer is a malignant neoplasm that forms in the tissues of the cervix. Worldwide, cervical cancer is the second most common type of cancer in women. It is much less common in the United States because of the routine use of cervical cytological screening. However, the American Cancer Society (2014) estimates that in this country, 12,360 women will be diagnosed with invasive cervical cancer and 4,020 women will die of cancer of the cervix in 2014. Cervical cancers originate in the cells on the surface of the cervix, which are composed of squamous and columnar epithelium.

❋ Nursing Insight— *The uterine cervix and cervical cancers*

Approximately 80% to 90% of cervical cancers are squamous cell carcinomas—neoplasms that originate in the squamous cells that cover the surface of the exocervix. Most of the remaining cervical cancers are adenocarcinomas, which are becoming increasingly more common in women born in the past 20 to 30 years. Cervical adenocarcinoma develops from the mucus producing gland cells of the endocervix. Less commonly, cervical cancers have features of both squamous cell carcinomas and adenocarcinomas and are called adenosquamous carcinomas or mixed carcinomas (ACS, 2014).

The development of cervical cancer, which is typically a very slow process, begins as dysplasia, a precancerous condition. Dysplasia, which can be detected by a Pap test, is 100% treatable. Most women who are diagnosed with cervical cancer today have not had regular Pap tests or they have not followed up on abnormal results. Undetected, precancerous changes can develop into cervical cancer and spread to the bladder, intestines, lungs, and liver (ACS, 2014).

❋ Collaboration in Caring— *The Pearl of Wisdom Campaign to Prevent Cervical Cancer*

The Pearl of Wisdom Campaign to Prevent Cervical Cancer is a united, global effort to raise awareness of the opportunities now available to prevent cervical cancer. The campaign reaches women, health-care providers, policy makers, health advocates, and the media in an effort to increase awareness of the new means of preventing cervical cancer, encourage women to take full advantage of these methods, and advocate for the implementation of these tools for girls and women everywhere. The Pearl of Wisdom Campaign was started by the European Cervical Cancer Association, which includes 100 organizations from across Europe, including cancer charities, cancer treatment centers, medical associations, university teaching hospitals, and health education organizations. The campaign promotes the "Pearl of Wisdom" as the global symbol for cervical cancer prevention in the same way as the pink ribbon serves the breast cancer campaign. Launched in the United States in 2009, the campaign is led by the national nonprofit organization Tamika and Friends, Inc. All profits from purchases of the Pearl of Wisdom pin go to the U.S. Pearl of Wisdom Campaign Fund to support cervical cancer prevention activities. Campaign partners, which include more than 24 national as well as local women's health and advocacy organizations, distribute simple, consistent key messages about cervical cancer to ensure that their collective voices effectively reach women. Additional information about the Pearl of Wisdom Campaign to Prevent Cervical Cancer may be found at the organization Web site: http://www.pearlofwisdom.us/about_us.

RISK FACTORS

Although the exact mechanism for the progression of cervical cancer is unknown, several key contributing factors have been identified (Box 6-6). Nurses must remain up to date about cancer risk factors so that they can appropriately identify and screen individuals at risk and provide accurate, culturally centered patient counseling and education. As is true in other areas of health promotion, it is useful to focus

Box 6-6 Cervical Cancer Risk Factors

- HPV infection (the most important risk factor)
- Cigarette smoking (causes damaging cellular changes within the cervix; doubles the risk for cervical cancer)
- Immunosuppression (HIV increases the likelihood for infection with HPV, which increases the risk for cervical cancer. Also, the immune system normally destroys/slows the growth of cancer cells.)
- Coinfection with other STDs (e.g., *Chlamydia trachomatis,* herpes simplex virus)
- Diet (low in fruits and vegetables increases the risk; obesity increases the risk of cervical adenocarcinoma)
- Early onset of sexual activity (before age 18) (During adolescence, the process of metaplasia is heightened, increasing the likelihood of HPV-related cellular changes.)
- Clinical history of condyloma acuminata (Infection with a low-risk HPV type increases the likelihood for coinfection with a high-risk type.)
- Inadequate cervical screening
- Male sexual partner who has had other partners, especially if a previous partner had cervical cancer
- Multiple sexual partners (three or more in a lifetime)
- An uncircumcised sexual partner
- Oral contraceptives (Long-term use [>5 years] increases the risk; however, the risk returns to normal after discontinuation.)
- Multiple full-term pregnancies (Three or more full-term pregnancies are associated with an increased risk; reasons unknown.)
- Young age at first full-term pregnancy (Women younger than 17 years with first full-term pregnancy are almost two times more likely to get cervical cancer later in life than those who postpone pregnancy until 25 years or older; this is attributed to the combination of pregnancy-induced hormonal effects on the cervix and the presence of HPV, both of which contribute to neoplastic changes.)
- Poverty (most likely related to lack of cervical cancer screening)
- In utero exposure to diethylstilbestrol (DES) (increased risk for clear-cell adenocarcinoma of the vagina or cervix; risk is greatest if DES exposure occurred during the first 16 weeks of pregnancy; there may also be an increased risk of squamous cell cancers and precancers of the cervix linked to HPV)
- Family history of cervical cancer (If the mother or a sister had cervical cancer, the woman's chances of developing the condition are two to three times higher.)
- Alcoholism

Sources: Adams & Carnright (2013); ACS (2014); McCormish (2012); Whyte (2012).

teaching efforts on risk factors such as lifestyle choices (e.g., tobacco and alcohol use, diet, sexual practices, HPV exposure) over which the woman has some control.

Cultural Diversity: Cervical Cancer

Cervical cancer disproportionately affects low-income women and women of color. The CDC (2013b) estimates that the costs for treating cervical cancer nationwide range from $300 to $400 million each year. In this country, from 2006 to 2010, the median age at diagnosis was 49 years. During that time frame, cervical cancer occurred most often in Hispanic women, at a rate of 10.9 per 100,000 women; in African American women, the rate was 9.6 per 100,000, as compared with 7.9 per 100,000 white women; and in American Indian/Alaska Native women, the rate was 7.3 per 100,000. In white women in the United States, the

rate of new-onset cervical cancer peaks in the middle of the fourth decade of life and then decreases. The peak incidence in Hispanics is in the mid- to late-60s, and for women of Asian or Pacific Island ethnicity, the incidence peaks in the early 70s. The incidence of cervical cancer continues to increase throughout life in African American women in the United States (Howlader et al., 2013). Factors that may influence cervical screening behaviors for these populations of women include a lack of a health promotion/disease prevention perspective, a lack of knowledge about Pap tests, financial barriers, and failure of health-care providers to recommend screening.

SYMPTOMS

Most of the time, early cervical cancer produces no symptoms. In fact, patients with cervical cancer usually do not experience any problems until the cancer is advanced and has spread. An important nursing role in cervical cancer education centers on emphasizing the importance of routine cervical cancer screening and teaching women about symptoms that may be associated with cancer of the cervix.

Optimizing Outcomes— Teaching about symptoms of cervical cancer

Nurses should emphasize that although early cervical cancer usually produces no symptoms, patients should remain alert to the following signs and symptoms that may be associated with the disease:

- Continuous vaginal discharge, which may be pale, watery, pink, brown, bloody, or foul smelling
- Abnormal vaginal bleeding between menstrual periods, after intercourse, or after menopause
- Menstrual periods that become heavier and last longer than usual
- Any vaginal bleeding after menopause

Signs and symptoms that may be associated with advanced cervical cancer include:

- Loss of appetite
- Weight loss
- Fatigue
- Pelvic pain
- Back pain
- Leg pain
- Single swollen leg
- Heavy vaginal bleeding
- Leaking of urine or feces from the vagina
- Bone fractures

Optimizing Outcomes— With a computer-based tool to predict cervical cancer risk

A tool for assessing cervical cancer risk may offer health-care professionals a simpler method for making treatment decisions. Katki and colleagues at the National Cancer Institute have developed a tool that uses cervical precancer (i.e., CIN 3 or higher) as a common treatment threshold. The tool, which is based on the established predictability of cervical precancer, allows clinicians to use their tablets or computers to accurately calculate a patient's current, 1-year,

3-year, and 5-year risk of developing cervical precancer based on the woman's age, current test results, and available past test results. This information can then be used to guide development of an appropriate plan of care.

DIAGNOSTIC WORK-UP AND TREATMENT OF CERVICAL CANCER

Once a diagnosis of cervical cancer has been made, the physician orders additional tests to determine whether the cancer is confined to the local area or has spread to distant organs. This process is termed *staging*. Tests that may be appropriate include x-ray computed tomography (CT scan), magnetic resonance imaging (MRI), positron emission tomography (PET scan), cystoscopy, chest x-ray, and intravenous pyelogram (IVP). The cancer stage is based on where the cancer is found (Box 6-7).

Treatment for cervical cancer depends on the stage of the cancer—whether it is localized or has spread to surrounding tissues or distant organs. A high-grade, preinvasive lesion (i.e., carcinoma in situ [CIS]) is removed to prevent progression to invasive disease. A conization procedure is usually recommended, although hysterectomy may be advised, depending on the individual situation (ACOG, 2012a).

🌼 *Nursing Insight*— *Factors that influence cervical cancer prognosis*

A number of factors influence the prognosis for a woman who has received a diagnosis of cervical cancer. These factors include the type of cancer, the stage of the disease, and the woman's age and general physical condition. Precancerous conditions are completely curable when followed up and treated properly. The 5-year survival rate for cancer that has not spread beyond the cervical area is 90.9%. However, the 5-year survival rate falls steadily as the cancer extends to other areas in the body (NCI, 2013).

Box 6-7 Stages of Invasive Cervical Cancer

STAGE I
The tumor has invaded the cervix beneath the top layer of cells. Cancer cells are located only in the cervix.

STAGE II
The tumor extends to the upper part of the vagina. It may extend beyond the cervix into nearby tissues toward the pelvic wall. The tumor does not invade the lower third of the vagina or the pelvic wall.

STAGE III
The tumor extends to the lower part of the vagina. It may also have invaded the pelvic wall. If the tumor blocks the flow of urine, one or both kidneys may not be working well.

STAGE IV
The tumor invades the bladder or rectum, or the cancer has spread to other parts of the body.

RECURRENT CANCER
The cancer was treated but has returned after a time during which it could not be detected. The cancer may show up again in the cervix or in other parts of the body.

Source: NCI (2013).

🌼 **Collaboration in Caring**— *Using a team approach to facilitate treatment of cervical cancer*

Depending on the cervical cancer stage, the health-care provider may wish to refer the woman to the care of a gynecological oncologist, a surgeon who specializes in treating gynecological cancers. Other members of the health-care team who may be involved in the patient's treatment plan include medical oncologists, radiation oncologists, oncology nurses, mental health professionals, and registered dieticians.

RADIATION THERAPY

Radiation therapy (RT) uses high-energy x-rays to destroy cancer cells. Cancers that extend beyond the cervix into the pelvis, lower vagina, and urinary tract typically receive radiation. RT may be combined with surgery or chemotherapy to treat early cervical cancers and more invasive stages of the disease; it can also be used to relieve symptoms caused by advanced cancer. Radiation may be delivered by external beam, by radioactive implants placed directly at the cancerous site ("internal therapy"), or by a combination of these two therapies.

External Therapy

External beam radiation, administered the same way as a diagnostic x-ray, is usually given five times a week for 5 or 6 weeks, with an extra boost of radiation at the end of that time. With this treatment modality, the entire pelvic area is irradiated, including the rectum, large intestine, small intestine, bone, and skin. Providing education and emotional support are key components of nursing care for women receiving external beam radiation. The nurse can encourage the patient to remain as active as possible throughout the course of therapy. Patients should be counseled that they might experience certain side effects in the treatment target area, such as hair loss, dry or irritated skin, or permanent darkening of the skin. While undergoing external RT, patients are cautioned not to remove any skin markings made by the radiologist (NCI, 2013).

🌼 **Complementary Care:** *Strategies to promote comfort during external radiation therapy*

Nurses can teach women who are undergoing external beam RT about various strategies to promote comfort and healing. For example, the nurse can suggest that the patient:

- Practice good personal hygiene
- Use lotions or creams only with the physician's approval, and remain vigilant about skin care and the condition of the treatment area
- Wear loose clothing over the treatment area
- Wear cotton underwear
- Expose the treatment area to air whenever possible
- Avoid exposing the treatment area to temperature extremes
- Avoid the use of adhesive tape in the treatment area
- Consider meditation and other stress reduction modalities
- Consider acupuncture for persistent nausea and vomiting

After completion of the external RT, patients are taught about self-care strategies to promote comfort and healing, and they are advised that side effects from the therapy may persist for weeks after the therapy has ended.

"What to say" — *Teaching about self-care strategies after external radiation therapy*

Nurses can empower women with self-care strategies to promote comfort and healing after the completion of external RT. For example, the nurse may advise the patient to do the following:

- Be sure to consume a nutritious diet.
- Drink plenty of fluids.
- Obtain adequate rest, and take naps as needed.
- Take medications as prescribed; check with your health-care provider before taking any nonprescribed medications.
- Maintain good oral and skin care.
- Anticipate that the effects from the radiation may persist for 10 days to 2 weeks after the last treatment.
- Anticipate that signs of healing will occur in about 3 weeks after the last treatment.
- Avoid infection; report any symptoms of infection to your health-care provider.
- Promptly report symptoms of complications, such as gastrointestinal symptoms (e.g., continued nausea, vomiting, anorexia, diarrhea) or skin symptoms (e.g., redness, swelling, pain, pruritus at the radiation site) to your health-care provider.

Internal Therapy

Implant radiation, also known as brachytherapy ("slow therapy"), involves placement of the radioactive material as close to the tumor as possible while sparing the adjacent healthy tissue. The radioactive material is either placed in a capsule and inserted into the cervix or placed in thin needles that are inserted directly into the tumor. This method of treatment takes place in the hospital setting. The patient stays in the hospital for 1 to 3 days while the implants remain in place; during this time, the patient is considered radioactive. The device is removed before discharge. Brachytherapy is then repeated several times over a period of 1 to 2 weeks. Once the radioactive material has been removed, no radioactivity remains in the body. In some situations, the internal radiation therapy is delivered during a brief treatment session, and the patient is able to go home afterward. In premenopausal women, sterility and cessation of menstruation usually occur after brachytherapy. Patients should be advised to promptly report signs of infection (i.e., vaginal or rectal bleeding, hematuria, foul-smelling vaginal discharge, fever, abdominal distention or pain) to their health-care provider (Carter & Downs, 2011; NCI, 2013).

Optimizing Outcomes— **Monitor and limit personal radiation exposure**

Nurses and other health-care providers who come in direct contact with patients receiving internal radiation therapy should monitor their personal radiation exposure by wearing a film badge or other device to determine the amount of exposure received. When providing direct patient care, isolation techniques (i.e., good hand washing technique, wearing gloves when handling bodily fluids) are observed, and time spent in proximity to the patient is limited to 30 minutes or less per 8 hours to avoid exposure to gamma rays. It is important to use the principles of time, distance, and shielding to protect from personal radiation exposure and to explain to the patient and her family why nursing care is focused on providing only essential care during the course of internal radiation therapy. Also, the nurse explains that pregnant women and children younger than 16 years should not visit the patient. If the radiation source becomes dislodged, a radiation specialist uses special long-handled tongs to remove the device and place it in a lead container. All linens and dressings are considered contaminated (Venes, 2013).

Along with physical care, education and emotional support remain central in the nursing care for all patients undergoing radiation therapy. Understandably, patients experience considerable emotional distress related to their diagnosis, fear of the anticipated treatment (e.g., pain, perceived personal radioactivity, adverse effects on bodily functions), and concerns about the impact of their treatment on family members. Potential nursing diagnoses for patients undergoing radiation therapy for the treatment of cervical cancer are presented in Box 6-8.

Nurses can advise patients undergoing external RT that although the affected area may look and feel sunburned, the treated tissues usually regain their normal appearance within 6 to 12 months. It is also important that all patients be counseled about common RT side effects, such as fatigue; diarrhea; frequent or uncomfortable urination; loss of hair in the genital area; and vaginal dryness, itching, and burning. Patients should also be advised to abstain from intercourse until a few weeks following completion of the

---

Box 6-8 Potential Nursing Diagnoses for Patients Undergoing Radiation Therapy for Cervical Cancer

Knowledge Deficit related to planned treatment procedures
Fear and Anxiety related to
- diagnosis
- pain
- interference with sexual functioning
- concerns about personal radioactivity
  responses of family members and significant others
Disturbed Sensory Perception related to
- internal radiation therapy
- restricted contact with visitors and health-care professionals
Risk for Skin Integrity Impairment related to
- external radiation exposure
- immobility and bedrest (with internal radiation therapy)
Risk for Physical Injury related to dislodgment of the radiation source (with internal RT)
Acute Pain related to internal radiation applicators

Sources: Bulechek, Butcher, Dochterman, & Wagner (2013); Johnson, Moorhead, Bulechek, Maas, & Swanson (2012); Moorhead, Johnson, Maas, & Swanson (2013).

RT. In general, patients who are treated with internal RT may resume intercourse in 7 to 10 days. Altered patterns of sexuality related to RT side effects are not unusual. Patients may experience a decrease in vaginal secretions and sensation, as well as vaginal stenosis (narrowing). These aftereffects can cause coital pain and discomfort and can contribute to diminished sexual desire. Depending on the specific problem, the nurse may offer suggestions such as applying water-based lubricants for vaginal dryness and/or the regular use of a vaginal dilator for vaginal stenosis; patient/partner referral to other resources may be appropriate (NCI, 2013). Other complications of external beam radiation and brachytherapy are listed in Box 6-9.

Surgery

For invasive cancer, radiation therapy can be used alone or in combination with some form of surgery. Surgery options range from cervical conization to radical hysterectomy. A radical trachelectomy involves removal of the cervix, part of the vagina, and the lymph nodes in the pelvis. This surgery is reserved for a small number of women with small tumors who desire pregnancy in the future. Total hysterectomy involves removal of the cervix and the uterus. Radical hysterectomy involves removal of the uterus, cervix, parametrium (tissue surrounding the uterus), ovaries, fallopian tubes, upper vagina, and some or all of the local lymph nodes (Carter & Downs, 2011; NCI, 2013).

Nursing Insight— *Understanding pelvic exenteration*

Pelvic exenteration is a rare, extreme procedure that is used to treat recurrent cervical cancer that has spread to surrounding organs. This surgery, which involves removal of the same organs and tissues as radical hysterectomy, may also include removal of the bladder, rectum, part of the colon, and/or the vagina.

Chemotherapy

Chemotherapy may be used for cervical cancer that has either metastasized too far from its origin to be treated by surgery or radiation or that has recurred. It may also be used to relieve pain associated with advanced cervical cancer or

---

Box 6-9 Complications of External Beam Radiation and Brachytherapy

Anemia and/or bruising

Cystitis (inflammation of the bladder)

Increased risk of infection

Premature menopause

Proctitis (inflammation of the rectum)

Sexual difficulties

Skin rash, inflammation, pruritus

Thrombophlebitis, pulmonary embolism, pneumonia (related to immobility associated with internal radiation therapy)

Vaginal scarring and stenosis

Vesicovaginal fistula (development of an abnormal connection between the vagina and the bladder or rectum)

Source: NCI (2013).

---

to shrink cancer to an operable size before surgery is performed. This treatment modality is termed *neoadjuvant chemotherapy*, and it can help to prevent cervical cancer from spreading. Chemotherapeutic agents approved to treat advanced or recurrent cervical cancer include cisplatin (Cis-Platinum, Platinol), bleomycin (Blenoxane), and topotecan hydrochloride (Hycamtin). The medications are either administered by mouth or via IV infusion. Chemotherapy treatments are usually alternated with "recovery periods" that allow the patient a rest time before beginning a new cycle of therapy (NCI, 2013).

Combination chemotherapy, which involves the combination of two or more chemotherapy medications, may be more effective than any single agent. When used in association with surgery or radiation, chemotherapy can help to prevent the spread or recurrence of cervical cancer. Nurses can counsel patients undergoing chemotherapy about common side effects associated with these medications, which include nausea and vomiting, change in appetite, oral lesions, vaginal sores, temporary hair loss, fatigue, bruising and bleeding, skin rash, joint pain, swelling in the legs and feet, susceptibility to infection, anemia, menstrual cycle changes, onset of early menopause, and infertility. In most situations, women who undergo chemotherapy for cervical cancer are already infertile as a result of surgery or RT. Physicians may prescribe hormones to help offset the symptoms associated with premature menopause (NCI, 2013).

Optimizing Outcomes— **Biological therapy to boost cervical cancer treatment**

Biological therapy, designed to repair, stimulate, or enhance the immune system's responses, may be used to treat cancer that has metastasized to other body organs. Interferon alfa, a cell protein that provides immunity to viral infections, is the type of biological therapy most often used. Biological therapy is usually administered on an outpatient basis and is sometimes combined with chemotherapy. Nurses can counsel women about possible side effects associated with this treatment modality, including:

- Flu-like symptoms: fever and/or chills; muscle aches; weakness; diarrhea, nausea, or vomiting
- Rash
- Loss of appetite
- Easy bleeding or bruising (NCI, 2013)

Optimizing Outcomes— **Supportive care for cancer patients**

Nurses can inform women who have received a diagnosis of cancer about supportive care that is available at any stage of the disease. Patients may find information about relief from the side effects of treatment, tips to help to control pain and other symptoms, and emotional support to help them cope with the feelings associated with a diagnosis of cancer. Resources for coping are available on the NCI Web site at http://www.cancer.gov/cancertopics/coping and from NCI's Cancer Information Service at 1-800-4-CANCER or LiveHelp Online Chat (https://livehelp.cancer.gov/app/chat/chat_launch).

Nurses are perfectly situated to provide women with factual information about cervical cancer screening, HPV, and cervical cancer. For example, nurses can explain that although HPV is the cause of cervical cancer, most HPV infections resolve without treatment and do not progress to cervical cancer, especially when regular screening is performed. Most new HPV infections occur in women in their 20s, but the most common decades of life for cervical cancer to be diagnosed is in the 40s and 50s, and 25% of new diagnoses occur in women over age 60. Sharing this information empowers patients with the essential knowledge they need to make informed choices about seeking continued screening at the recommended intervals (Kahn et al., 2011; Lowe, 2012).

Teaching women about risk factors for cervical cancer may motivate them to stop smoking or seek regular cervical cancer screening, if they have not done so in the past. Sharing information about strategies to reduce exposure to HPV (e.g., using condoms, limiting sexual partners, practicing monogamy) may assist in making decisions about intimate relationships. Women of all ages should be educated about the HPV vaccine—although the upper age limit for the vaccine is 26, they may be mothers, grandmothers, aunts, or sisters of preteen or teen girls. Because one concern about the HPV vaccine centers on a potential for patient and care provider complacency about cervical cancer screening, it is imperative that nurses continue to emphasize the importance of routine screening according to current early-detection guidelines (Kahn et al., 2011).

Nurses who care for pregnant women can use prenatal visits as an opportunity to counsel patients about the HPV vaccine and cervical cancer prevention and encourage them to begin the series during the postpartum visit. Nurses can support funding for programs that increase access to Pap testing and HPV vaccination for economically disadvantaged women. Finally, through age-appropriate, culturally sensitive educational efforts, nurses can empower patients to make informed choices about the HPV vaccine and, if they do choose to initiate the vaccine, encourage completion of the series.

✿ Nursing Insight— *Cancer screening and the Affordable Care Act*

According to a study conducted by Levy, Bruen, and Ku (2012), full implementation of the Patient Protection and Affordable Care Act of 2010 (ACA) could enable more than 1 million low-income women to obtain screening for breast and cervical cancers by expanding health insurance coverage. Approximately 6.8 million low-income women would gain health insurance, potentially increasing the annual demand for cancer screenings initially by about 500,000 mammograms and 1.3 million Papanicolaou tests.

⟳ Now Can You— Discuss aspects of cervical cancer?

1. Identify at least 15 risk factors for cervical cancer?
2. Teach a woman how to recognize symptoms of cervical cancer?
3. Describe the various treatment modalities for cervical cancer?
4. Discuss the nursing role in caring for patients undergoing treatment for cervical cancer?

Summary Points

- Cervical cancers originate in the cells on the surface of the cervix, which are composed of squamous and columnar epithelium.

- Cytological screening for cervical cancer should begin at age 21 years, regardless of the woman's sexual history.

- An important nursing role in cervical cancer education centers on emphasizing the importance of compliance with recommended cervical cancer screening and teaching women about symptoms that may be associated with cancer of the cervix.

- Infection with human papillomavirus (HPV) is known to be the primary cause of cervical cancer.

- An essential area for nurses in HPV awareness and prevention centers on education and counseling for adolescents and teens and their parents.

- The HPV vaccines are indicated for the prevention of cervical cancer, genital warts, and dysplastic or precancerous cervical lesions caused by several of the HPV virus types.

- Routine Pap test screening is recommended for women regardless of whether they have received the HPV vaccine.

- Nurses are perfectly situated to provide women with factual information about cervical cancer screening, HPV, and cervical cancer.

Review Questions

Multiple Choice

1. The squamocolumnar junction of the cervix:
   A. Is shed during menstruation
   B. Is devoid of cellular growth and replacement
   C. Is the area where the squamous epithelium and the columnar epithelium come together
   D. Surrounds the vaginal introitus

2. The nurse teaches the patient that she can enhance the accuracy of her Pap test screening by:
   A. Avoiding intercourse for 48 hours before the test
   B. Douching 24 hours before the test
   C. Scheduling the appointment to occur during menstruation
   D. Using lubricants with intercourse 24 hours before the test

3. The liquid-based process for cervical cytology screening can also be used to test for:
   A. HIV
   B. Syphilis
   C. Bacterial vaginosis
   D. *Chlamydia trachomatis*

4. If an abnormal Pap test result requires further evaluation, a procedure that allows for a close-up visualization of the vagina and cervix is:
   A. Colposcopy
   B. Cryosurgery
   C. Endocervical curettage
   D. Conization

5. The nurse teaches about risk factors for cervical cancer, which include:

A. Initiation of sexual activity after age 26

B. A history of three or more sexual partners

C. A history of infection with the varicella virus

D. Nulliparity

REFERENCES

Adams, H.P., & Carnright, E.L. (2013). HPV infection and cervical cancer prevention. *Clinician Reviews, 23*(9), 42–50.

American Cancer Society (ACS). (2013). *Human papillomavirus, cancer, HPV testing, and HPV vaccines*. Retrieved from http://www.cancer.org/cancer/cancercauses/othercarcinogens/infectiousagents/hpv/humanpapillomavirusandhpvvaccinesfaq/hpv-faq-hpv-risk-factors

American Cancer Society (ACS). (2014). *Cervical cancer: Prevention and early detection*. Retrieved from http://www.cancer.org/cancer/cervicalcancer/detailedguide/cervical-cancer-key-statistics

American College of Obstetricians and Gynecologists (ACOG). (2008). Management of abnormal cervical cytology and histology. Practice Bulletin No. 99. (Reaffirmed 2010). *Obstetrics & Gynecology, 112*(5), 1419–1444).

American College of Obstetricians and Gynecologists (ACOG). (2010). Cervical cancer in adolescents: Screening, evaluation, and management. Committee Opinion No. 463. *Obstetrics and Gynecology, 116*(8), 469–472.

American College of Obstetricians and Gynecologists (ACOG). (2012a). Screening for cervical cancer. Practice Bulletin No. 131. *Obstetrics & Gynecology, 120*(11), 1222–1238.

American College of Obstetricians and Gynecologists (ACOG). (2012b). Well-woman visit. Committee Opinion No. 534. *Obstetrics & Gynecology, 120*(8), 421–424.

American College of Obstetricians and Gynecologists (ACOG). (2013). Management of abnormal cervical cancer screening test results and cervical cancer precursors. Practice Bulletin No. 140. *Obstetrics & Gynecology 122*(6), 1338–1366.

American College of Obstetricians and Gynecologists (ACOG). (2014). Human papillomavirus vaccination. Committee Opinion No. 588. *Obstetrics and Gynecology, 123*(3), 712–718.

Association of Women's Health, Obstetric, and Neonatal Nurses (AWHONN). (2010). HPV vaccination for the prevention of cervical cancer. AWHONN Position Statement.*Journal of Obstetric, Gynecologic, & Neonatal Nursing, 39*(11), 129–130. doi:10.1111/j.1552-6909.2009.01097.x

Brewer, N.T., & Fazekas, K.I. (2007). Predictors of HPV vaccine acceptability: A theory-informed, systematic review. *Preventive Medicine, 45*(2/3), 107–114.

Buitrago, R. (2011). Adolescents need HPV shots early. *The Clinical Advisor, 14*(9), 119–120.

Burchell, A.N., Tellier, P.P., Hanley, J., Coutlee, F., & Franco, E.L. (2010). Human papillomavirus infections among couples in new sexual relationships. *Epidemiology, 21*(1), 31–37.

Burkman, R.T. (2010). New screening recommendations: Benefits and harms are in the eye of the beholder. *Female Patient, 35*(3), 12–13.

Burns, J.L., Walsh, L.J., & Popovich, J.M. (2010). Practical pediatric and adolescent immunization update. *Journal for Nurse Practitioners, 6*(4), 254–266.

Carlos, R.C., Dempsey, A.F., Patel, D.A., & Dalton, V.K. (2010). Cervical cancer prevention through human papillomavirus vaccination. *Obstetrics & Gynecology, 115*(4), 834–838.

Carter, J.S., & Downs, L.S. (2011). Cervical cancer tests and treatment. *The Female Patient, 36*(1), 34–37.

Center for Adolescent Health and the Law (CAHL). (2014). *State minor consent laws*. Retrieved from http://www.cahl.org./

Centers for Disease Control and Prevention (CDC). (2009). *New vaccination criteria for U.S. immigration*. Retrieved from http://www.cdc.gov/immigrantrefugeehealth/laws-regs/vaccination-immigration/revised-vaccination-immigration-faq.html

Centers for Disease Control and Prevention (CDC). (2010). FDA licensure of bivalent human papillomavirus vaccine (HPV2, Cervarix) for use in females and updated HPV vaccination recommendations from the Advisory Committee on Immunization Practices (ACIP). *Morbidity and Mortality Weekly Report (MMWR), 59*(20), 626–629.

Centers for Disease Control and Prevention (CDC). (2012). *Fact sheet for vaccine information statements*. Retrieved from http://www.cdc.gov/vaccines/pubs/vis/vis-facts.htm

Centers for Disease Control and Prevention (CDC). (2013a). *Cervical cancer*. Retrieved from http://www.cdc.gov/cancer/cervical/

Centers for Disease Control and Prevention (CDC). (2013b). Cervical cancer screening among women by hysterectomy status and among women ≥ years—United States, 2000–2010. *Morbidity and Mortality Weekly Report (MMWR), 61*(51), 1043–1047.

Centers for Disease Control and Prevention (CDC). (2013c). *Genital HPV infection—Fact sheet*. Retrieved from http://www.cdc.gov/std/HPV/STDFact-HPV.htm

Centers for Disease Control and Prevention (CDC). (2014). *Genital HPV infection—fact sheet*. Retrieved from http://www.cdc.gov/std/HPV/STDFact-HPV.htm

Chelmow, D., Waxman, A., Cain, J., & Lawrence, H.C. (2012). The evolution of cervical screening and the specialty of obstetrics and gynecology. *Obstetrics & Gynecology, 119*(4), 695-699. doi:10.1097/AOG.0b013e31824b2ed8

Chou, B., Krill, L.S., Horton, B.B., Barat, C.E., & Trimble, C.L. (2011). Disparities in human papillomavirus vaccine completion among vaccine initiators. *Obstetrics & Gynecology, 118*(1), 14–20. doi:10.1097/AOG.0b013e318220ebf3

Cox, J.T., Huh, W., Mayeaux, E.J., Randell, M., & Taylor, M. (2011). Management of external genital and perianal warts (EGW): Proceedings of an expert panel meeting. *The Female Patient, 36*(11), S1–S13.

Crane, A.M. (2010). Cervical cancer in lesbians. *Advance for NPs & PAs, 1*(4), 29–30.

Darragh, T.M., Colgan, T.J., Cox, J.T., Heller, D.S., Henry, M.R., Luff, R.D., . . . Wilbur, D.C., & Members of LAST Project Work Groups. (2012). The lower anogenital squamous terminology standardization project for HPV-associated lesions: Background and consensus recommendations from the College of American Pathologists and the American Society for Colposcopy and Cervical Pathology. *Journal of Lower Genital Tract Disease, 16*(3), 205–242.

Dillon, P.M. (2007). *Nursing health assessment: A critical thinking, case studies approach* (2nd ed.). Philadelphia, PA: F.A. Davis.

Dorell, C.G., Yankey, D., Santibanez, T.A., & Markowitz, L.E. (2011). Human papillomavirus vaccination series initiation and completion, 2008–2009. *Pediatrics, 128*(4), 830–839.

D'Souza, G., & Dempsey, A. (2011). The role of HPV in head and neck cancer and review of the HPV vaccine. *Preventive Medicine, 53*(Suppl. 1), S5–S11.

Einstein, M.H., & Cox, J.T. (2013). Cervical disease. *OBG Management, 25*(5), 43–50.

Fazekas, K., Brewer, N., & Smith, J. (2008). HPV acceptability in a rural Southern area. *Journal of Women's Health, 17*(6), 539–547.

Fisher, M., Alderman, E., Kreipe, R., & Rosenfeld, W. (Eds.). (2011). *Textbook of adolescent health care*. Elk Grove Village, IL: American Academy of Pediatrics.

Fonseca-Moutinho, J.A. (2011). Smoking and cervical cancer. *ISRN Obstetrics and Gynecology, 2011*, 1–6. doi:10.5402/2011/847684

Food and Drug Administration (FDA). (2014). FDA approves first human papillomavirus test for primary cervical cancer screening. Retrieved from http://www.fda.gov/newsevents/newsroom/pressannouncements/ucm394773.htm

Frey, M.K., & Gupta, D. (2011). Evaluation of women with atypical glandular cells on cervical cytology. *The Female Patient, 36*(8), 23–29.

Gattoc, L.D., Flowers, L., & Ault, K. (2012). Anal intraepithelial neoplasia and anal cancer: Who should be screened? *Contemporary OB/GYN, 57*(4), 36–45.

Gisvold, C. (2013). HPV's new targets. *Advance for NPs & PAs, 4*(3), 31–33.

Gottlieb, S.L., & Brewer, N.T. (2009). Disparities in how parents are learning about the human papillomavirus vaccine. *Cancer Epidemiology, Biomarkers & Prevention, 18*(2), 363–372.

Gravitt, P.E. (2011). The known unknowns of HPV natural history. *The Journal of Clinical Investigation, 121*(12), 4593–4599. doi:10.1172/JXI57149

Guimond, M.E., & Salman, K. (2013). Modesty matters: Cultural sensitivity and cervical cancer prevention in Muslim women in the United States. *Nursing for Women's Health, 17*(3), 211–217. doi:10.1111/1751-486X.12034

Harmanli, O., & Jones, K.A. (2010). Using lubricant for speculum insertion. *Obstetrics & Gynecology, 116*(2), 415–417.

Hill, D.A., & Lamvu, G. (2012). Effect of lubricating gel on patient comfort during vaginal speculum examination. *Obstetrics & Gynecology, 119*(2), 227–231.

Howlader, N., Noone, A.M., Krapcho, M., Garshell, J., Neyman, N., Altekruse, S.F., . . . Cronin, K.A. (Eds). (2013). *SEER CANCER STATISTICS REVIEW, 1975–2010*. Bethesda, MD: National Cancer Institute. Retrieved from http://seer.cancer.gov/statfacts/html/cervix.html

Hrivnak, J. (2013). Health issues in lesbian patients. *Advance for NPs & PAs, 4*(10), 17–20.

Institute of Medicine. (2011). *The health of lesbian, gay, bisexual, and transgender people: Building a foundation for better understanding*. Retrieved from http://www.iom.edu/Reports/2011/The-Health-of-Lesbian-Gay-Bisexual-and-Transgender-People.aspx

Kahn, J.A., Feemster, K., & Hillard, P.J. (2011). HPV vaccination: Do your patients get the message? *Contemporary OB/GYN, 56*(3), 24–31.

Katki, H.A., Wacholder, S., Solomon, D., Castle, P.E., & Schiffman, M. (2009). Risk estimation for the next generation of prevention programmes for cervical cancer. *Lancet Oncology, 10*(11), 1022–1023.

Klein, N.P., Hansen, J., Chao, C., Velicer, C., Emery, M., Slezak, J., . . . Jacobsen, S.J. (2012). Safety of quadrivalent human papillomavirus vaccine administered routinely to females. *Archives of Pediatrics & Adolescent Medicine, 166*(12), 1140–1148. doi:10.1001/archpediatrics.2012.1451

Lemieux, M.L. (2010). Primary screening for cervical cancer: Incorporating new guidelines and technologies into clinical practice. *The Journal for Nurse Practitioners, 6*(6), 417–426.

Levy, A.R., Bruen, B.K., & Ku, L. (2012). Health care reform and women's insurance coverage for breast and cervical cancer screening. *Preventing Chronic Disease, 9*(10), 16–26. doi:http://dx.doi.org/10.5888/pcd9.120069

Linton, D.M. (2013). Primary care prevention of cervical cancer. *The Clinical Advisor, 16*(3), 32–37.

Lowe, N.K. (2012). Cervical cancer screening guidelines 2012. *Journal of Obstetric, Gynecologic & Neonatal Nursing, 42*(1), 1–2.

McCormish, E. (2012). Cervical cancer: Who's at risk? *Nursing for Women's Health, 15*(6), 474–483. doi:10.1111/j.1751-486X.2011.01675.x

McGuire, L. (2011). Who should be vaccinated against HPV? *Advance for NPs & PAs, 2*(8), 33–35.

Marshall, H., Phillip, R., Don, R., & Peter, B. (2007). A cross-sectional survey to assess community attitudes to introduction of human papillomavirus vaccine. *Australian and New Zealand Journal of Public Health, 31*(3), 235–242.

Markowitz, L.E., Hariri, S., Lin, C., Dunne, E.F., Steinau, M., McQuillan, G., & Unger, E.R. (2013). Reduction in human papillomavirus (HPV) prevalence among young women following HPV vaccine introduction in the United States, National Health and Nutrition Examination Surveys, 2003–2010. *The Journal of Infectious Diseases.* Advance online publication. doi:10.1093/infdis/jit192

Massad, L.S., Einstein, M.H., Huh, W.K., Katki, H.A., Kinney, W.K., Schiffman, M., . . . Lawson, H.W. (2013). 2012 Updated consensus guidelines for the management of abnormal cervical cancer screening tests and cancer precursors. *Obstetrics & Gynecology, 121*(4), 829–846. doi:10.1097/AOG.0b013e3182883a34

Mayo Clinic. (2014). *HPV infection.* Retrieved from http://www.mayoclinic.org/diseases-conditions/hpv-infection/basics/risk-factors/con-20030343

Mehta, N.R., Julian, P.J., Meek, J.I., Sosa, L.E., Bilinski, A., Hariri, S., . . . Niccolai, L.M. (2012). Human papillomavirus vaccination history among women with precancerous cervical lesions. *Obstetrics & Gynecology, 119*(3), 575–581. doi:10.1097/AOG.0b013e3182460d9f

Montgomery, K., Bloch, J.R., Bhattacharya, A., & Montgomery, O. (2010). Human papillomavirus and cervical cancer knowledge, health beliefs, and preventative practices in older women. *Journal of Obstetric, Gynecologic, & Neonatal Nursing, 39*(3), 238–249. doi:10.1111/j.1552-6909.2010.01136.x

National Cancer Institute (NCI). (2012). *HPV and cancer.* Retrieved from http://m.cancer.gov/topics/factsheets/HPV

National Cancer Institute (NCI). (2013). *Cervical cancer treatment.* Retrieved from http://www.cancer.gov/cancertopics/pdq/treatment/cervical/HealthProfessional/page1

Nelson, A.L. (2011). Current and emerging options for treating external genital warts. *The Female Patient, 36*(Suppl. 7), S3–S8.

Policar, M.S. (2011). Female genital tract cancer screening. In R.A. Hatcher, J. Trussell, A.L. Nelson, W. Cates, D. Kowal, & M.S. Policar (Eds.), *Contraceptive technology* (20th ed., pp. 621–650). Decatur, GA: Bridging the Gap Communications.

Porterfield, S.P. (2011). Vertical transmission of human papillomavirus from mother to fetus: Literature review. *The Journal for Nurse Practitioners—JNP, 7*(8), 665–670. doi:10.1016/j.nurpra.2011.05.003

Pruitt, B. (2012). For all the right reasons: The HPV vaccine to prevent cervical cancer. *The American Journal for Nurse Practitioners, 16*(5/6), 31–34.

Royer, H.R., & Falk, E.C. (2011). Young women's beliefs regarding human papillomavirus. *Journal of Obstetric, Gynecologic, & Neonatal Nursing, 41*(1), 92–102. doi:10.1111/j.1552-6909.2011.01309.x

Saslow, D., Solomon, D., Lawson, H.W., Killackey, M., Kulasingam, S.L., Cain, J., . . . Myers, E.R., & ACS-ASCCP-ASCP Cervical Cancer Guideline Committee. (2012). *CA–A Cancer Journal for Clinicians, 62*(3), 147–172. doi:10.3322/caac.21139

Schiffman, M., & Wentzensen, N. (2010). From human papillomavirus to cervical cancer. *Obstetrics & Gynecology, 116*(1), 177–185.

Schwartz, T.M. (2011). Squamous cell carcinoma of the anus: A need for action. *The American Journal for Nurse Practitioners, 15*(9/10), 37–42.

Small, S.L., & Patel, D.A. (2012). Impact of HPV vaccine availability on uptake. *The Journal for Nurse Practitioners—JNP, 8*(1), 61–66.

Solomon, D., Davey, D., Kurman, R., Moriarty, A., O'Connor, D., Prey, M., . . . Young, N. (2002). The 2001 Bethesda System: Terminology for reporting results of cervical cytology. *Journal of the American Medical Association, 287*(16), 2114–2119.

Somerall, D.W. (2013). Screening for breast and cervical cancer: Understanding the different recommendations. *Nursing for Women's Health, 17*(4), 331–335. doi:10.1111/1751-486X.12052

Teitelman, A.M., Stringer, M., Nguyen, G.T., Hanlon, A.L., Averbuch, T., & Stimpfel, A.W. (2011). Social cognitive and clinical factors associated with HPV vaccine initiation among urban, economically disadvantaged women. *Journal of Obstetric, Gynecologic, & Neonatal Nursing, 40*(6), 691–701. doi:10.1111/j.1552-6909.2011.01297.x

Thomas, T.L., Stephens, D.P., & Blanchard, B. (2010). Hip hop, health, and human papillomavirus (HPV): Using wireless technology to increase HPV vaccination uptake. *The Journal for Nurse Practitioners—JNP, 6*(6), 464–470.

U.S. Department of Health and Human Services (USDHHS). (2013). *Healthy People 2020: Topics & objectives: Sexually transmitted disease.* Retrieved from http://www.healthypeople.gov/2020/topicsobjectives2020/objectiveslist.aspx?topicId=37

U.S. Food and Drug Administration (FDA). (2014). *FDA approves Gardasil 9 for prevention of certain cancers caused by five additional types of HPV.* Retrieved from http://www.fda.gov/NewsEvents/Newsroom/PressAnnouncements/ucm426485.htm

U.S. Department of Health and Human Services Health Resources and Services Administration. (2013). *Cervical cancer screening.* Retrieved from http://www.hrsa.gov/quality/toolbox/measures/cervicalcancer/part4.html

U.S. Preventive Services Task Force (USPSTF). (2012). Screening for cervical cancer—U.S. Preventive Services Task Force recommendation. Retrieved from http://www.uspreventiveservicestaskforce.org/uspstf11/cervcancer/cervcancerrs.htm

Venes, D. (2013). *Taber's cyclopedic medical dictionary* (22nd ed.). Philadelphia, PA: F.A. Davis.

Walter, E.B., & Chung, R.J. (2013). Immunizations for preteens. *North Carolina Medical Journal, 74*(1), 66–72.

Warren, D.M., & Thomas, E. (2011). The relationship between limited English proficiency and cervical cancer screening in Hispanic women. *Women's Health Care: A Practical Journal for Nurse Practitioners, 10*(9), 31–35.

Waxman, A.G., Chelmow, D., Darragh, T., Lawson, H., & Moscicki, A. (2012). Revised terminology for cervical histopathology and its implications for management of high-grade squamous intraepithelial lesions of the cervix. *Obstetrics & Gynecology, 120*(6), 1465–1472. doi:10.1097/AOG.0b013e31827001d5

Watts, L.A., Joseph, N., Wallace, M., Rauh-Hain, J.A., Muzikansky, A., Growdon, W.B., & del Carmen, M.G. (2009). HPV vaccine: A comparison of attitudes and behavioral perspectives between Latino and non-Latino women. *Gynecologic Oncology, 112*(3), 577–582.

Whyte, J. (2012). HPV and cervical cancer: Latest developments. *Consultant, 52*(8), 555–560.

Wilson, R.T., Giroux, J., Kasicky, K.R., Fatupaito, B.H., Wood, E.C., Crichlow, R., . . . Cobb, N. (2011). Breast and cervical cancer screening patterns among American Indian women at IHS clinics in Montana and Wyoming. *Public Health Reports, 126*(6), 806–815.

Woodson, S.A. (2010). *HPV counseling: A clinician resource, Updated 2010.* Washington, DC: Association of Women's Health, Obstetric and Neonatal Nurses (AWHONN).

CONCEPT MAP

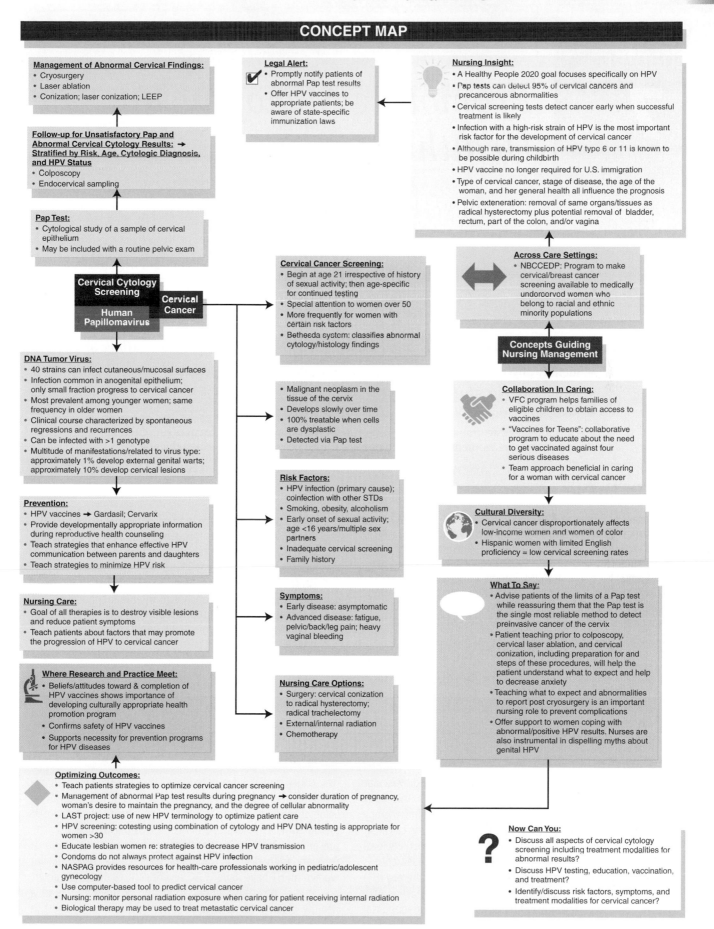

Management of Abnormal Cervical Findings:
- Cryosurgery
- Laser ablation
- Conization; laser conization; LEEP

Follow-up for Unsatisfactory Pap and Abnormal Cervical Cytology Results: → Stratified by Risk, Age, Cytologic Diagnosis, and HPV Status
- Colposcopy
- Endocervical sampling

Pap Test:
- Cytological study of a sample of cervical epithelium
- May be included with a routine pelvic exam

Cervical Cytology Screening

Human Papillomavirus

Cervical Cancer

DNA Tumor Virus:
- 40 strains can infect cutaneous/mucosal surfaces
- Infection common in anogenital epithelium; only small fraction progress to cervical cancer
- Most prevalent among younger women; same frequency in older women
- Clinical course characterized by spontaneous regressions and recurrences
- Can be infected with >1 genotype
- Multitude of manifestations/related to virus type: approximately 1% develop external genital warts; approximately 10% develop cervical lesions

Prevention:
- HPV vaccines → Gardasil; Cervarix
- Provide developmentally appropriate information during reproductive health counseling
- Teach strategies that enhance effective HPV communication between parents and daughters
- Teach strategies to minimize HPV risk

Nursing Care:
- Goal of all therapies is to destroy visible lesions and reduce patient symptoms
- Teach patients about factors that may promote the progression of HPV to cervical cancer

Where Research and Practice Meet:
- Beliefs/attitudes toward & completion of HPV vaccines shows importance of developing culturally appropriate health promotion program
- Confirms safety of HPV vaccines
- Supports necessity for prevention programs for HPV diseases

Legal Alert:
- Promptly notify patients of abnormal Pap test results
- Offer HPV vaccines to appropriate patients; be aware of state-specific immunization laws

Cervical Cancer Screening:
- Begin at age 21 irrespective of history of sexual activity; then age-specific for continued testing
- Special attention to women over 50
- More frequently for women with certain risk factors
- Bethesda system: classifies abnormal cytology/histology findings

- Malignant neoplasm in the tissue of the cervix
- Develops slowly over time
- 100% treatable when cells are dysplastic
- Detected via Pap test

Risk Factors:
- HPV infection (primary cause); coinfection with other STDs
- Smoking, obesity, alcoholism
- Early onset of sexual activity; age <16 years/multiple sex partners
- Inadequate cervical screening
- Family history

Symptoms:
- Early disease: asymptomatic
- Advanced disease: fatigue, pelvic/back/leg pain; heavy vaginal bleeding

Nursing Care Options:
- Surgery: cervical conization to radical hysterectomy; radical trachelectomy
- External/internal radiation
- Chemotherapy

Nursing Insight:
- A Healthy People 2020 goal focuses specifically on HPV
- Pap tests can detect 95% of cervical cancers and precancerous abnormalities
- Cervical screening tests detect cancer early when successful treatment is likely
- Infection with a high-risk strain of HPV is the most important risk factor for the development of cervical cancer
- Although rare, transmission of HPV type 6 or 11 is known to be possible during childbirth
- HPV vaccine no longer required for U.S. immigration
- Type of cervical cancer, stage of disease, the age of the woman, and her general health all influence the prognosis
- Pelvic exenteration: removal of same organs/tissues as radical hysterectomy plus potential removal of bladder, rectum, part of the colon, and/or vagina

Across Care Settings:
- NBCCEDP: Program to make cervical/breast cancer screening available to medically underserved women who belong to racial and ethnic minority populations

Concepts Guiding Nursing Management

Collaboration In Caring:
- VFC program helps families of eligible children to obtain access to vaccines
- "Vaccines for Teens": collaborative program to educate about the need to get vaccinated against four serious diseases
- Team approach beneficial in caring for a woman with cervical cancer

Cultural Diversity:
- Cervical cancer disproportionately affects low-income women and women of color
- Hispanic women with limited English proficiency = low cervical screening rates

What To Say:
- Advise patients of the limits of a Pap test while reassuring them that the Pap test is the single most reliable method to detect preinvasive cancer of the cervix
- Patient teaching prior to colposcopy, cervical laser ablation, and cervical conization, including preparation for and steps of these procedures, will help the patient understand what to expect and help to decrease anxiety
- Teaching what to expect and abnormalities to report post cryosurgery is an important nursing role to prevent complications
- Offer support to women coping with abnormal/positive HPV results. Nurses are also instrumental in dispelling myths about genital HPV

Optimizing Outcomes:
- Teach patients strategies to optimize cervical cancer screening
- Management of abnormal Pap test results during pregnancy → consider duration of pregnancy, woman's desire to maintain the pregnancy, and the degree of cellular abnormality
- LAST project: use of new HPV terminology to optimize patient care
- HPV screening: cotesting using combination of cytology and HPV DNA testing is appropriate for women >30
- Educate lesbian women re: strategies to decrease HPV transmission
- Condoms do not always protect against HPV infection
- NASPAG provides resources for health-care professionals working in pediatric/adolescent gynecology
- Use computer-based tool to predict cervical cancer
- Nursing: monitor personal radiation exposure when caring for patient receiving internal radiation
- Biological therapy may be used to treat metastatic cervical cancer

Now Can You:
- Discuss all aspects of cervical cytology screening including treatment modalities for abnormal results?
- Discuss HPV testing, education, vaccination, and treatment?
- Identify/discuss risk factors, symptoms, and treatment modalities for cervical cancer?

7

Promoting Menopausal Health

You can't turn back the clock.
But you can wind it up again.

—Bonnie Pruden

LEARNING TARGETS *At the completion of this chapter, the student will be able to:*

◆ Identify physiological changes that occur during the menopausal period.

◆ Identify self-care strategies to promote health during midlife and the later years.

◆ Recognize various risk factors for cardiovascular disease and osteoporosis.

◆ Develop an educational program for perimenopausal women that focuses on potential health threats and empowers women with strategies to optimize physical and emotional well-being.

PICO(T) Questions

The intent of Evidence-Based Practice (EBP) is to provide nursing care that integrates the best available evidence. An initial step in EBP is to write a PICO(T) question that effectively guides the research. A PICO(T) question is an acronym that stands for population (P), intervention or issue (I), comparison of interest (C), outcome (O), and time frame (T). Depending on the question, all or some of the question components are used in the research process. Use these

PICO(T) questions to spark your thinking as you read the chapter.

1. Do (P) postmenopausal women of normal weight (BMI 19–25) report (O) less frequent (I) hot flashes compared with (C) postmenopausal women of above normal weight (BMI >25)?

2. Do (P) women who use complementary and alternative medicine (CAM) approaches to treat menopausal or postmenopausal symptoms report (O) a lower level of (I) anxiety related to menopausal health compared with (C) women who do not?

Evidence-Based Practice

Weinberg, N., Young, A., Hunter, C.J., Agrawal, N., Mao, S., & Budoff, M.J. (2012). Physical activity, hormone replacement therapy, and the presence of coronary calcium in midlife women. *Women & Health, 52,* 423–436.

Atherosclerotic calcification is a risk factor for cardiovascular events, independent of other traditional risk factors. This study examined the relationship between the use of hormone therapy (HT) and the incidence and severity of atherosclerotic calcification, independent of lifestyle factors (i.e., physical activity level and diet) in postmenopausal women. Previous research has revealed controversy regarding the use of hormone therapy (HT) relative to the risk-benefit for coronary artery disease (CAD). One large, randomized study of HT use among postmenopausal women demonstrated no significant increased cardiovascular

risk. Other studies have noted less impact in women with delayed initiation of HT. Several investigations have explored the value of coronary artery calcium (CAC) scanning (via computed tomography) as a sensitive marker for cardiovascular risk; the presence of calcium in the coronary arteries is indicative of coronary artery disease. Additional research has revealed that women on HT have lower CAC severity scores. To date, numerous studies have also underscored the positive effects of a healthy lifestyle (e.g., physical activity, and healthy diet) in reducing risk for CAD.

Evidence-Based Practice (continued)

Study participants included 544 asymptomatic postmenopausal women with no history of CAD who underwent physician-referred outpatient CAC scanning to measure cardiovascular risk. Of the 544 participants, 252 (46.3%) were HT users. Data collected included the following: age, race/ethnicity, weight, height, blood pressure, calculated body mass index (BMI), present cholesterol level, stress level, diet type, medication use, and frequency of sweating during exercise. Risk factors included the following: current cigarette smoking, diabetes, hypertension, hypercholesterolemia, hypertension, family history of CAD, and history of premature CAD in a first-degree relative. Physical activity (PA) was quantified through the use of the self-administered Baecke Questionnaire of Habitual Physical Activity, an instrument that assesses habitual PA in units per week.

The mean age of the 544 participants was 60.1 years (range 50–80). The HT users' mean age was 59.6 years; the HT nonusers' mean age was 60.7 years. A significantly greater proportion of HT users were Caucasian (68%), 14% were black, 13% were Hispanic, and 4% were Chinese. Among the HT nonusers, 60% were Caucasian, 18% were black, 17% were Hispanic, and 5% were Chinese.

The mean BMI was higher in the HT users, although none of the other cardiovascular risk factors was significantly different. On average, HT was initiated at 54 years; the mean number of years of use was 2.2 years (range 0–33).

For HT users, the mean CAC score was 56.8; for HT nonusers, the mean CAC score was 96.4, a finding that was consistent with results reported in other studies. A strong correlation was noted between participant age and the presence of CAC.

The mean amount of PA was 22.7 units/week for all participants: For HT users, PA was 23.9 units/week; for HT nonusers, the PA was 21.7 units/week. A higher score is equated to increased PA units per week. There was a significant relationship among PA, CAC, and HT: The severity of CAC was less with increasing levels of PA. A personal history of hypertension, high cholesterol, stress, and a positive family history were not found to be significant.

Study findings demonstrated a protective association of HT and physical activity. HT users had a significantly lower prevalence of any coronary artery calcium (defined as CAC score >0; 37%) than nonusers (50%). Interestingly, participants who reported adherence to a high-protein or vegetarian diet had nearly a twofold increased odds of CAC as compared with those who reported a regular, mixed, or low-fat diet.

Based on their findings, the investigators suggested that physical activity and diet should be taken into account in prospective studies of the relation of hormone therapy use to coronary artery calcium.

1. How is this information useful to clinical nursing practice?

2. Based on these findings, what are implications for further research?

See Suggested Responses for Evidence-Based Practice on Davis *Plus*.

Introduction

This chapter explores the years surrounding the menopausal transition. By 2025, 1.1 billion women worldwide will be postmenopausal. In 1900, the average age of menopause was 46 years and the average life expectancy was 51 years, although many women lived well beyond this age. In contemporary times, American women, on average, can expect to live to be 80 years old and spend close to one-third of their lives as postmenopausal women. For the modern woman, menopause does not mark the end of life. Instead, it represents a transition into another phase, with a potential life span of another 30 to 50 years (The North American Menopause Society [NAMS], 2010b).

A healthy lifestyle that balances optimal nutrition and regular exercise with mental and social stimulation helps women to lead productive, enriched lives well into the ninth decade. The period surrounding menopause offers a unique time for women to evaluate their physical and emotional health, make plans for the future, and prepare for many, many healthy years ahead. With evidence-based information about menopause and the normal aging process, as well as various health issues such as cardiovascular disease and osteoporosis, nurses can empower women with the tools they need to prepare for and embrace the coming years with energy, enthusiasm, and strategies for optimizing their health and well-being. Armed with factual information, women can actively partner with their health-care provider in the decision-making process. Nurses are perfectly positioned to provide ongoing menopausal education and counseling to assist women in making fully informed choices.

Although menopause is a natural, inevitable process, women do have control over how they pass through this special time of life. They can engage in strategies to ease uncomfortable symptoms and minimize their risks of chronic disease. For example, refraining from smoking, maintaining appropriate weight through exercise and diet, limiting alcohol intake, reducing stress, remaining socially active, and recognizing that happiness and long-term health come about through a personalized approach are tools that help women to enjoy good health during the later years of life. As a noted author observed, "The wise woman achieves menopause, it does not overcome her" (Weed, 2002). During this special time in their lives, many women describe an enhanced sense of well-being, hard-won individuality, and a positive attitude for living life to its fullest.

The Climacteric, Premenopause, Menopause, Perimenopause, and Postmenopause

The *climacteric* is a transitional time in a woman's life marked by declining ovarian function and decreased hormone production. The climacteric begins at the onset of ovarian decline and ends with the cessation of postmenopausal symptoms. *Menopause,* a term derived from Latin *mensis* for "month" and Greek *pausis,* meaning "to cease," refers to the last menstrual period and can be dated with certainty only 1 year after menstruation ceases. Menopause is defined as the permanent cessation of menses resulting from reduced ovarian hormone secretion that occurs naturally or is induced by surgery, chemotherapy, or radiation. The average age at menopause in the United States is 51.4 years; the normal age at menopause ranges from 40 to 58 years (American College of Obstetricians and Gynecologists [ACOG], 2014).

Premenopause is the time up to the beginning of perimenopause, but the term is also used to define the time up to the last menstrual period. *Perimenopause* is the period of time preceding menopause, usually between 2 and 8 years before menopause. The age at onset of perimenopause ranges from 39 to 51 years. Although perimenopause may last as few as 2 or as many as 10 years, on average, it lasts 4 years. During this time of transition, levels of estrogen and progesterone increase and decrease at uneven intervals, causing the menstrual cycle to become longer, shorter, and eventually absent. Ovulation is sporadic. Symptoms of perimenopause, including irregular menses, hot flashes, vaginal dryness, dyspareunia, and mood changes, are associated with the fluctuation and decline in hormone levels. *Postmenopause* begins when ovarian estrogen terminates, ovulation ceases, and menstrual periods have stopped for 12 consecutive months. During postmenopause, estrogen is produced solely by the adrenal glands. Women typically enter postmenopause between the ages of 40 and 58; the average age is 51 (ACOG, 2014).

Nursing Insight— *Perspectives on the perimenopausal period*

Every woman travels her own unique course through perimenopause. Interestingly, the term *perimenopause* is a relatively new concept—the word was not even listed in a medical dictionary until after 1989. The term "menopausal transition" describes the years from the onset of the loss of ovarian cycling to the last menstrual period. Menopause occurs regardless of a woman's age when the number of remaining ovarian follicles falls below a critical level of about 1,000. The health habits established during the perimenopausal and early postmenopausal years can determine the woman's health status and quality of life for her critical elderly years after age 75, when serious health problems are greatest (ACOG, 2014).

Throughout the menopausal transition, changes take place in both the physiological and emotional domains. Hormone levels shift, readjust, and reach new balances, and the tissues and organs whose function is influenced by these hormones also change structurally and functionally. At the same time, mental and emotional alterations occur as well. Although some of the changes are physiological in nature, others involve various dimensions of self-perception and self-concept as women are challenged to deal with this natural passage into a new phase of life.

Cultural Diversity: *Views on Menopause*

Cross-cultural studies have revealed that the menopausal experience is greatly influenced by the attitudes of the culture and community in which women reside. In the United States, owing in part to the present-day graying of the baby boom generation, attitudes toward menopause and aging are undergoing change. For many traditional cultures throughout the world, menopause represents a time for women to assume leadership roles in the community and a time for honor and recognition as one of the tribal members with an accumulation of wisdom. American women are embracing this broad cultural perspective as an opportunity to shift self-perception and create a positive cultural image of women during this stage of life. Today, the majority of American women do not believe that menopause interferes with their quality of life (National Institutes of Health [NIH], 2005; The North American Menopause Society [NAMS], 2010b).

Signs and Symptoms of Menopause

A number of signs and symptoms typically herald the physical changes that take place during the menopausal transition. During this time, nurses can empower women with various strategies to promote mental and physical well-being. Potential nursing diagnoses for women experiencing the perimenopausal period are presented in Box 7-1.

Nursing Insight— *Body systems affected by the natural decline in estrogen*

Estrogen secretion naturally declines as women age. Estrogen receptors are plentiful throughout the female body. During the childbearing years, estrogen is a dominant hormone that regulates the menstrual cycle and exerts important effects on the reproductive and urinary tracts, the heart and blood vessels, bones, breasts, skin, hair follicles, mucous membranes, pelvic muscles, and the brain. Loss of estrogen is associated with a multitude of acute symptoms, including hot flashes, sleep disruptions, and mood changes. For many women, menopause-related estrogen depletion is also associated with longer-term manifestations such as urogenital symptoms (Allmen & Moore, 2010; NAMS, 2010b).

MENSTRUAL CYCLE CHANGES

It is rare for a woman to cease menstruation all at once. Most often, the menstrual periods become progressively more irregular. The volume of blood flow is variable as well

---

Box 7-1 Potential Nursing Diagnoses for Perimenopausal Women

- Knowledge deficit related to menopause and its management
- Risk for injury related to osteoporosis and coronary heart disease
- Sexual dysfunction related to physiological changes associated with declining estrogen levels
- Readiness for enhanced family coping related to the menopausal transition
- Risk for situational low self-esteem related to the physical and emotional changes during the menopausal transition

Sources: Bulechek, Butcher, Dochterman, & Wagner (2013); Johnson, Moorhead, Bulechek, Maas, & Swanson (2012); Moorhead, Johnson, Maas, & Swanson (2013).

and may be accompanied by midcycle spotting. Changes in bleeding patterns largely result from a lack of ovulation. The absence of ovulation interrupts the production of progesterone, the hormone that stabilizes the endometrium, or uterine lining. Under the influence of prolonged, continuous estrogen, the endometrium continues to proliferate and may only be irregularly sloughed off. When bleeding does occur, it may be heavier or more prolonged. The endometrial lining may also develop irregular or thickened areas; it may not slough off evenly or in its entirety, and these events cause the menses to stop and start again.

Although irregular menses is usually a normal part of the perimenopausal process, any heavy bleeding should be investigated. Uterine fibroids, a frequent cause of increased bleeding, are common in perimenopausal women. Cervical or uterine cancer should also be considered as a possible cause of this symptom. If heavy bleeding is an ongoing problem and cancer has been ruled out, hormonal intervention in the form of low-dose oral contraceptives, progesterone alone, or another form of hormone therapy (HT) may be suggested. If fibroids are the cause of heavy bleeding, medical or surgical intervention may be advised. (See *Women's Health Companion* [WHC] Chapter 4 for a discussion of uterine cancer and fibroid tumors, and WHC Chapter 6 for a discussion of cervical cancer.) It is important to remember that although fertility declines during this transitional period, it does not disappear until menopause is complete. Menopause is signaled by the passage of 1 full year without menstruation. For most women, birth control remains an important consideration during the perimenopausal period (Nelson, 2011).

HORMONAL CHANGES

During the perimenopausal period, hormone levels are frequently erratic, with highs and lows occurring without the usual synchronicity. A common hormonal pattern that occurs when ovulation becomes unpredictable is an elevated estrogen level throughout the cycle with low progesterone levels during the second half of the cycle, when progesterone is normally at its peak. Some women develop very low levels of estrogen as well. At this time, ovarian function declines and the ovaries lose their ability to manufacture large amounts of sex hormones. The physiological feedback loops between the ovaries, the hypothalamus, and the pituitary glands also lose their synchronized pattern. Progesterone undergoes the most dramatic drop during menopause because its production depends on ovulation and the development of the corpus luteum.

Small amounts of estrogen continue to be produced by the ovaries for up to 10 years following cessation of menses. The body has other means of estrogen production, however. The woman's fat cells convert androgens produced by the adrenal glands to estrogens. Androgens are female forms of "male-type" hormones that are produced by the ovaries and the adrenal glands. Androgens are responsible for the maintenance of muscle strength and the sex drive. As estrogen and progesterone levels fall, the effects of the androgens often become relatively more pronounced. For example, these hormones can produce an increase in facial hair often noted after menopause. For some women, androgen levels (including testosterone) fall as well, producing symptoms of low libido or decrease in muscle mass with a relative increase in the amount of adipose (fat) tissue (NAMS, 2010b).

SKIN AND HAIR CHANGES

Declining levels of estrogen affect many tissues throughout the body. The skin and mucous membranes become dry. The fatty layer beneath the skin tends to shrink, and this change is associated with an overall decrease in elasticity and moisture. The skin feels rougher to the touch, and the outer skin may be looser than the deeper layers, which results in wrinkling. The skin produces less melanin, and it can burn more easily. The increasing predominance of androgens often causes a darker, thicker, more wiry hair to appear on the symphysis pubis, underarm area, chest, lower abdomen, and back. Some women experience an increase in facial hair, and the hair on the head may become dry. Pubic and axillary hair often thins. Genetically susceptible women may experience female pattern (scalp) hair loss, a condition most likely related to the altered estrogen-to-androgen ratio that accompanies menopause (Grimes, Blankenship, Kremer, Reese, & Sonstein, 2011; NAMS, 2010b; Scheinfeld, 2011).

BREAST CHANGES

Glandular tissues in the breasts shrink during the menopausal period. The breasts may lose their fullness, flatten, and drop. The nipples may become smaller and flatter.

UROGENITAL CHANGES

Vaginal changes may accompany the perimenopausal period, or they may not occur for several years after menopause. The mucous membranes, previously supported by estrogen stimulation, become thin, dry, and fragile. The vagina loses its rough texture and dark pink coloration and becomes smooth and pale. The vagina also shortens and narrows. Women may experience vaginal itching, burning, bleeding, or soreness. The vagina lubricates more slowly, and there is a diminished amount of cervical mucus produced. Owing to these changes, intercourse often becomes painful. Bleeding and/or pain may occur following minimal trauma, such as that occurring during intercourse or a pelvic examination. Vulvar changes may also make activities such as riding a bicycle uncomfortable. There is also an alteration in the normal vaginal flora, which results in a decrease in the normal protective mechanisms of the vagina. Declining estrogen secretion is accompanied by a corresponding reduction in the lactobacilli needed to maintain a healthy acidic vaginal environment. With these changes in pH, normally harmless pathogens may colonize the more alkaline vagina, potentially leading to infection. When the vaginal mucosa becomes inflamed, the condition is termed "atrophic vaginitis," a condition characterized by burning, leukorrhea, and malodorous yellow discharge (NAMS, 2010b; Nelson, 2011; Pearson, 2011).

A & P review **Estrogen Deficiency and Urogenital Atrophy**

Estrogen plays a critical role in maintaining the structure and function of the vagina. The layers of the vaginal mucosa, which is estrogen sensitive, are composed of parabasal (the least mature), intermediate or basal (larger and polygon shaped), and superficial squamous cells (the most mature). Prior to menopause, the matured vaginal epithelium has more superficial cells than parabasal cells, indicating the presence of estrogenic stimulation. In menopausal women, systemic declines in estrogen levels correspond to decreased cellular maturation. The proportion of superficial cells present on cytological examination is expressed as the vaginal maturation index (VMI). The VMI is a ratio of parabasal, intermediate, and superficial squamous cells found on a cytological smear of cells taken from the upper one-third of the vagina (Fig. 7-1). Although infrequently used in clinical practice today, the maturation index of vaginal cells is useful in evaluating the qualitative response of the vaginal tissue to estrogen. Under the influence of estrogen, mature superficial cells predominate; when estrogen levels are low, parabasal cell numbers fall, leading to gradual atrophic changes in the tissues of the vagina and vulva, as well as in the urethra and trigone area of the bladder (Allmen & Moore, 2010; Freeman, 2010, 2012; NAMS, 2010b).◆

Menopause-induced changes in the genitourinary tract can produce symptoms that include urinary urgency, increased frequency, stress or urge incontinence and recurrent urinary tract infections. Unlike other symptoms associated with menopause, such as hot flashes, those of urogenital atrophy often worsen with advancing age. Vulvovaginal or urinary atrophic symptoms in postmenopausal women can cause significant reductions in quality of life, avoidance of sexual intercourse, and emotional distress. More than one-third of women over the age of 60 in the United States have some form of urinary incontinence.

The most common types of urinary incontinence are "urge" incontinence, "stress" incontinence, and "mixed" incontinence. Urge incontinence is the sudden onset of urinary leakage caused by the bladder contracting (e.g., from infection, bladder irritants, or bladder spasms). Stress incontinence is the sudden onset of urinary leakage caused by increased pressure on the bladder; it may occur with coughing, sneezing, laughing, or running. Mixed incontinence is a combination of both stress and urge incontinence (Spencer, 2012).

The prevalence of incontinence appears to increase gradually during young adult life, peak around middle age, and then steadily increase during the later years. Risk factors for urinary incontinence in women include history of pregnancy, pelvic surgery, or cesarean birth; diet high in bladder irritants (e.g., alcohol, caffeinated or carbonated beverages); smoking; advancing age; and obesity. The estimated annual direct cost of urinary incontinence in women

in this country is around $12.43 billion. Therapies for urinary incontinence / overactive bladder include behavioral treatment (e.g., pelvic floor muscle training and exercise; behavioral modification such as reduction in consumption of bladder irritants and scheduled voiding), medications, and other approaches such as pessaries, onabotulinumtoxinA (Botox), and sacral neuromodulation (use of an implantable device that stimulates the S3 sacral nerve root). Pelvic floor muscle rehabilitation focuses on strengthening the levator ani muscles in order to help the patient suppress bladder contractions (ACOG, 2005; Hamlin & Robertson, 2013; Kenton, 2014; Muffly & Paraiso, 2012; O'Dell, 2014; Seidel, 2011; Woods, 2013).

A & P review Estrogen Deficiency and Urogenital Changes

In the urinary tract, estrogen deficiency causes urethral and bladder mucosal thinning, urethral shortening, weakening of the sphincter, decreased bladder capacity, increased postvoid residual urine volume, and uninhibited detrusor muscle contractions. After menopause, the urethral mucosa atrophies, and the collagen content in the connective tissue surrounding the urethra decreases; blood flow in the urethra is also reduced. These changes may cause dysuria, urinary frequency, and stress incontinence; estrogen-deficient women may also be susceptible to recurrent urinary tract infections. Owing to a decrease in collagen and elastin, declining estrogen levels also contribute to loss of mechanical support of the pelvic diaphragm (Freeman, 2010; Kellogg-Spadt, 2012).◆

Nursing Insight— *Menopause, pelvic floor dysfunction, and urinary incontinence*

Pelvic organ support is provided by the physiologically complex interactions between the vagina, the levator ani muscles and their fascial coverings, the connective tissue attachments to the bony pelvis (including the uterosacral ligaments), the arcus tendineus fascia pelvis, and the perineal body and perineal membrane. The pelvic floor muscles atrophy after menopause, becoming weak and unable to adequately support the pelvic structures and organs. As the pelvic organs shift position, they begin to press against the vagina, resulting in prolapse, usually of the vagina or bladder. A prolapse can result in pain during intercourse and urinary incontinence.

Exercises can strengthen the muscles; however, muscle damage cannot be reversed. Surgery is the primary treatment for pelvic prolapse; the timing of the surgery depends on the woman's symptoms and their effect on her daily activities. Some symptoms can be medically managed until surgery is appropriate. Many treatment options are available for urinary incontinence, especially if it is not accompanied by a cystocele, which results when the bladder herniates into the vagina (Evans & Karram, 2011; Jones, Bryson, & Harmanli, 2010; Muffly & Paraiso, 2012).

Urinary incontinence has been shown to affect women's social, clinical, and psychological well-being. It is estimated that fewer than one-half of all incontinent women seek medical assistance for this problem, even though urinary incontinence can often be treated (ACOG, 2005). Loss of estrogen supply to the estrogen-dependent tissues of the

Vaginal Epithelial Cells

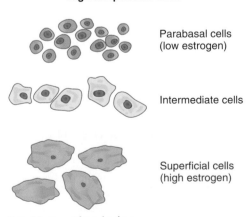

Parabasal cells (low estrogen)

Intermediate cells

Superficial cells (high estrogen)

Figure 7-1 Maturation index.

genitourinary tract results in a decrease in muscle tone and control in the bladder and urethra. Stress urinary incontinence (SUI) is a disturbance in urinary control (e.g., loss of urine) due to sudden increases in intra-abdominal pressure that often occurs during sneezing, coughing, or laughing. SUI is more likely to occur in women who have given birth. For most women, pelvic floor muscle exercises, also known as Kegel exercises, can be very effective in strengthening the pelvic floor and in improving symptoms associated with SUI. Some practitioners provide patients with "Kegel beads" to encourage and remind them to perform the exercises. Patients are instructed to slide the beads from one side of the chain to the other until all sets (10) are performed for the day (Jones et al., 2010; Keilman, 2011).

❝What to say❞ — *Teaching patients how to perform pelvic floor (Kegel) exercises*

To teach patients about pelvic floor exercises, the nurse may provide the following information:

These exercises strengthen the pelvic floor and should help decrease your urinary symptoms. To perform the pelvic floor exercise,

- First, contract the vaginal opening as if you are trying to stop the flow of urine; if you are able to contract the muscles to stop the stream, you are using the correct muscles
- Now hold to a count of six
- Relax to a count of 10, then repeat these steps 10 more times
- Perform five to 10 sets of pelvic floor exercises each day

For patients who are unable to isolate the levator ani, electrical stimulation and/or muscle biofeedback may be helpful. Electrical stimulation during pelvic floor exercises expands and contracts the pelvic muscles in a manner similar to the Kegels. This approach, conducted in the health-care practitioner's office, may be helpful for women who have difficulty contracting the pelvic muscles voluntarily. It involves the use of a device that delivers current to the pudendal nerve through a vaginally placed probe (Elliott & Sokol, 2011; Evans & Karram, 2011; Jones et al., 2010; Spencer, 2012).

Biofeedback therapy has been used to assist the reeducation of patients with pelvic floor spasms and has been shown to result in significant symptomatic improvement after several months of therapy. Biofeedback uses a vaginal sensor that measures the level of muscle activity generated by voluntary pelvic floor contraction. With biofeedback, the patient is taught to voluntarily control the pelvic muscles and bladder. With an electrode attached to the skin, biofeedback machines measure the electrical signals elicited when the pelvic muscles and urinary sphincter are contracted. Through the visual cues from the graph shown on the monitor, patients can learn to control these muscles voluntarily (Jones et al., 2010).

Vaginal cones, which may also be vaginal weights, can be used to strengthen the vaginal muscles as well. The woman is instructed to insert the tampon-shaped cone into the vagina while in a standing position, beginning with the lightest weight. Once the cone has been inserted, the patient should contract the levator ani muscles in an effort to keep the cone in place for 15 to 20 minutes. As the muscles strengthen, the patient then transitions, one at a time, to the next heaviest cone. It is helpful to use the cone while doing pelvic floor exercises as well. As the pelvic muscles strengthen, patients can use the cones while engaging in exercise (Jones et al, 2010).

Some women choose to use a pessary, which is a device inserted into the vagina to support the prolapsed bladder or uterus. This device must be fitted by a health-care practitioner, and needs to be removed and cleaned regularly with soap and water to reduce the risk of infection. Surgical intervention for a prolapsed bladder usually involves an anterior repair (colporrhapy). This procedure involves shortening of the pelvic muscles to provide better support for the bladder (Culligan, 2012; Tam & Davies, 2013).

Urinary urgency and/or frequency combined with an involuntary loss of urine are common signs of an overactive bladder. Pharmacological management of incontinence is aimed at relaxing the involuntary contractions that occur at the bladder. For overactive bladder, medications frequently used include tolterodine (Detrol), oxybutynin (Ditropan), and solifenacin (VESIcare). Common side effects associated with these medications include dry mouth, nausea, dizziness, drowsiness, and constipation. Low-dose vaginal estrogen creams, tablets, or rings may also be prescribed to provide relief of urinary symptoms (Evans & Karram, 2011).

? **Global Health Case Study** Adelita

Stress Urinary Incontinence

Adelita is a 45-year-old native of Mexico City, Mexico, who visits the Well Woman Clinic for her initial examination. During the interview, she confides in the nurse that she frequently leaks urine when she laughs or sneezes and finds this symptom, which has been present for approximately 6 months, to be embarrassing. She denies any symptoms of a urinary tract infection. Adelita states that she routinely wears a panty liner "just in case" she has an accident but would like to know whether this is "normal" and whether anything can be done.

Adelita has given birth to five children and underwent a postpartum bilateral tubal ligation after her youngest child was born 10 years ago. Her last menstrual period was 2 months ago; Adelita explains that lately she may "skip a month" and therefore doesn't know when to expect a period. The remainder of her medical history is unremarkable. Today's laboratory findings and physical examination (including pelvic exam) are within normal limits.

critical thinking questions

1. Based on Adelita's history and present symptoms, what is the most likely diagnosis?

2. What condition should first be ruled out?

3. The nurse anticipates what first-line approach for Adelita's stress urinary incontinence?

4. What teaching does the nurse provide Adelita?

5. What other information does the nurse provide?

Promoting Sexual Health During the Menopausal Years

Years ago, researchers Masters and Johnson studied sexuality in menopausal women and found that there is a general reduction in the four phases of the sexual response cycle with increasing years after menopause. However, they also discovered that women who maintained regular sexual activity experienced vaginal lubrication similar to levels expected in women who were premenopausal, and these women continued to be capable of full sexual response and enjoyment. Sexual activity is also beneficial in improving tone and blood flow to the pelvic floor.

Nursing Insight— *Sexual responsiveness in older women*

Sexual responsiveness reaches a peak for women in their late 30s and can remain on a high plateau into the 60s. Some women report an increased sexual desire after menopause. The fear of unwanted pregnancy often frees women to be much more sexually expressive and responsive than they were in their premenopausal years. When caring for midlife women, the nurse should never assume that sexual activity stops at age 65, or that a person without a partner is not sexually active (Halloran, 2012).

The two most important influences on older women's sexual activity are the strength of the relationship and the health status of each partner. The lack of an available partner can have a negative effect on sexual intimacy for many midlife and older women. When discussing sexuality issues with older women, it is important for nurses to provide safe sex counseling and accurate information, and offer support and nonjudgmental guidance. The nurse can reassure the woman that the desire for sex into old age is a natural one and the body continues to have the capacity for sexual satisfaction (Katz, 2011; Maes & Louis, 2011).

Many women do, however, experience changes in libido (sex drive), reduction in vaginal lubrication, discomfort during intercourse, and changes in orgasmic response in the years after menopause. The use of various oils (e.g., vegetable, vitamin E, olive) or vaginal lubricants that are specifically formulated for menopausal vaginal discomfort allows many older women to continue to enjoy sexual intercourse. Lengthening the foreplay time may promote enhanced vaginal lubrication as well.

"What to say" — *Initiating dialogue about menopausal sexual difficulties*

When discussing menopause-related problems, it is important to use patient-friendly terms such as *vaginal dryness, discomfort,* or *irritation* rather than *sexual dysfunction.* Owing to the fact that the patient may be reluctant to initiate dialogue about sexual or urinary problems, the nurse may enhance the woman's comfort level with questions such as

- "Many women come to our office with various complaints such as vaginal dryness, itching, and pain with sex. Have you experienced any of these problems?"

- "Have you had any problems with frequent urination, leaking urine, not making it to the bathroom on time, or burning during urination?"

- "Have you tried any vaginal lubricants or other products to enhance comfort during intercourse?" (Allmen & Moore, 2010; Kellog-Spadt, 2012).

Nurses can empower perimenopausal women with strategies to help combat vaginal dryness. Depending on the situation, the nurse may offer the following suggestions:

- Remain sexually active—sexual activity increases blood flow to the vagina, increases elasticity and lubrication of the vaginal tissues, and maintains muscle tone. Orgasm, achieved by any means, helps to decrease vaginal atrophy.

- Consume phytoestrogen-containing foods and herbs.

- Consider vitamin E, which has an estrogenic effect—apply vitamin E oil to the vagina; take vitamin E supplements (contraindicated in women with hypertension).

- Consider the use of vegetable or olive oil, which is more soothing to the genital tissue than the commercially available alcohol-based products, but be aware that the oils can degrade latex condoms.

- Consider vitamin C and bioflavonoids, substances that increase estrogen levels.

If natural remedies and interventions do not alleviate the discomfort associated with vaginal dryness, several nonprescription, nonhormonal products are available. For example, depending on the specific product used, Replens, Me Again, Vagisil Feminine Moisturizer, Feminease, Luvena, and KY Liquibeads may assist with moisture, lubrication, coital comfort, and normalization of vaginal pH. The duration of effectiveness is generally 24 to 48 hours. However, nonhormonal lubricants and moisturizers do not restore the integrity of the vagina. Nurses should caution women to avoid the use of Vaseline and other petroleum-based products, which can denigrate latex condoms and also increase the chance for infection. Also, some over-the-counter products have an alcohol base and can have an undesirable drying effect (Andelloux, 2011; Barbieri, 2013; Kellogg-Spadt, 2011, 2012).

For women who experience a significant decrease in sex drive along with intolerable vaginal symptoms, the use of estrogen therapy, delivered in the form of a vaginal cream or tablet or via a silastic device, may be helpful (ACOG, 2013a). Currently, FDA guidelines recommend the use of a vaginal hormonal preparation for menopausal women whose only symptom is vaginal atrophy (NAMS, 2010b). According to a position statement from The North American Menopause Society (2013), the choice of therapy for vulvovaginal atrophy depends on the severity of symptoms, the effectiveness and safety of therapy for the individual patient, and patient preference. Although estrogen therapy is the most effective treatment for moderate to severe symptoms, the safety of local estrogen in women with breast cancer is not known (NAMS, 2013).

Optimizing Outcomes— With the therapeutic effects of vaginal estrogen therapy

Vaginal estrogen therapy promotes a healthy vaginal ecology by restoring vaginal pH to premenopausal levels and normalizing vaginal cytology. Treatment also leads to substantial subjective relief and marked improvement of vulvovaginal atrophy manifestations. Restoration of the vaginal mucosa with subsequent improvement in symptoms associated with vaginal atrophy is likely to improve sexual function by facilitating intercourse. Vaginally delivered estrogen therapy may also reduce urinary urge incontinence and diminish the recurrence of urinary tract infections (Allmen & Moore, 2010; Minkin & Guess, 2012; Woods, 2013).

Low-dose vaginal estrogen cream (e.g., Premarin, Estrace) has been shown to significantly improve symptoms associated with vaginal dryness and reduce the incidence of urinary tract infections. Because systemic absorption of estrogen is minimal, most experts do not recommend the concomitant use of progestins to prevent endometrial hyperplasia in women who have a uterus. Typically, the woman is instructed to insert the estrogen cream into her vagina every day for the first 3 weeks, and then twice a week or as needed. Nurses need to instruct patients to discontinue local estrogen therapy for several days before a Pap screening so as not to obscure the cytology slide. A tablet that contains a low dose of estradiol (e.g., Vagifem) is also available; it is inserted in the vagina twice a week. Nurses should counsel all women who use estrogen therapy to promptly report any vaginal bleeding or breast pain (Nelson, 2011; Woods, 2013).

Hormonal vaginal rings, which are silastic devices impregnated with estrogen (estradiol), offer another option. The vaginal rings Estring and Femring are designed to deliver a slow release of estrogen (estradiol) locally to the vagina. The vaginal ring is inserted for a period of 3 months and then replaced by the patient or health-care provider. The Estring is formulated with an ultra-low dose of estradiol (7.5 micrograms released per day) and is associated with minimal systemic absorption. No concomitant progestin therapy (to prevent endometrial hyperplasia in women who have a uterus) is necessary. The Femring is formulated with a higher dose of estradiol (available to deliver 0.05 mg per day or 0.1 mg per day), and women with an intact uterus who use this product should almost always receive a progestin to avoid endometrial hyperplasia. Vaginal rings can be displaced by a rectocele (bulging of the front wall of the rectum into the back wall of the vagina) or cystocele (herniation of the bladder into the vagina). Some older women with limited dexterity may experience difficulty positioning the vaginal ring, and the ring may become dislodged with intercourse, douching, or defecation. If a woman is unable to self-insert the ring, she can visit her health-care provider every 3 months for a replacement and continue to receive ongoing local therapy (Minkin, 2013; Minkin & Guess, 2012; Nelson, 2011; Pearson, 2011; Woods, 2013).

In 2013, the FDA approved a new oral drug for vulvar and vaginal atrophy. Ospemifene (Osphena) is a tissue-selective estrogen agonist/antagonist (i.e., acts as an estrogen agonist in some tissues and an estrogen antagonist in others) designed for the treatment of dyspareunia caused by vulvar and vaginal atrophy in menopausal women. In clinical trials, ospemifene (administered in a once-daily oral 60 mg dose) was found to reduce pain with sexual intercourse and increase vaginal mucosal maturation and vaginal pH to a greater extent than placebo. According to package labeling, clinicians should consider adding a progestin to prevent endometrial neoplasia in women with an intact uterus using ospemifene; also, endometrial monitoring should also be considered in long-term users. The use of vaginal or systemic estrogen is contraindicated in women with breast cancer; other contraindications include venous thromboembolism (VTE) (current or personal history), stroke, and myocardial infarction (or a history of it). Adverse reactions to the medication include hot flushes, vaginal discharge, and muscle spasms (Portman, Bachmann, & Simon, 2013).

Nursing Insight— Lichen sclerosis et atrophicus and vulvovaginal symptoms

Lichen sclerosis et atrophicus (LS&A) is a rare, benign, chronic, and progressive skin condition that usually affects the vulva in postmenopausal women. Lesions of vulvar LS&A appear as thin, white, finely scaly patches with diffuse borders affecting the labia majora and minora. Diagnosis is made by the histological examination of a vulvar punch biopsy. Hormonal factors, genetics, immunological abnormalities, and local factors such as infection have been suggested possible causes, although the actual etiology of LS&A is unknown. Most patients complain of nonspecific vulvar irritation or discomfort of variable intensity. Interestingly, some women are completely asymptomatic; others with severe disease and related symptoms (e.g., intense pruritus, pain, ulceration) may develop dysuria, dyspareunia, and vaginal or meatal stenosis. Treatment usually consists of the nightly application of a topical corticosteroid such as clobetasol (Temovate, Clobex) or halobetasol propionate (Ultravate). Because patients with genital LS&A are at an increased risk for the development of squamous cell cancer, routine follow-up is essential (Monroe, 2012).

HOT FLUSHES, FLASHES, NIGHT SWEATS, AND SLEEP DISTURBANCES

One of the hallmarks of menopause is the occurrence of the vasomotor symptoms hot flushes, hot flashes, and night sweats. A *hot flush* is a visible red flush of skin and perspiration. A *hot flash* is a sudden warm sensation in the neck, head, and chest; heat may be radiated from all parts of the body. During a hot flash, skin temperatures rise as a result of peripheral vasodilation and sweating begins primarily on the upper body. Most women describe a sudden sweeping wave of heat sensation that spreads over the body. An increase in the heart rate of about 7 to 15 beats per minute occurs at approximately the same time as the peripheral vasodilation and sweating. It may take up to 30 minutes or longer for skin temperatures to return to normal. Hot flashes can occur infrequently (e.g., monthly; weekly) or frequently (hourly), although there is usually an individual pattern. A circadian rhythm has been observed, with hot flash frequency peaking in the early evening hours—about 3 hours after the peak in core body temperature (NAMS, 2010b).

Night sweats are characterized by profuse perspiration and heat radiating from the body during the night. The woman's sleep may be interrupted each night because her nightclothes and bed linens become soaked with perspiration. Hot flashes constitute the most common symptom reported by women experiencing menopause and are present in 68% to 90% of women. They can occur often throughout the day and create anxiety, distress, and a significantly decreased quality of life (NAMS, 2010b).

Nursing Insight— *Vasomotor symptoms and NAMS terminology*

The terms "vasomotor symptoms," "hot flash," and "hot flush" are often used to describe the same phenomenon. The North American Menopause Society (NAMS) defines vasomotor symptoms as a global term that encompasses both hot flashes and night sweats. NAMS prefers the term "hot flash" rather than "hot flush" (NAMS, 2010b).

For some women, hot flashes are only a significant problem for 1 to 2 years; others experience vasomotor symptoms that can persist for up to 15 years. Approximately 10% to 15% of women characterize their hot flashes as "debilitating." In many non-Westernized cultures, hot flashes either do not occur or are so minimal they are barely noticed. In this country, hot flashes cause women to seek medical advice more than any other symptom of menopause (Freeman, Sammel, Lin, Liu, & Gracia, 2011; NAMS, 2010b; Nelson, 2011).

The cause of the alternating vasodilation and vasoconstriction associated with hot flashes is not well understood, but it is known that this symptom is related to hormonal changes that affect the temperature-regulating centers in the hypothalamus. Low levels of estrogen alone are not responsible. It is believed that the presence of estrogen, followed by its withdrawal, triggers an imbalance in the body's temperature control center, which subsequently decreases the core body temperature. The body then attempts to activate heat centers to readjust the body's thermostat. Other problems that may be associated with vasomotor instability include dizziness, numbness, or tingling in the fingers and toes and headaches. Environmental and lifestyle factors such as being in a crowded or warm room, consuming hot drinks, nitrates, alcohol or spicy foods, and stress can precipitate or aggravate an episode of vasomotor symptoms (Hauser, 2012).

Optimizing Outcomes— Consider alternate causes for various vasomotor symptoms

The nurse should be aware of other conditions that may cause vasomotor symptoms in women. These include thyroid disease, epilepsy, infection, pheochromocytoma (a rare tumor of the adrenal gland), leukemia, pancreatic tumors, autoimmune disorders, new onset hypertension, and mast-cell disorders. Also, some medications, such as tamoxifen (Nolvadex) and raloxifene (Evista), can cause hot flashes. Night sweats may be associated with more serious diseases, such as tuberculosis and lymphoma (NAMS, 2010b).

Sleep disturbance is associated with menopausal symptoms (e.g., hot flashes, night sweats) and, most important, with comorbidities (e.g., obesity, diabetes, depression, esophageal reflux) and stress. Some menopausal women experience depressive symptoms, which may be related to a lack of restorative sleep. However, clinical depression is not a part of the perimenopausal period for most women, and routine screening for depression should be a component of well-woman visits for all ages. Sleep disorders in midlifewomen should not be attributed solely to the menopausal symptom experience. Referral for clinical evaluation to assess for primary sleep disorders such as restless legs, insomnia, or sleep-disordered breathing may be appropriate (Chichester & Ciranni, 2011; Edelman, 2012; NAMS, 2010b; Rajki, 2011).

Now Can You— Discuss Certain Aspects of Menopause?

1. Differentiate among the terms "climacteric," "premenopause," "perimenopause," and "postmenopause"?
2. Identify menstrual cycle changes, hormonal changes, skin and hair changes, and urogenital changes that typically accompany menopause?
3. Describe four strategies for maintaining and promoting sexual health and enjoyment during the menopausal transition and later years?
4. Identify and describe various vasomotor symptoms that frequently accompany menopause?

Promoting Comfort During the Menopausal Transition

COMPLEMENTARY AND ALTERNATIVE MEDICINE

Complementary and alternative medicine (CAM) includes a broad base of healing philosophies, approaches, and therapies that conventional medicine has not commonly understood or used. In general, a therapy is termed "complementary" when it is used *in addition to* conventional treatment, and it is called "alternative" when it is used *instead of* conventional treatment (NAMS, 2010b).

Many women use CAM approaches such as stress management, guided imagery, biofeedback, massage therapy, yoga, chiropractic care, acupuncture, and dietary supplements to relieve various menopausal symptoms. Other nonmedicinal interventions for the relief of mild vasomotor symptoms include engaging in regular exercise; consuming cool, refreshing foods such as cabbage, cucumbers, and pineapple; minimizing the intake of alcohol, fatty foods, sugar, and caffeine; avoiding "triggers" such as hot drinks, alcohol, or spicy foods; and dressing in layers to keep cool. Wearing clothing made of cotton, washable linen, or fabrics that wick perspiration away from the skin and increase air movement can increase comfort. Synthetic fabrics such as polyester should be avoided, as they can trap body heat and trigger hot flashes. Nurses can also counsel women to drink eight to 10 glasses of water each day and perform deep-breathing or paced-respiration exercises at the beginning of a hot flash to diminish its effects (NAMS, 2010b; Nelson, 2011).

❊ Complementary Care: *Paced respiration may help relieve hot flashes*

Paced respiration, a pattern of slow, deliberate deep breathing sustained over a specific period of time, has been used to reduce hot flashes in healthy midlife women. One simple technique involves the following instruction: Breathe deeply. Inhale deeply, then exhale and try to make the exhalation last as long as the inhalation; repeat this several times as needed. Current evidence suggests that paced respiration at six to eight breaths per minute, when practiced 15 minutes twice a day, and initiated at the onset of hot flashes, can be beneficial (Burns & Carpenter, 2012).

Daily aerobic exercise helps to reduce the frequency and severity of hot flashes by assisting in body-temperature regulation. Exercise is also beneficial in reducing cardiovascular disease and osteoporosis risk and helps to maintain normal glucose levels and weight. Midlife women who engage in regular exercise report a higher quality of life, and routine exercise can help to improve depression, muscular soreness or stiffness, palpitations, memory, and sleep quality (Nelson, 2011).

In 1998, the U.S. Congress established the National Center for Complementary and Alternative Medicine (NCCAM) at the National Institutes of Health to stimulate, develop, and support research on CAM for the benefit of the public. NCCAM was charged with providing the American public with reliable information about the safety and effectiveness of CAM practices. NCCAM groups CAM therapies into the following five major domains: Alternative Medical Systems; Mind-Body Medicine; Manipulative and Body-Based Methods; Energy Medicine; and Biologically-Based Treatment (NAMS, 2010b).

Alternative Medical Systems

Alternative medical systems include complete systems of theory and practice that have evolved independent of and often prior to the conventional biomedical approach. Many are traditional systems of medicine practiced by individual cultures throughout the world. Alternative Medical Systems, Mind-Body Medicine, Manipulative and Body-Based Methods, and Energy Medicine are briefly described in Box 7-2.

❊ Nursing Insight— *Traditional Chinese medicine and menopause*

Traditional Chinese Medicine (TCM) includes menopause as part of a phenomenon that involves an imbalance of body energy. The TCM practitioner may use herbs, meditative or breathing exercises, massage, or diet to help a woman restore and balance the energy, and therefore, reduce menopausal symptoms. TCM practitioners may also use acupuncture for treating symptoms associated with menopause (NAMS, 2010b).

Biologically Based Treatments

Biologically based complementary and alternative medicines include biologically based practices, interventions, and products, many of which overlap with conventional medicine's use of dietary supplements. Botanical therapies

---

Box 7-2 Alternative Medical Systems, Mind-Body Medicine, Manipulative and Body-Based Methods, and Energy Medicine

ALTERNATIVE MEDICAL SYSTEMS

Traditional Chinese Medicine (TCM)

Traditional Chinese Medicine is a system of healing that dates back to 200 BC in written form. TCM emphasizes the proper balance of two opposing and inseparable forces: yin and yang. Yin represents the cold, slow, or passive principle, and yang represents the hot, excited, or active principle. An imbalance of these two forces is thought to lead to blockage in the flow of qi (pronounced "chee" and meaning "vital energy") and of blood along pathways known as meridians. TCM consists of a group of techniques and methods, including acupuncture, herbal medicine, oriental massage, and qi gong, to bring the body back into harmony and balance (NAMS, 2010b).

Ayurveda

Meaning "science of life," Ayurveda is India's traditional system of medicine. Ayurvedic medicine is a comprehensive system of medicine that places equal emphasis on body, mind, and spirit and strives to restore the innate harmony of the individual. Some of the primary Ayurvedic treatments include diet, exercise, meditation, herbs, massage, exposure to sunlight, and controlled breathing (NAMS, 2010b).

Homeopathic Medicine

Homeopathy is an unconventional Western system that is based on the principle that "like cures like" (i.e., large doses of a particular substance may produce symptoms of an illness, very small doses will cure it). Very small doses of specially prepared plant extracts and minerals are used to stimulate the body's defense mechanisms and healing processes to treat illness. The homeopathic approach focuses on the links among an individual's physical, emotional, and mental symptoms (NAMS, 2010b).

Naturopathic Medicine

In naturopathic medicine, disease is viewed as a manifestation of alterations in the processes by which the body naturally heals itself, and emphasis is placed on health restoration rather than on disease treatment. Practitioners of naturopathic medicine employ a variety of healing practices, including diet and clinical nutrition, homeopathy, acupuncture, herbal medicine, hydrotherapy, spinal and soft-tissue manipulation, physical therapies involving electric currents, ultrasound and light therapy, therapeutic counseling, and pharmacology (NAMS, 2010b).

MIND-BODY MEDICINE

Mind-body medicine focuses on the interactions among the brain, mind, body, and behavior and the powerful ways in which emotional, mental, social, spiritual, and behavioral factors can directly affect health. Mind-body medicine is an approach that respects and enhances each person's capacity for self-knowledge and self-care and emphasizes techniques that are grounded in this approach. Hypnosis, dance, music and art therapy, prayer and mental healing, relaxation and visual imagery, meditation, and yoga are typical techniques used with this approach (NAMS, 2010b).

MANIPULATIVE AND BODY-BASED METHODS

These methods are based on manipulation and/or movement of structures and systems of the body, including bones and joints, the soft tissues, and the circulatory and lymphatic systems. While there is considerable variation in the training and approaches of manipulative and body-based providers, they all share certain principles, such as the belief that the human body is self-regulating and has the ability to heal itself. Practitioners of manipulative and body-based methods include osteopathic physicians (DOs), massage therapists, and reflexologists (NAMS, 2010b).

ENERGY MEDICINE

Energy therapies focus on either energy fields originating within the body (putative energy fields [biofields], which cannot be measured), or those from other sources (veritable energy fields that involve the use of measurable wavelengths and frequencies, also called "electromagnetic fields"). Examples of putative energy medicine include qi gong, Reiki, intercessory prayer, and therapeutic touch (NAMS, 2010b).

are complex mixtures of preparations made from the whole plant or plant part, such as root, leaves, gum, resin, or essential oil. Most botanical therapies are medicinal herbs. A medicinal herb is a plant or plant part that produces and contains chemical substances that act on the body (NAMS, 2010b).

✤ Complementary Care: *Herbal therapies: modes of administration*

Herbal therapies intended for ingestion may be administered in a variety of ways, such as:

- Tea infusions (soft, aromatic parts of the plant are steeped, not boiled, in water)
- Tea decoctions (barks and roots, boiled in water)
- Essential oils (highly concentrated)
- Tinctures and fluid extracts (herbs macerated into water-alcohol mixtures)
- Dried standardized extract (these typically contain part of a plant but can contain the whole plant; extracts are standardized to one ingredient only)
- Homeopathic preparations (extremely diluted)

(NAMS, 2010b)

The most studied of the botanicals for menopause-related conditions are compounds often termed *phytoestrogens* (sometimes called "dietary estrogens"). Phytoestrogens are a diverse group of naturally occurring nonsteroidal plant compounds that have a structural similarity with estradiol and are able to exert estrogenic and/or antiestrogenic effects. There are three principal groups of phytoestrogens: isoflavones, coumestans, and lignans. Because herbal compounds containing phytoestrogens are not FDA regulated, there is no proof of the efficacy, safety, or overall quality of the products. Until such information becomes available, these remedies should be considered to have the same issues as traditional menopausal hormone therapy (discussed later in this chapter) (NAMS, 2010b).

⑤ legal alert— Advise women to use isoflavones with caution

Isoflavones (e.g., red clover, soy) are the most widely used phytoestrogens for menopause. Isoflavones comprise a class of organic compounds, often naturally occurring, related to the isoflavonoids. Some isoflavones and isoflavone-rich foods possess activity against cancer, including certain types of breast and prostate cancers. Isoflavones are produced almost exclusively by members of the bean family, and soybeans are the most common source of isoflavones in human food. Soy and other isoflavone supplements are regulated in the United States as dietary supplements; their effectiveness has not been well established, and they are not monitored for purity, amount of active ingredient, or health claims. Possible adverse effects associated with these products include constipation, diarrhea, belching, bloating, nausea, and insomnia; conflicting data exist concerning breast cancer risk (NAMS, 2010b; Reed & Guiltinan, 2010).

Phytoestrogens interact with estrogen receptors in the body. Foods that contain phytoestrogens include wild yams, cashews, peanuts and almonds, dandelion greens,

apples, cherries, alfalfa sprouts, sage, black beans, and soy products (e.g., beans, flour, milk, sauce). The use of soy-rich foods has also been investigated as an alternative to hormone therapy for menopausal symptoms. According to the Natural Standard database, there is good evidence for sage and soy for menopause symptom management (http://www.naturalstandard.com/). The North American Menopause Society (NAMS) concedes that soy products may have small benefits in the treatment of vasomotor symptoms in the short term (12 weeks), but not for longer periods (6–12 months). According to NAMS, there is strong evidence that soy is nonbeneficial in the prevention of postmenopausal bone loss, but may be useful in maintaining cognitive function; however, additional studies are needed (NAMS, 2010b; Sego, 2012).

An important role for nurses centers on counseling women to become informed about any herbal preparations they are considering, and to consult with their health-care providers before using any of them. Nurses should explain that before using any substance, it is important to understand the mechanisms of action, contraindications, and potential adverse effects. Herbs may be beneficial in resolving physical symptoms, as well as mood swings and depression. To obtain current information about various dietary supplements, health professionals and consumers may consult various Internet sites such as those offered by the U.S. National Library of Medicine and the National Institutes of Health (http://www.nlm.nih.gov/medlineplus/dietarysupplements.html), and (http://www.nlm.nih.gov/medlineplus/druginformation.html), and the U.S.D.A. National Agricultural Library (http://nal.usda.gov/).

Nurses may also inform patients who wish to use soy, herbs, or other dietary supplements about ConsumerLab (http://www.consumerlab.com/), an independent company that tests and provides objective reviews of many over-the-counter consumer supplements; there is an annual subscription fee to access the information.

Oriental herbal teas composed of licorice, ginseng, sage, coptis, red raspberry leaf, and Chinese rhubarb may provide some relief for hot flashes. Dong quai and black cohosh have been used for various menopausal discomforts. Dong quai, the most commonly prescribed Chinese herbal medicine for "female problems," purportedly regulates and balances the menstrual cycle and is said to "strengthen the uterus." It is also purported to exert estrogenic activity. However, dong quai has not been found to be useful in reducing hot flashes and is not recommended for this symptom. Also, dong quai can trigger heavy uterine bleeding and should never be used in women who have fibroids, hemophilia, or other blood-clotting problems; it is contraindicated for use with anticoagulants (ACOG, 2014; NAMS, 2010b).

Black cohosh (*Cimicifuga racemosa*) may be helpful in the short-term (less than 2 years) treatment of menopausal symptoms including hot flashes, sleep disorders, anxiety, and depression. There have been case reports of possible hepatotoxicity associated with black cohosh, but no serious liver-related diseases were observed or reported in trials. Both dong quai and black cohosh have been investigated for effectiveness, with varying results. According to the National Center for Complementary and Alternative Medicine (NCCAM) (http://nccam.nih.gov/), there is very little high-quality scientific evidence about the effectiveness and long-term safety of complementary and alternative medicine for menopausal symptoms (ACOG, 2014; Anastasi, Chang, & Capili, 2011; McCracken & Dunaway, 2011; NAMS, 2010b; Reed & Guiltinan, 2010; Teschke, 2010).

Complementary Care: *St. John's wort, valerian, chasteberry, and ginseng*

St. John's wort and valerian root have been used for mood disturbances during menopause. The flower hypericum perforatum, known as St. John's wort, has been used for centuries to treat mild to moderate depression. Commercial preparations typically contain the generally recommended doses and one capsule is taken three times a day. Side effects are similar to but much less than those associated with standard antidepressant medications and include fatigue, dry mouth, dizziness, and constipation. St. John's wort should not be used concomitantly with psychotropic medications. Valerian root (*Valeriana officinalis*) has traditionally been used as a tranquilizer and soporific. Valerian improves subjective experiences of sleep when taken nightly for 1 to 2 weeks. Although it has no demonstrable toxicity, there have been reports of adverse reactions and visual disturbances. Little is known about the actions, effects, or potential interactions of valerian with other medications (ACOG, 2014; NAMS, 2010b).

Some practitioners have recommended chasteberry and ginseng for menopausal loss of libido. Chasteberry, or vitex, is also known as chaste tree, Monk's pepper, agnus castus, Indian spice, sage tree hemp, and tree wild pepper. It has been used for vaginal dryness at menopause and also for depression and to enhance libido in menopausal women. Asian ginseng (Panax ginseng) is promoted as an "adaptogen" that helps one cope with stress and boost immunity. Ginseng is also reputed to be an aphrodisiac, although this claim has not been substantiated by medical evidence (ACOG, 2014; NAMS, 2010b). According to the Natural Standard database, there is poor evidence for ginseng and chasteberry for the treatment of menopausal symptoms. However, there is good evidence for both sage and soy for menopause symptom management.

Now Can You— Discuss various CAM therapies for menopausal symptoms?

1. Identify and briefly describe three alternative medical systems?
2. Describe the major focus of mind-body medicine and identify six examples of typical techniques used with this approach?
3. Briefly explain the techniques of intercessory prayer and healing touch?
4. Provide appropriate counseling to a woman who wishes to use herbal products?

HORMONAL THERAPIES

Estrogen is the only pharmacological therapy that is government approved in the United States and Canada for treating menopause-related symptoms. Estrogen-containing drugs for menopausal use are divided into two categories: estrogen therapy (ET) and combined estrogen-progestogen therapy (EPT) (NAMS, 2010b).

Nursing Insight— *NAMS menopausal hormone therapy terminology*

Estrogen therapy (ET)—unopposed estrogen prescribed for postmenopausal women who have had a hysterectomy.

Estrogen plus progestogen (EPT)—a combination of estrogen and progestogen (either progesterone or progestin, synthetic forms of progesterone). Although the available data suggest that the benefits of EPT are almost exclusively the result of estrogen, progestogen reduces the risk of endometrial adenocarcinoma in women with a uterus—and this risk is significantly increased in women who use unopposed estrogen.

Hormone therapy (HT)—encompasses both ET and EPT. The FDA refers to EPT as HT.

Local therapy—vaginal ET administration that does not result in clinically significant systemic absorption

Progestogen—encompasses both progesterone and progestin

Systemic therapy—HT administration that results in absorption in the blood high enough to provide clinically significant results

Timing of HT initiation—length of time after menopause when HT is initiated

(NAMS, 2010b)

Previously, the terms *estrogen replacement therapy* and *hormone replacement therapy* were used. However, according to the North American Menopause Society (NAMS), the term *replacement* is a misnomer because postmenopausal levels of HT provide only a small fraction of the estrogen the ovaries once produced. The FDA declared that the word *replacement* can no longer be used by marketers of products available in the United States. The FDA uses *ET* to describe unopposed estrogen therapy and *HT* to describe EPT. NAMS, however, prefers using *HT* to encompass all hormone therapy used for menopause, and *EPT* to more clearly describe combined therapy (NAMS, 2010b).

Menopause hormone therapy (HT) is a controversial issue. A brief review of the historical background, recent research, and current guidelines for use of HT can assist women and their health-care providers in making the appropriate decisions concerning this treatment option.

Historical Background

The widespread use of prescribing estrogen began in the 1960s. Estrogen was touted as a wonder drug that offered women the opportunity to age more slowly. By 1975, conjugated equine estrogen, marketed under the name of Premarin, was one of the most frequently prescribed drugs in the United States. Premarin is derived from the urine of pregnant mares. For many years, animal rights activists have promoted public awareness of cruelty to these animals and their offspring involved in the production of Premarin (National Women's Health Network, 2000).

In 1975, two studies were published that showed a two- to eightfold increase in the rate of uterine cancer among nonhysterectomized women receiving estrogen therapy. The risk was linked to estrogen dosage and the duration of treatment. In response to this finding, a number of women's organizations sought to heighten public awareness of the risks associated with estrogen use, claiming that women were not given adequate information to make informed choices. As this information became more widespread, use of estrogen in this country declined. Later studies were conducted to investigate combinations of estrogen and a progestin (a synthetic form of progesterone). Results of these studies revealed that the estrogen-progestin combination protected against precancerous changes of the uterine lining. Based on these findings, a shift to the use of estrogen-progestin combinations occurred (National Women's Health Network, 2000).

By the late 1980s, results of several studies had shown that women who received estrogen were less likely to suffer heart attacks than those who did not receive estrogen. Although the FDA refused to grant approval to the manufacturer for prescribing estrogen to healthy women as a heart disease preventive, many clinicians were recommending estrogen for this purpose. Without long-term data, the combination of estrogen along with a progestin began to be prescribed for this same purpose, even though the combination had not been in use long enough to evaluate its effect on heart disease. The Postmenopausal Estrogen/Progestin Interventions (PEPI) study was published in 1995. The results from this trial showed that the most commonly used progestin, medroxyprogesterone acetate (Provera), greatly interfered with the positive effect of estrogen alone on high-density lipoprotein (HDL) levels. Natural progesterone (i.e., oral micronized progesterone), also used in the study, did not negate the positive effects of estrogen on HDL levels (National Women's Health Network, 2000). Major findings from other studies, including the Heart and Estrogen/Progestin Replacement Study (HERS I and II), the Nurse's Health Study, the Women's Health Initiative (WHI), and the Kronos Early Estrogen Prevention Study (KEEPS), are summarized in Box 7-3.

Where Research and Practice Meet: Considerations of the WHI Research Results

Findings from the WHI research may be used to guide patient education and counseling. Nurses should consider the following points (Chlebowski et al., 2010; Ribowsky, 2011; Rossouw, Manson, Kaunitz, & Anderson, 2013):

- The HT arm of the WHI trial was stopped because the rate of breast cancer crossed a predetermined boundary set at the initiation of the trial. However, breast cancer rates had not reached a statistical significance when the trial was halted.
- The fact that that the slight increase in invasive breast cancer was noted during the fourth year of the study, along with the trend toward a later decrease in the total number of breast cancer cases, suggests that HT promotes the growth of existing breast cancer, rather than causes breast cancer. No increased risk in breast cancer was seen among women on estrogen therapy for an average of 7.1 years. Estrogen plus progestin therapy, but not estrogen therapy, increased the risk of breast cancer with a suggestion of greater risk when initiated close to the menopause. Estrogen-progestin therapy, and to a lesser extent, estrogen therapy, increases breast cell proliferation, breast pain, and mammographic density. Hormone therapy may impede the diagnostic interpretation of mammograms. Women with risk factors for breast cancer (e.g., positive family history, early puberty, late parity) should be individually assessed before initiating HT for the relief of moderate to severe vasomotor symptoms.
- For the first time for any therapy, findings from the WHI study indicated that HT reduces hip fractures and colon cancer.

Box 7-3 Major Findings From the HERS, WHI, and KEEPS Studies

The *Heart and Estrogen/Progestin Replacement Study (HERS)* (1998), the *Heart and Estrogen/Progestin Replacement Study Follow-up (HERS II)* (2002), and the *Nurse's Health Study* (1976, 1989)

- These studies are designed to assess the relationship between HT and coronary artery disease events among postmenopausal women.
- Although findings from the HERS II study showed that HT did not provide cardiac protection in women who had previously been diagnosed with heart disease, reanalysis of data indicated that certain women (e.g., women on statin medications to lower cholesterol) experienced fewer problems associated with thromboembolic events (Alexander, 2007).

THE WOMEN'S HEALTH INITIATIVE (WHI) (1991)

- A long-term primary prevention trial conducted over 15 years with more than 160,000 healthy postmenopausal women aged 50 to 79.
- Purpose: to evaluate the safety and effectiveness of estrogen as well as an estrogen/progestin combination given to healthy women over a 9-year period beginning in 1993, with final analysis planned for 2005.
- Designed to assess the major benefits and risks of hormone therapy with regard to coronary heart disease, venous thrombotic events, breast cancer, colon cancer, and fractures.
- Quality of life issues, such as a reduction in hot flashes and vaginal dryness, were not included.
- In July 2002, after approximately 5 years of follow-up, the estrogen and progestin arm of the WHI trial was halted because the predetermined boundary for invasive breast cancer was exceeded. At this time, it was concluded that the risks outweighed the benefits for the indicators that were being studied.
- The risk of cardiovascular disease (CVD), coronary heart disease (CHD), stroke, and venous thromboembolism (VTE) was increased as well (Writing Group for the Women's Health Initiative Investigators, 2002).
- There was a 37% and a 24% decrease in colorectal cancer and total fractures, respectively.
- Of importance, there was no difference in rates of mortality between the two groups (i.e., those who did receive HT and those who did not receive HT).
- In 2004, the estrogen-only trial was also halted because the risk with the conjugated equine estrogen (Premarin) for stroke was elevated and the other endpoints were unlikely to change with continuation of the trial.
- Later analysis of the findings suggested that timing of hormone therapy use has an effect: In the age 50 to 59 cohort, coronary heart disease was decreased. Based on this information, it is believed to be safest to begin hormone therapy within 10 years of menopause.
- Another follow-up study of the WHI participants demonstrated that women aged 50 to 59 that were on estrogen therapy had lower amounts of calcium deposits in their coronary arteries (Rossow, Maanson, Kaunitz, & Anderson, 2013; Williams & Brownlee, 2010; Writing Group for the Women's Health Initiative Investigators, 2002).

THE KRONOS EARLY ESTROGEN PREVENTION STUDY (KEEPS) (2012)

- Goal was to explore the effects of oral and transdermal HT in a younger (aged 42–58), newly menopausal (within 3 years after menopause) population.
- Favorable effects of HT: relief of menopausal symptoms (i.e., improved sleep and quality of life, improved dyspareunia, preservation of bone mineral density).
- Improved libido and reduced insulin resistance (transdermal formulation only).
- No increase in blood pressure (with oral or transdermal formulation).
- Mood, depression, anxiety, and tension improved (oral formulation only).

Source: Manson (2013).

Menopausal Hormone Therapy: Considerations and Choices

Owing to the findings from large-scale prospective clinical trials such as the WHI, which demonstrated that hormone therapy is not without risks, the FDA and several professional organizations recommend prescribing the lowest effective dose for the shortest duration of time consistent with treatment goals for the individual patient. Growing evidence indicates that the benefits and risks vary with the type of estrogen and progestogen prescribed, as well as the route of administration, timing of therapy, baseline risk of disease, chronological age, age at menopause, cause of menopause, time since menopause, and previous use of any hormone (Rassouw et al., 2013). A summary of NAMS (2012) recommendations concerning HT for the treatment of various menopausal symptoms is presented in Box 7-4.

Recommendations for duration of use differ between estrogen therapy (ET) and estrogen-progestin therapy (EPT). Owing to the fact that ET is associated with a more favorable safety profile, it is generally considered for longer duration of therapy in the absence of adverse effects and risk factors. Women who experience a premature menopause are at an increased risk of osteoporosis and possibly cardiovascular disease, and they frequently experience more intense symptoms than do women who reach menopause at the median age. Hence, HT is frequently advised for these young women until the median age of menopause when treatment should be reassessed (NAMS, 2012).

Today, clinicians have a wide variety of estrogen products from which to choose, including oral tablets; transdermal patches; and topical sprays, gels, and lotions, as well as vaginal creams, tablets, and rings. The choice of therapy is often based on patient preference. Examples of estrogen and progestogen products for menopause-related symptoms are presented in Box 7-5; The North American Menopause Society has prepared charts for health-care providers that include information about all estrogen and progestogen products that are currently available in the United States and Canada. The charts may be viewed at http://www.menopause.org/publications/clinical-practice-materials/hormone-therapy-charts.

The Nursing Role in Menopausal Hormone Therapy Counseling

When counseling women about HT benefits and risks, it is helpful to consider a number of factors, such as cardiac protection, osteoporosis prevention, short- and long-term hormone use, and alternatives to HT. Women who are taking or considering HT only for the prevention of cardiovascular disease should be counseled about other strategies to lower their risks of heart disease.

Nursing Insight— *Hormone therapy and heart disease*

According to the American College of Obstetricians and Gynecologists (ACOG) (2013a) and The North American Menopause Society (NAMS) (2010b), menopausal HT should not be used for the primary or secondary prevention of coronary heart disease at present. Findings from a recent (2013) Cochrane review suggest that treatment with HT for either primary or secondary prevention of CVD events is not effective and causes an increase in the risk of stroke and venous thromboembolic events. Hormone therapy use should be limited to the treatment of menopausal symptoms at the lowest effective dosage over the shortest duration possible, and continued use should be reevaluated on a periodic basis. Treatment should be used with caution in women with predisposing risk factors for CVD events (Main et al., 2013).

Box 7-4 Summary of NAMS 2012 Recommendations for HT Use

Breast cancer: Diagnosis of breast cancer increases with EPT use longer than 3 to 5 years; women who start EPT shortly after menopause may have a greater risk than women who start more than 5 years afterward. Because risk for breast cancer does not appear to increase during an average of 7 years of ET use, there is more flexibility in duration of ET treatment. ET use in breast cancer survivors has not been proved to be safe and may be associated with an increased risk of recurrence.

Cognitive aging and dementia: Available data do not adequately address whether HT used soon after menopause increases or decreases the rate of cognitive decline or later dementia risk. HT is not recommended at any age for preventing or treating cognitive aging or dementia.

Coronary heart disease: HT is not recommended as a sole or primary indication for coronary protection at any age; starting ET alone soon after menopause may slow development of calcified atherosclerotic plaque and lower CHD risk.

Diabetes mellitus: Inadequate evidence to recommend HT as the sole or primary indication for preventing diabetes in perimenopausal or postmenopausal women.

Endometrial cancer: Women with an intact uterus taking systemic ET should take concomitant progestogen to counteract the risk of endometrial cancer; HT is not recommended for women with a history of endometrial cancer.

Mood and depression: Although HT might have a positive effect on mood and behavior, HT is not an antidepressant and should not be considered as such; evidence is insufficient to support HT use for the treatment of depression.

Osteoporosis: Extended HT is an option for women with decreased bone mass; benefits decrease quickly once therapy has ended; standard-dose HT reduces postmenopausal osteoporotic fractures, even in women without osteoporosis, and low doses are effective in maintaining or improving bone mineral density. However, no HT product currently has government approval for the treatment of osteoporosis.

Ovarian cancer: Data on HT and ovarian cancer conflict; the association between ovarian cancer and HT beyond 5 years is rare.

Stroke: HT is not recommended for primary or secondary prevention of stroke.

Vasomotor symptoms: Moderate to severe vasomotor symptoms (e.g., hot flashes, night sweats) remain the primary indication for HT; also best treatment for moderate to severe vulvar and vaginal atrophy; local vaginal ET is recommended for treating urogenital atrophy alone; systemic or local ET can relieve dyspareunia. The most effective treatment for menopausal vasomotor symptoms and associated quality of life is ET or EPT.

Venous thromboembolism (VTE): Most likely an increased risk of VTE with oral HT, especially in women with a history of VTE or factor V Leiden (a hypercoagulability disorder).

Sources: ACOG (2013a, 2014); Main et al. (2013); NAMS (2012); Rossouw et al. (2013); Shifren & Schiff (2010).

Box 7-5 Examples of Estrogen and Progestogen Products for Menopause-Related Symptoms

ESTROGEN ONLY

Estrace, Premarin (oral tablet, vaginal cream)

Femtrace, Ogen (oral tablet)

Alora, Climara, Estraderm, Menostar, Minivelle, Vivelle, (transdermal patch)

Divigel, Elestrin, EstroGel, Estrasorb (transdermal gel, emulsion)

Femring, Estring (vaginal ring)

Vagifem (vaginal tablet)

Evamist (topical spray)

PROGESTOGEN ONLY

Provera (oral tablet)

Prometrium (oral tablet)

ESTROGEN-PROGESTOGEN COMBINATIONS

CombiPatch (transdermal patch)

Climara Pro (transdermal patch)

health (ACOG, 2013a; Fantasia & Sutherland, 2014; NAMS, 2010b).

Estrogens do not cause endometrial cancer, as long as an appropriate dosage of progestogen (either as progestin or progesterone) is added to the hormonal regimen. Individual regimens and formulations differ and include both synthetic and natural formulations. Each route and type of progestogen carries different effects, risks, and benefits. The estrogen-progesterone combinations are available in oral and transdermal patch formulations. It has been shown that women who use combined HT are no more likely than those who have never used HT to develop overgrowth (hyperplasia) of the endometrium or endometrial cancer (ACOG, 2013b; NAMS, 2010b).

"**What to say**" — *Counseling patients about bleeding symptoms when systemic HT is first initiated*

Nurses should educate women who plan to initiate HT about certain symptoms, such as vaginal spotting and unscheduled bleeding, that often occur as the body adapts to a new hormonal symptom. Nurses may offer the following information:

- Vaginal bleeding and spotting are most likely to occur in the first 3 months after initiation of therapy.
- Follow-up visits should be scheduled at 1 and 3 months—and improvement in symptoms should be noted at that time.
- It is important to promptly report the following symptoms: persistent bleeding; bleeding that stops but then starts again; or the presence of blood clots in the vaginal discharge.

Evidence that the risk of depression is higher in early menopause is mixed. Although two small randomly controlled trials found that short-term estrogen therapy is effective for the treatment of affected perimenopausal women, another trial found no such benefit for depressed older postmenopausal women. At present, there is insufficient evidence for using hormone therapy to treat depression in general (Khouzam, 2012).

Also, despite earlier findings, no evidence has been generated to support the use of hormone therapy to prevent dementia or cognitive decline. Beginning estrogen-progestogen therapy after age 65 for these reasons may actually increase the risk of dementia within the subsequent 5 years. Studies that investigated whether dementia can be prevented in women who begin hormone therapy during the menopause transition or early postmenopausal period provided insufficient evidence of help or harm. Estrogen therapy does not appear to have any effect on Alzheimer's disease. The U.S. Preventive Services Task Force (USPSTF) and the American College of Obstetricians and Gynecologists (ACOG) advise against the use of HT to improve cognition or to prevent or treat dementia (ACOG, 2004; Alexander, 2007; Henderson, 2011; USPSTF, 2012).

Educating Patients About Hormone Therapy Options

In general, transdermal estrogen (estradiol) provides the same relief of menopausal symptoms as do the oral preparations but without the side effects of breast tenderness or

Women who are taking HT only for the prevention of osteoporosis should be assessed for their personal osteoporosis risk and should be advised to consult with their health-care provider about continuing HT for this purpose. There are other alternatives for the prevention of osteoporosis that should be considered in women whose only need for HT is in the prevention of osteoporosis (ACOG, 2012a; National Osteoporosis Foundation [NOF], 2013a). (See discussion of osteoporosis later in this chapter.)

For women who seek short-term (1–4 years) relief of menopausal symptoms, the benefits of HT most likely outweigh the risks. Although certain symptoms such as hot flashes and night sweats tend to be of short duration for most women, other menopausal symptoms such as vaginal dryness generally continue throughout the postmenopausal period. Also, many women believe that estrogen helps them to feel, think, and sleep better. These women may conclude that for them, the added benefits of fracture prevention and colon cancer reduction associated with HT outweigh the risks. Nurses may share information about alternatives to HT, such as the use of vaginal lubricants, and strategies for relief from sleep disturbances (Ruhl, 2010). However, the decision to continue with long-term HT is one that must be made on an individual basis following consideration of each woman's benefits and risks, including those benefits and risks that were not addressed in the WHI (Kaunitz, Pinkerton, & Simon, 2014).

Large randomized controlled trials, including the WHI, have suggested that hormone therapy reduces the incidence of diabetes among postmenopausal women. The reason for this benefit is unknown, although it may be related to lower weight gain or reduced insulin resistance among women using HT. However, there is inadequate evidence to recommend hormone therapy solely for diabetes prevention in perimenopausal women. Also, it is important to bear in mind that the WHI studied only one preparation of HT. Hence, data generated from the WHI study cannot be applied to all HT therapies. An important role for nurses who care for midlife women involves providing them with current evidence-based information about HT along with culturally appropriate resources for promoting menopausal fluid retention. Transdermal estradiol delivery systems (i.e., patches, gels, sprays) have been shown to be safer than oral administration in reducing certain markers of cardiovascular risk. Because the hormones bypass the liver and are directly absorbed into the bloodstream, transdermal administration is more effective in maintaining stable blood levels of estrogen. Also, because the transdermal estradiol is absorbed directly into the body, first-pass metabolism by the gastrointestinal tract and liver is avoided. When given orally, larger doses of estrogen are required to achieve therapeutic levels and to offset metabolism by the liver and inactivation by the gut wall. In addition, when compared with the transdermal formulations, oral estrogen therapy has been shown to increase the risk of venous thromboembolic disease. With trandsdermal estradiol preparations, serum hormone levels remain constant, and rapid cessation of drug administration is possible with removal of the transdermal system (Durham, 2012; Fantasia & Sutherland, 2014; Shoupe, 2012).

No large studies have compared the advantages and disadvantages of the different transdermal formulations. The patch, applied one or two times a week to a hairless area of the skin, is considerably more irritating to the skin than either the gel or emulsion. Also, the gel and the emulsion are more discrete than the patch. To use the gel or emulsion, the patient is taught to apply the product to clean, dry, intact skin at the same time each day. The emulsion is applied to the complete surface of both legs once a day; the gel is applied to one upper arm and shoulder once a day. The gels are messy and must dry before a woman dresses or washes. An estradiol transdermal spray is also available. The spray is applied to a small area on the inner forearm once daily; the dose can be increased to two or three sprays as needed for symptom control. Patients are taught to allow the application site to dry for 2 minutes before it is covered with clothing and to avoid washing the site for 30 minutes after applying. When using two or three sprays, the applicator cone should be placed adjacent to, but not overlapping, the area of the previous administration. Because all gels and sprays are alcohol based, patients must be cautioned to avoid fire, flame, or smoking until they have dried. Also, gels and sprays may have specific instructions regarding the application of sunscreen. All of these products should be used for the shortest possible period of time and require 4 to 12 weeks before relief of symptoms is obtained. Nonoral delivery methods are recommended for women with CVD; clotting abnormalities; thromboembolic history; pronounced obesity; or prolonged hypertension, diabetes, or immobilization (ACOG, 2013b; Buster, 2010; Liu & Minkin, 2013; Minkin, 2010; Shoupe, 2012).

Nurses can empower women with current, evidence-based information about contraindications, risks, and side effects of various hormone therapies. Providing this information helps guide patients to make appropriate, informed decisions. The risks and side effects of estrogen and progestogen are presented in Box 7-6.

legal alert— Be knowledgeable of the contraindications to estrogen

Nurses who care for patients who use estrogen therapy must be knowledgeable of the absolute contraindications to estrogen. These include the following:

- Known or suspected estrogen-dependent cancer
- Known, suspected, or history of breast cancer except in appropriately selected patients being treated for metastatic disease
- Undiagnosed abnormal genital bleeding
- Active or history of deep venous thrombosis, pulmonary embolism
- Active or recent (within the past year) arterial thromboembolic disease (e.g., stroke, myocardial infarction)
- Liver dysfunction or disease
- Known or suspected pregnancy
- Known hypersensitivity to ET/EPT
 (NAMS, 2010b, 2012; Shifren & Schiff, 2010)

Box 7-6 Risks and Side Effects of Estrogen and Progestogen

RISKS OF ESTROGEN

Breast cancer

Deterioration of liver function in women with severe liver disease

Endometrial cancer

Increased risk of stroke

Possible small increase in the risk of coronary events

Possible worsening of gallbladder disease

Small increase in the risk of venous thromboembolism

Worsening of edema in women with severe cardiac disease

Worsening of hypertriglyceridemia

Worsening of pain from benign breast disease

SIDE EFFECTS OF ESTROGEN

Increased risk of gallbladder disease

Worsening of estrogen-dependent conditions, such as uterine fibroids and endometriosis

Increase in fibrocystic breast problems

Vaginal bleeding

Hypertension

Nausea and vomiting

Headaches, jaundice, and fluid retention

Impaired glucose tolerance

Changes in the shape of the cornea (sometimes leading to contact lens intolerance)

SIDE EFFECTS OF PROGESTOGEN

Fluid retention

Breast tenderness

Jaundice

Nausea

Insomnia

Depression

Menstrual bleeding

Source: NAMS (2010b).

Optimizing Outcomes— Using the NAMS 2012 Position Statement to guide care

The North American Menopause Society's evidence-based 2012 Position Statement emphasizes recent data on breast cancer, cognitive aging/decline and dementia, coronary heart disease, stroke, and discontinuation of therapy. The updated position statement further distinguishes the emerging differences in the therapeutic benefit-risk ratio between ET and combined EPT in women of various ages and with various intervals since the onset of menopause. The full text is available at http://www.menopause.org/docs/default-document-library/psht12.pdf?sfvrsn=2. Also, NAMS provides a downloadable patient education tool on the subject of hormone therapy; this is available at http://www.menopause.org/docs/default-document-library/psht12patient.pdf?sfvrsn=2.

Cultural Diversity: Declines in Postmenopausal Hormone Use

Sprague, Trentham-Dietz, and Cronin (2012) examined data from the National Health and Nutrition Examination Survey that included over 10,000 women aged 40 and older to evaluate national trends in the prevalence of hormone use and patient characteristics. In 1999–2000, the prevalence of oral postmenopausal hormone use was 22.4% overall. A sharp decline in use of all hormonal formulations occurred in 2003–2004, when the overall prevalence decreased to 11.9%. The decline was initially limited to non-Hispanic whites; use among non-Hispanic blacks and Hispanics did not decline substantially until 2005–2006. Hormone use continued to decline through 2009–2010 across all patient demographic groups, with the current (2012) prevalence at 4.7% overall. Although the findings were consistent with previous studies that demonstrated ethnic disparities in the diffusion of new medical information, the investigators noted that a primary limitation in interpretation of the study results centered on the self-reported nature of the hormone use data (Sprague et al., 2012).

Bioidentical Compounds

The term "bioidentical hormones" was introduced by Jonathan Wright, MD, a practitioner who used the term to communicate his still-unsubstantiated claim that plant-derived hormones are "identical" in molecular structure to human hormones. When used to describe hormones, the term "bioidentical" simply means chemically indistinguishable from the hormones produced in a woman's body (i.e., estradiol-17ß and progesterone). "Bioidentical" is a marketing term generally accepted to mean a hormone that is chemically identical to the hormone produced in the body during women's reproductive years. Numerous FDA-approved drugs contain these hormones and therefore are also "bioidentical" (Box 7-7) (ACOG, 2012a, 2014; NAMS, 2010b).

Compounded bioidentical hormones are plant-derived (i.e., from wild yam or soy) hormones that are prepared by a pharmacist and can be custom made for a patient according to a physician's specifications. The use of bioidentical compounds has been promoted as a natural approach because these substances claim to replace specific hormones

---

Box 7-7 FDA- Approved Pharmaceutical Bioidentical Hormone Preparations

- Estradiol - injections (Delestrogen, Depot-Estradiol)
- Estradiol - oral (Estrace, Femtrace)
- Estradiol - spray (Evamist)
- Estradiol - topical emulsion (Estrasorb)
- Estradiol - transdermal gel (Divigel, Elestrin, EstroGel)
- Estradiol - transdermal patches (Alora, Climara, Esclim, Estraderm, Menostar, Vivelle, Vivelle-Dot)
- Estradiol - vaginal cream (Estrace)
- Estradiol - vaginal ring (Estring, Femring)
- Estradiol - vaginal tablets (Vagifem, Vagifem LD)
- Progesterone as oral micronized progesterone (Prometrium), vaginal cream (Crinone),* and ovules (Endometrin)*

*FDA approved for infertility; not menopausal hormone therapy.
Sources: Minkin (2010); Moore (2010); Pinkerton (2012).

---

that are naturally present in a woman's body. Because the only truly natural source of human estradiol is the human ovary, all plant sources must be processed to synthesize estradiol. Therefore, all bioidentical products are, in actuality, synthetic (ACOG, 2012a, 2014; NAMS, 2010b).

Many bioidentical replacement hormones are compounded in private laboratories or pharmacies as individualized made-to-order products. Bioidentical hormones prepared by a compounding pharmacist are not regulated and approved by the U.S. Food and Drug Administration. Women need to be made aware of the limitations and poor results that may be associated with this therapy (ACOG, 2012a, 2014; Minkin, 2010; NAMS, 2010b; Shoupe, 2012).

Certain bioidentical preparations of estrogen or progestin are approved by the FDA for oral, intravaginal, transdermal, or percutaneous applications. These particular medications have undergone strenuous testing for safety, efficacy, and quality control. However, *compounded* bioidentical formulations are not FDA-regulated in the same way. These products are not subject to rigorous testing or quality control standards. Also, the compounded products do not carry a package insert that lists important contraindications, warnings, and precautions—which may make them appear to be safer than traditional therapy medications. These products lack standardization, and in many cases, the specific active ingredients and minimally effective dosages are not known (ACOG, 2012a, 2014; NAMS, 2010b; Pinkerton, 2012; Shoupe, 2012).

Nursing Insight— Wariness of compounded bioidentical hormone formulations is warranted

Custom-made HT formulations, called "bioidentical hormone therapy," or BHT, are compounded for an individual according to a health-care provider's prescription. Often touted to be "natural," in actuality, bioidentical hormones are all synthesized, making terms such as "natural" and "nonsynthetic" inaccurate and meaningless. The American College of Obstetricians and Gynecologists (ACOG) and The North American Menopause Society (NAMS) consider the bioidentical hormone preparations to have the same safety risks as traditional hormone therapy and assert that they may carry additional risks associated with the compounding process. In addition, evidence-based data supporting the efficacy of bioidentical compounded preparations are lacking. The risks, benefits, and quality of these products have not been evaluated through rigorous testing, a standard requirement for traditional hormone therapy medications (ACOG, 2012a, 2014; NAMS, 2010b).

These products are custom compounded to "normalize" a woman's hormone levels. However, natural levels of estrone, estradiol, and other hormones are in constant flux, so they are impossible to normalize. Practices such as having personal hormone levels measured via blood tests or saliva tests as a basis for compounding "individualized" HT products are expensive and useless; no scientific data exist to indicate what these levels should be (ACOG, 2012a; NAMS, 2010b).

NONHORMONAL PRESCRIPTION MEDICATIONS

Women who experience debilitating vasomotor symptoms and wish to avoid traditional hormone therapy (HT) may be willing to try certain prescription medications including antidepressants, belladonna alkaloid preparations, anticonvulsants, or antihypertensive agents.

> ✿ **Nursing Insight**— *Nonhormonal medications for vasomotor symptoms*
>
> Various nonhormonal medications have been prescribed for the relief of severe vasomotor symptoms. Antidepressant agents known as selective serotonin reuptake inhibitors (SSRIs), including fluoxetine (Prozac), paroxetine* (Paxil), citalopram (Celexa), escitalopram (Lexapro), and sertraline (Zoloft), and serotonin/norepinephrine reuptake inhibitors (SNRI), including venlafaxine (Effexor) and desvenlafaxine (Pristiq), may reduce hot flashes. However, studies that compared the efficacy of venlafaxine with that of medroxyprogesterone acetate (MPA, a progestational agent) found that a single dose of MPA alleviated hot flashes more effectively than did daily use of the antidepressant (Barbieri, 2013; NAMS, 2010b; Pinkerton, Constantine, Hwang, & Cheng, 2013). A recent randomized controlled trial comparing venlafaxine to acupuncture therapy (Walker et al., 2010) found equivalent efficacy between the two therapies in treating hot flashes, depressive symptoms, and other quality-of-life symptoms, and acupuncture therapy was associated with fewer side effects.
>
> Bellergal-S (Bellamine-S) is a combination of phenobarbital, ergotamine, and belladonna. This medication may be useful for certain women with sleep-related vasomotor symptoms. However, this agent is contraindicated with a number of other medications and may interact with many other substances including acetaminophen, alcohol, antacids, certain antibiotics, digoxin, metronidazole, and warfarin (Nelson, 2011).
>
> In some women, clonidine (Catapres), an antihypertensive medication, and gabapentin (Neurontin), an anticonvulsant, have been useful in controlling hot flashes. Transdermal clonidine therapy is preferred over oral clonidine; gabapentin frequently causes nausea and other gastrointestinal side effects (Barbieri, 2013; Nelson, 2011). Gabapentin, taken 1 to 2 hours before bedtime, is useful for sleep disorders in hypoestrogenic women; other therapies for sleep difficulties include eszopiclone (Lunesta), zolpidem (Ambien), and strategies to improve sleep hygiene such as keeping the bedroom cool, avoiding naps,

exercising daily, maintaining a regular sleep-wake schedule, keeping the bedroom dark and quiet, dimming ambient lighting in the evening, avoiding caffeine after lunch and alcohol late in the evening, stopping smoking, and limiting fluids before bedtime (Barbieri, 2013).

---

*In late 2013, paroxetine mesylate (Brisdelle) received FDA approval as the first nonhormonal medication for hot flashes associated with menopause.

> ⊜ **Now Can You**— **Discuss certain aspects of menopausal hormone therapy?**
>
> 1. Identify the NAMS recommendations for HT use for the following conditions: vasomotor symptoms, osteoporosis, coronary heart disease, diabetes mellitus, and cognitive functioning?
> 2. Explain why a progestogen may be appropriate for a patient who wishes to use HT?
> 3. Counsel a patient about the proper use of various transdermal formulations?
> 4. Explain what is meant by the term "bioidentical hormones"?

Cardiovascular Disease

Cardiovascular disease (CVD) is the number one killer of older American women, and the diagnosis of heart disease presents a greater challenge in women than in men. This disease includes coronary heart disease (CHD), stroke, congestive heart failure (CHF), hypertension, and other diseases of the heart and vascular system. Over the past few decades, improved prevention and treatment have reduced the annual number of CVD deaths in men, but not in women. Cardiovascular disease is a particularly important problem among minority women. The death rate due to CVD is substantially higher in African American women than in Caucasian women. Despite the heightened public awareness of cardiovascular disease in women, the majority of women in this country continue to underestimate their risk of dying as a result of CVD (American Heart Association [AHA], 2013a; Carey & Gray, 2012).

> ✿ **Nursing Insight**— *Women and cardiovascular disease*
>
> Compared with men, many women before the age of menopause appear to be partly protected from coronary heart disease, heart attack, and stroke. As women age, their risk of heart disease and stroke begins to rise and keeps rising. The reasons for the lower incidence of coronary heart disease and stroke in younger women are not clear. Results from clinical trials have shown that estrogen therapy alone or in combination with progestin does not protect from heart disease or stroke. The American Heart Association does not advise women to take postmenopausal hormone therapy to reduce the risk of coronary heart disease or stroke (AHA, 2013a).

Cardiovascular disease is a chronic, degenerative disease. Although the exact mechanisms are not well understood, it is known that there is deterioration in arterial wall elasticity due to the deposition of plaque containing cholesterol and other compounds. The plaque formation may result from attempts by the body to repair damage to the lining of blood vessels. Blood flow is slowed through the narrowed areas, and clots tend to form around the deposits, causing further occlusion of the vessels (AHA, 2013a).

According to the American Heart Association, the risk of heart disease and stroke increases with age. CVD ranks first among all disease categories in hospital discharges for women and nearly 38% of all female deaths in this country occur from coronary heart disease, hypertension, stroke, congestive heart failure, and other cardiovascular diseases. At present, an estimated 43 million women in the United States are affected by heart disease, and 90% of women have one or more risk factors for developing CVD. However, only one in five U.S. women believes that heart disease is her greatest health threat. More women than men die of stroke. Interestingly, low blood levels of "good" cholesterol (high-density lipoprotein, or HDL) appear to be a stronger predictor of heart disease death in women than in men in the over-65 age group. High blood levels of triglycerides (another type of fat) may be a particularly important risk factor in women and the elderly (AHA, 2013a).

Cultural Diversity: Heart Disease and Hispanic and African American Women

Hispanic women are more likely to develop heart disease 10 years earlier than Caucasian women, and only one in three Hispanic women is aware that heart disease is the number one killer in their demographic group. CVD is the leading cause of death for African American (AA) women, and the AHA estimates that only one in five AA women thinks she is personally at risk. Nearly 47% of AA women aged 20 and older have CVD, and only 43% of AA women know that heart disease is their greatest health risk (AHA, 2013a). Women of color with low socioeconomic and educational levels who reside in rural areas in southern states are at significantly increased risk for developing CVD (McSweeney, Pettey, Souder, & Rhoads, 2011).

THE AMERICAN HEART ASSOCIATION GUIDELINES FOR WOMEN

The AHA *2011 Effectiveness-Based Guidelines for the Prevention of Cardiovascular Disease in Women* emphasize that health-care professionals should focus on women's lifetime heart disease risk, rather than just the short-term risk. This approach underscores the importance of healthy lifestyles in women of all ages to reduce the long-term risk of heart and blood vessel diseases. The new guidelines for risk assessment include personal risk factors and family history, as well as the Framingham Risk Score, which estimates the risk of developing coronary heart disease within 10 years. Expanded recommendations on lifestyle factors such as physical activity, nutrition, and smoking cessation, as well as specific recommendations on drug treatments for blood pressure and cholesterol control, are included (Mosca et al., 2011).

Nursing Insight— The Framingham Risk Score (FRS) and the Reynolds Risk Score (RRS)

Some experts have expressed concerns about the utility of the Framingham Risk Score (FRS) in women, including the fact that it does not reflect the risk for developing "soft" endpoints that are more common in women, such as stroke, angina, or need for coronary revascularization. Furthermore, the 10-year risk projection in the FRS may underestimate a woman's risk for developing CHD since women tend to live longer than men, resulting in an increased lifetime risk even if one risk factor is left untreated. To address these concerns, the Reynolds Risk Score (RRS) has recently been introduced and may be a superior indicator of CVD risk, especially in postmenopausal women. This score combines the same risk factors as the FRS, but also includes family history, glycosylated hemoglobin value, and high sensitivity C-reactive protein levels (a biomarker associated with subclinical inflammation). Patients and health-care providers may learn more about the RRS by visiting http://health.drgily.com/reynolds-risk-score-women-heart-attack-risk.php.

The updated guidelines state that the use of unregulated dietary supplements is not a method proved to prevent heart disease. Research that has become available since the last guidelines were developed suggests that health-care providers should consider the use of aspirin in women over age 65 to prevent stroke. In women younger than age 55 years, routine use of aspirin is not recommended to prevent myocardial infarction (MI), owing to an increased risk of cerebral and gastrointestinal bleeding. The U.S. Preventive Services Task Force (USPSTF) (2009) recommendations for daily aspirin use are for men aged 45 to 79 to prevent myocardial infarction and for women aged 55 to 79 to prevent ischemic stroke when the potential benefit outweighs the potential harm from gastrointestinal hemorrhage. Evidence is insufficient to assess the benefits versus harms of aspirin in elders. Health-care providers should avoid the use of menopausal therapies such as hormone therapy or selective estrogen receptor modulators (SERMs) (i.e., raloxifene, tamoxifen) to prevent heart disease because they have been shown to be ineffective in protecting the heart and may, in fact, increase the risk of a stroke. Estrogen plus progestin can increase the risk of MI, breast cancer, venous thromboembolism, stroke, dementia, and ovarian cancer. In women who have undergone hysterectomy, estrogen alone confers a risk of stroke and dementia/memory loss. Likewise, no cardiovascular benefit has been shown for SERMs (AHA, 2013a; Mayhew, 2010; Roberts, 2010 USPSTF, 2009).

Optimizing Outcomes— With AHA guidelines for women's heart health

The AHA Guidelines for Women include the following:

- To help manage blood pressure, consider recommended lifestyle changes: weight control, increased physical activity, alcohol moderation, sodium restriction, and an emphasis on eating fresh fruits, vegetables, and low-fat dairy products.
- Do not smoke, and avoid environmental tobacco smoke. Consider counseling, nicotine replacement, or other forms of smoking cessation therapy.

- Accumulate at least 150 minutes/week of moderate exercise, 75 minutes/week of vigorous exercise, or an equivalent combination of moderate- and vigorous-intensity aerobic physical activity. Aerobic activity should be performed in episodes of at least 10 minutes, preferably spread throughout the week.
- Engage in muscle-strengthening activities that involve all major muscle groups performed on >2 days/week.
- To lose weight or sustain weight loss, include a minimum of 60 to 90 minutes of moderate-intensity activity (e.g., brisk walking) on most, and preferably all, days of the week.
- Reduce the intake of saturated fat, cholesterol, alcohol, sodium, and sugar and to avoid trans-fatty acids.
- Consume dark oily fish (e.g., salmon, tuna, herring) at least twice a week; women with hypercholesterolemia and/or hypertriglyceridemia should consider consumption of omega-3 fatty acids in the form of fish or in capsule form (e.g., EPA [eicosapentaenoic acid] 1,800 mg/day) for primary and secondary prevention.
- If at high risk for coronary heart disease, consider taking 75–325 mg of aspirin per day.
- Do not use antioxidant supplements such as vitamin E, vitamin C, and beta-carotene for primary or secondary prevention of CVD.
- Do not use folic acid to prevent CVD.
(AHA, 2013a; Manson & Bassuk, 2011; Mosca et al., 2011)

 Across Care Settings: Go Red for Women, WISEWOMAN, and the Heart Truth

In 2004, the American Heart Association launched its multitiered cause marketing the "Go Red for Women" movement to raise women's awareness of their risk for heart disease and empower them to take charge of their heart health. In 2010, the AHA set a strategic goal of reducing death and disability from cardiovascular disease and strokes by 20% while improving the cardiovascular health of all Americans by 20% by the year 2020. Nurses and patients can obtain accurate, up-to-date information about heart disease and stroke and the Go Red for Women movement by calling 1-888-MY-HEART or by visiting http://www.goredforwomen.org./

The WISEWOMAN (Well-Integrated Screening and Evaluation for WOMen Across the Nation) program, located at the CDC, provides screening and lifestyle interventions for many low-income, uninsured, or underinsured women aged 40 to 64. Information is available at the WISEWOMAN Web site http://www.cdc.gov/wisewoman/.

Sponsored by the National Heart, Lung, and Blood Institute, the Heart Truth is a campaign whose goal is to give women a personal and urgent wake-up call about their personal risk of heart disease. Women can learn more about the Heart Truth by visiting http://www.nhlbi.nih.gov/educational/hearttruth/.

Where Research and Practice Meet: Constipation and Risk of Cardiovascular Disease

Salmoirago-Blotcher and colleagues (2011) conducted a secondary analysis of more than 73,000 participants in the Women's Health Initiative to explore the possibility of constipation as a marker for cardiovascular risk in older women. Constipation was associated with increased age, African American and Hispanic descent, smoking, diabetes, high cholesterol, family history of myocardial infarction, hypertension, obesity, lower physical activity levels, lower fiber intake, and depression. After adjustments were made for demographics, risk factors, dietary factors, medications, frailty, and other psychological variables, the heightened risk for cardiovascular events remained only in the severely constipated group. Based on their findings, the investigators concluded that constipation in postmenopausal women is a marker for increased cardiovascular risk. Because constipation is easy to assess, nurses may wish to incorporate this information to assist in the identification of women at risk for cardiovascular disease.

Optimizing Outcomes— Teach women about heart attack warning signs

As with men, women's most common heart attack symptom is chest pain or discomfort. But women are somewhat more likely than men to experience some of the other common symptoms, particularly shortness of breath; nausea and vomiting; and back, neck, throat, tooth, or jaw pain. Atypical symptoms that have been reported include fatigue, fainting, weakness of the arms or shoulders, dizziness or vision changes, gaslike pain, indigestion, loss of appetite, pain between the shoulder blades, restlessness, and a feeling of impending doom (AHA, 2013a; DeVon, Saban, & Garrett, 2011; Johnson & Seibert, 2011).

RISK FACTORS FOR CVD

Women are considered to be at high risk for cardiovascular disease if they have established CVD or CHD, peripheral artery disease, cerebrovascular disease, chronic renal disease, or diabetes mellitus. Other traditional risk factors for coronary disease are listed in Box 7-8.

The 2011 updated AHA evidence-based guidelines provided a new algorithm for risk classification in women that stratifies women into three categories—high risk, at risk, and optimal risk; the new classifications are presented in Box 7-9 (Mosca et al., 2011).

Fortunately, many of the major CVD risk factors can be significantly modified through therapeutic lifestyle changes and pharmacotherapy. Modifiable risk factors include smoking, hyperlipidemia, diabetes mellitus (DM), hypertension (HTN), and obesity. Educating women about strategies to control these five risk factors can empower them to make changes that can greatly reduce their lifetime risk for CVD.

Complementary Care: *IZI LLC sponsors Self I-Dentity through Ho'oponopono (SITH) for hypertension*

An ancient Hawaiian problem-solving process, *IZI LLC sponsors Self I-Dentity through Ho'oponopono* (SITH), aims to promote peace, balance, and a new meaning of life by helping one identify and correct stress actively and preventively. With the physical, mental, and spiritual SITH process, the self is freed from memories that replay as problems within the subconscious mind. Taught by trained instructors at conference centers throughout the world, the SITH process is carried out in three steps: repentance, forgiveness, and transmutation. Class attendees have

---

Box 7-8 Traditional Risk Factors for Cardiovascular Disease

- Increasing age (about 83% of people who die of CHD are 65 or older)
- Heredity (including race)—children of parents with heart disease are more likely to develop it themselves. African Americans have more severe high blood pressure than do Caucasians and a higher risk of heart disease. The highest coronary heart death rates and the highest overall CVD morbidity and mortality occur in black women. Heart disease is also higher among Mexican Americans, Native Americans, native Hawaiians, and some Asian Americans—and this is partly due to higher rates of obesity and diabetes in these populations.
- Premature menopause (<45 years)
- Cigarette smoking
- Obesity
- Dyslipidemia—in women >65 years, low HDL levels are associated with greater risk
- Elevated serum cholesterol levels
- Metabolic syndrome (a combination of medical disorders [e.g., elevated BP, triglycerides, and fasting plasma glucose, reduced HDL cholesterol, central obesity] that, when occurring together, increase the risk for developing CVD and diabetes)
- Hypertension (often related to the use of alcohol, cigarettes, excessive sodium, and obesity)
- Other modifiable factors such as a high-fat diet, sedentary lifestyle, stressful lifestyle

Sources: Arslanian-Engoren (2011); Johnson & Seibert (2011); Jones (2010); Mosca et al. (2011).

Box 7-9 2011 AHA CVD Risk Classifications for Women

High Risk	Clinically manifested congestive heart disease
	Clinically manifested cerebrovascular disease
	Clinically manifested peripheral arterial disease
	Abdominal aortic aneurysm
	End-stage or chronic kidney disease
	Diabetes mellitus
At Risk (at least one major risk factor)	Cigarette smoking
	Systolic BP >120 mm Hg, diastolic BP >80 mm Hg or treated hypertension
	Total cholesterol >200 mg/dL, HDL-C <50 mg/dL or treated for dyslipidemia
	Obesity, particularly central adiposity
	Poor diet
	Physical inactivity
	Family history of premature CVD occurring in first-degree relatives in women <65
	Metabolic syndrome
	Evidence of advanced subclinical atherosclerosis
	Poor exercise capacity on treadmill test and/or abnormal heart rate recovery after stopping exercise
	Systemic autoimmune collagen-vascular disease
	History of preeclampsia, gestational diabetes, or gestational hypertension
Optimal Risk	Total cholesterol <200 mg/dL (untreated)
	BP <120/80 mm Hg (untreated)
	Fasting blood glucose <100 mg/dL (untreated)
	Body mass index <25 kg/m^2
	Abstinence from smoking
	Physical activity at goal for adults >20 years of age: >150 min/week moderate
	intensity, >75 min/week vigorous intensity or combination
	Healthful diet (such as "DASH" diet)

Source: Mosca et al. (2011).

---

reported that use of the SITH process reduced stress; lowered BP readings; brought about improvement in chronic pain; and created feelings of peace, calm, and inner balance (Kretzer, 2011).

Smoking has been associated with early CVD events and doubles the risk of developing CVD by age 70. Nurses can encourage women to avoid both cigarette smoking and secondhand exposure to environmental tobacco smoke. When discussing smoking cessation strategies, it may be useful to identify and address barriers to smoking cessation such as a fear of weight gain, fear of an inability to deal with negative mood and anxiety, anticipated peer influence from other tobacco users, a lack of support, a lack of interest, and a longstanding use of smoking as a stress reliever (ACOG, 2011; Arslanian-Engoren, 2011).

Optimizing Outcomes— Medications to treat tobacco dependence

Patients may benefit from medications to treat tobacco dependence. Over-the-counter nicotine replacement products include chewing gum (Nicorette), lozenges (Commit, Nicorette mini lozenge), and patches (NicoDerm CQ, Habitrol). Prescription medications include nasal sprays (Nicotrol NS) and inhalers (Nicotrol). Non-nicotine prescription medications include bupropion hydrochloride (Wellbutrin, Zyban), nortriptyline (Aventyl, Pamelor), avarenicline (Chantix), and clonidine (Catapres). All of these agents significantly increase the rate of long-term smoking abstinence, especially varenicline and nicotine nasal spray (Nicotrol NS) (AHA, 2013b; Mayo Clinic, 2013).

Abnormal lipid levels—including elevated low-density lipoprotein cholesterol (LDL-C), low high-density lipoprotein cholesterol (HDL-C), elevated total cholesterol, and elevated triglycerides (TG)—are associated with an increased long-term likelihood of CVD. A fasting lipid profile should be obtained in women beginning at age 20 and then every 5 years thereafter. If a dyslipidemia is identified, secondary causes such as DM, hypothyroidism, obstructive liver disease, chronic renal failure, and medication-induced changes should be considered (Arslanian-Engoren, 2011; Bradley & Merz, 2011; Jones, Ansell, & Bloch, 2014).

Diabetes mellitus is a significant risk factor for CVD. In women, having DM confers a myocardial infarction (MI) risk equal to that in someone who has established coronary artery disease (CAD). Women with DM have a 57.3% risk for CVD by age 75, compared with a 16.3% risk in women without DM (Arslanian-Engoren, 2011).

Hypertension is also a significant risk factor for CVD, although the relative risk is closely correlated to how well women can control their blood pressure. Among U.S. women aged 20 years and older, 15.5% have been diagnosed with HTN. After age 65, HTN affects more women than men. Sadly, most of these women remain unaware that HTN constitutes a major risk factor for CVD (AHA, 2013a).

According to the American Heart Association (2013), 74.8 million women (aged 20 and older) in the United States are classified as overweight or obese. Obesity is more prevalent in women, especially in minorities and those with a lower socioeconomic status. Overweight and obesity are independent and contributory risk factors to CVD. Body mass index (BMI) >25 kg/m² is independently associated with an increased risk of CVD, with an even larger risk in persons with a BMI equal to or greater than 30. Those with a BMI of 40 kg/m² or greater tend to experience MI 12 years earlier than those with a normal BMI. Moreover, overweight and obesity are known contributors to other risk factors, such as DM, HTN, and dyslipidemia (AHA, 2013a).

> ### 🌸 *Nursing Insight*— *Understanding the term "cardiometabolic health"*
>
> "Cardiometabolic health" is a term, promoted by the American Diabetes Association (ADA) since 2006, to describe an individual's level of risk for developing diabetes and CVD; it's based on an assessment of all the factors that contribute to risk for these conditions. These factors can be called "cardiometabolic risk factors." The ADA's Cardiometabolic Risk Initiative is a national campaign to encourage health-care providers to focus on the prevention, recognition, and treatment of all risk factors (e.g., smoking, obesity, physical inactivity, psychological stress) for CVD and type 2 diabetes. Additional information is available at http://professional.diabetes.org/resourcesforprofessionals.aspx?cid=60379.

THE NURSING ROLE IN PROMOTING CARDIOVASCULAR HEALTH

The U.S. Preventive Services Task Force (USPSTF) 2012 recommendations for routine CHD screening for women include screening for hypertension, diabetes mellitus, obesity, lipid disorders, and tobacco use. Screening combined with individualized education and counseling about heart disease constitutes a central role for nurses in promoting cardiovascular health. Nurses can empower women with strategies to make lifestyle modifications to address the five major risk factors (smoking, dyslipidemia, DM, HTN, and obesity) for cardiovascular disease (Arslanian-Engoren, 2011; Association of Women's Health, Obstetric & Neonatal Nursing [AWHON], 2011; Roberts & Davis, 2013; USPSTF, 2012). Diets high in saturated fat, trans-fatty acids, cholesterol, calories, alcohol, and salt and low in fiber, fruits, and vegetables have been shown to contribute to HTN, DM, dyslipidemia, and obesity. Dietary changes to reduce blood pressure may include incorporation of the Dietary Approaches to Stop Hypertension (DASH) diet. The DASH diet emphasizes low sodium intake (2.3 g/d or less) and the consumption of fruits, vegetables, low-fat/nonfat dairy foods, whole grains, lean meat, fish, poultry, nuts, and beans. Nurses and patients may learn more about the DASH Diet Eating Plan by visiting the Web site at http://www.dashdiet.org/.

> ### 🌸 **Complementary Care:** *Olive oil to promote cardiovascular health*
>
> When counseling women about dietary modifications to promote CV health, nurses can encourage them to use olive oil in their cooking. In 2004, the U.S. Food and Drug Administration granted approval for labeling olive oil as a nonpharmaceutical product that reduces the risk of coronary heart disease. Olive oil has been shown to reduce after-meal lipemia and to promote more rapid metabolism of the damaging, oxidative chylomicrons formed after eating fats. Olive oil, a botanical product, may produce allergic reactions in sensitive individuals. Skin patch testing for patients with significant sensitivity histories is advised. Although there are no known drug interactions, highly antioxidant compounds can increase the potency of warfarin (Coumadin), so nurses should advise patients who use this anticoagulant to proceed with caution. Most studies are conducted with extra virgin olive oil using a daily intake of 1 to 2 ounces (30–60 mL). This is the amount typically found in salad dressings, cooking, and spreads.

A lack of physical activity is also known to contribute to CVD. Exercise inhibits atherosclerosis (a lifelong disease that results from a combination of genetic and environmental factors) (Fig. 7-2), reduces inflammatory responses, improves endothelial function, and reduces obesity, HTN, dyslipidemia, and insulin resistance (American Heart Association [AHA], 2013).

Normal artery

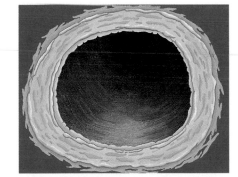

A

Atherosclerotic artery

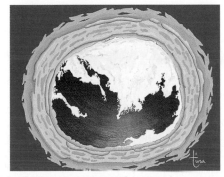

B

Figure 7-2 *A,* Cross section of normal coronary artery. *B,* Coronary artery with atherosclerosis narrowing the lumen. (Scanlon, V.C., & Sanders, T. [2007]. *Essentials of anatomy and physiology* [5th ed., p. 280]. Philadelphia, PA: F.A. Davis.)

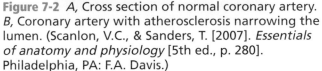

⊜ Optimizing Outcomes— With exercise to decrease CHD and DM risk

Exercise has been documented to decrease the risk of CHD by 40%, stroke by 30%, and type 2 diabetes mellitus by 30%. Nurses can encourage patients to exercise for a total of at least 30 minutes over the course of a day; 60 minutes is optimal, and 90 minutes is recommended for weight loss. According to the CDC (2011), 150 minutes of moderate-intensity aerobic activity each week lowers the risk for cardiovascular disease and type 2 diabetes. In its scientific statement *Interventions to Promote Physical Activity and Dietary Lifestyle Change for Cardiovascular Risk Factor Reduction in Adults,* the AHA recommends the use of behavioral interventions (e.g., goal-setting, self-monitoring, feedback, reinforcement) to motivate individuals to engage in physical activity on a regular basis. Community-based physical activity programs have been shown to be effective in reducing new cases of cancer (i.e., breast, colon), type 2 diabetes, and heart disease. Community-based interventions may include mass communication efforts, social support networks, provision of childcare during physical activity endeavors, online education programs, individualized physical activity goal setting and monitoring, and enhanced access to services such as fitness centers, bike paths, and walking trails (Artinian et al., 2010; Im et al., 2011; Im, Young et al., 2012; Roberts & Davis, 2013; Sherman, 2011). The AHA My Heart, My Life program offers a wealth of information and a variety of Web-based tools about physical activity and other topics including nutrition, weight management, stress management, and smoking cessation on its Web site at http://www.startwalkingnow.org/.

Nurses can also explore and address barriers to prevention and treatment of CVD. Barriers may be perceived or actual, mental or physical, or economic, geographical, or cultural. Exploring these barriers in a nonthreatening, culturally sensitive, therapeutic environment empowers women to identify and overcome them so that they may take action to improve their cardiovascular health. It is well established that women who have limited access to health care have more adverse health outcomes, including CVD (McSweeney et al., 2011).

✿ Nursing Insight— Barriers to CVD prevention and treatment

Nurses can help women identify barriers that can prevent actions to promote their cardiovascular health. Barriers may include:

- Confusion concerning information in the media
- The belief that a supreme being ultimately determines one's health
- The perception that one is not at risk for CVD
- A reluctance to make a change in lifestyle
- The belief that nothing can be done to prevent CVD
- A lack of time, energy, support, willpower
- An overwhelming feeling of stress that prevents participation in CVD prevention or treatment activities
- A lack of resources (financial, access to healthy foods, access to exercise space, family obligations)

(Doering & Eastwood, 2011; McSweeney et al., 2011; Mosca et al., 2011)

When counseling women about personal risk for CVD, nurses can inform them about the Reynolds Risk Score, developed by experts at Brigham and Women's Hospital in Boston. The interactive tool calculates the risk of having a heart attack, stroke, or other form of heart disease in the next 10 years. Nurses can also inform women about HeartHub (http://www.hearthub.org/), the American Heart Association's patient portal for information, tools, and resources about cardiovascular disease and stroke. This Internet resource offers a wealth of current information about various CV-related topics such as warning signs for heart attack, stroke, and cardiac arrest, and provides self-assessment activities for personal risk of diabetes, heart attack, and high blood pressure. On the HeartHub Internet site, heart health information is offered in Spanish, Vietnamese, and simplified and traditional Chinese.

✿ *Across Care Settings:* The National Coalition for Women With Heart Disease

For more than a decade, WomenHeart Champions have been educating, supporting, and advocating in communities nationwide for prevention, early detection, timely and accurate diagnosis and treatment, and effective health-care policy to help women better understand about heart disease. Often misdiagnosed and undertreated, more than 41 million American women are living with or at risk for developing heart disease. WomenHeart, the National Coalition for Women With Heart Disease, is the only national organization dedicated to promoting women's heart health. To learn more about this organization, women may visit the organization's Web site at www.womenheart.org.

Remaining up to date about current, evidence-based CVD information empowers nurses to offer care that promotes and optimizes women's cardiovascular health. Nurses can appropriately counsel patients about interventions that have been found harmful or are ineffective in preventing CVD in women. For example, both folic acid and antioxidant supplementation have been found ineffective in the primary and secondary prevention of CVD. Also, women younger than age 65 should not routinely use aspirin to prevent myocardial infarction. Finally, hormone therapy and estrogen-receptor modulators are no longer recommended for primary or secondary prevention of CVD in women (Bradley & Merz, 2011; Mosca et al., 2011).

An important goal in the *Healthy People 2020* national initiative addresses heart disease and stroke. A subgroup under this goal includes 24 standards that are key to monitoring cardiovascular health. As longstanding advocates for women's health, nurses are perfectly situated to help the nation achieve this goal through ongoing patient assessment and education. In addition, nurses can be instrumental in the development and implementation of creative programs designed to change lifestyles to promote cardiovascular health and in assuring that women at high risk receive timely, appropriate referral and follow-up (Moran & Walsh, 2013; U.S. Department of Health and Human Services [USDHHS], 2013b).

The American Heart Association (AHA) and American College of Cardiology Foundation (ACCF) have published guidelines to assist practitioners in the prevention of CVD. The AHA has released Evidence-Based Guidelines for Cardiovascular Disease Prevention in Women: 2011 Update, and the AHA and ACCF have jointly published *AHA/ACCF Secondary Prevention and Risk Reduction Therapy for Patients With Coronary and Other Atherosclerotic Vascular Disease: 2011 Update; A Guideline From the American Heart Association and American College of Cardiology Foundation.* This publication summarizes the highlights of these guidelines and serves as a rich resource for health-care professionals. Both sets of guidelines focus on major CVD risk factor reduction and the use of pharmacotherapy in patients with established CVD.

⊚ **Now Can You**— **Discuss certain aspects of cardiovascular disease?**

1. Discuss the utility of two tools specifically developed to determine risk for cardiovascular disease?
2. Identify at least five AHA guidelines for promoting heart health in women?
3. Develop a patient teaching program that focuses on five modifiable risk factors for cardiovascular disease?

Osteoporosis

As individuals age, there is a progressive decrease in bone density. Osteoporosis is a generalized, metabolic disease characterized by decreased bone mass and an increased incidence of bone fractures (Fig. 7-3). Osteopenia is a condition where bone mineral density (BMD) is lower than normal. Many clinicians consider osteopenia to be a precursor to osteoporosis. However, not every person diagnosed with osteopenia will develop osteoporosis. Osteoporosis is a largely preventable complication of menopause. Screening strategies and pharmacological interventions are available to prevent and treat osteoporosis.

🌸 *Nursing Insight*— *Appreciating the full impact of osteoporosis-related fractures*

Hip fractures (defined as fractures of the proximal femur), which occur on average at age 82, elicit a particularly devastating toll, resulting in higher cost, disability, and mortality than all other osteoporotic fracture types combined. In the United States, approximately 340,000 hip fractures occur in the elderly each year, resulting in annual health-care costs of more than $8 billion. It has been estimated that the associated health-care-related cost of osteoporotic fractures will reach $23.5 billion in 2025. Hip fractures cause up to a 25% increase in mortality within 1 year of the incident. Approximately 25% of women require long-term care after a hip fracture, and 50% will experience some long-term loss of mobility. Vertebral fractures may cause substantial pain as well as loss of height and exaggerated thoracic kyphosis (abnormal curvature of the

Normal bone

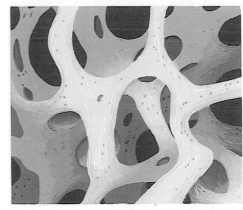

A

Osteoporosis

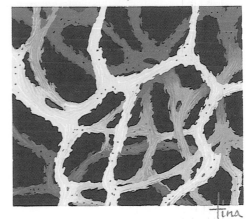

B

Figure 7-3 *A,* Normal spongy bone, as in the body of a vertebra. *B,* Spongy bone thinned by osteoporosis. (Scanlon, V.C., & Sanders, T. [2007]. *Essentials of anatomy and physiology* [5th ed., p. 113]. Philadelphia, PA: F.A. Davis.)

thoracic spine). Spinal pain and deformity can greatly restrict normal movement, including bending and reaching. Thoracic fractures may restrict lung function and cause digestive problems. Osteoporotic fractures exert a psychological toll as well. Pain, loss of mobility, change in body image, and loss of independence can exert a strong impact on self-esteem and mood (Droste, Holmes, Hernandez, & Mahdjoubi, 2010; NAMS, 2010a; NOF, 2013a; Sweitzer, Rondeau, Guido, & Rasmor, 2013).

NORMAL BONE PHYSIOLOGY

Bone is a living tissue. It is involved in a wide range of biochemical processes, which result in the constant breakdown and reformation of new bone. This process of remodeling replaces weakened areas with new, well-formed tissue. Bone is composed of two types of cells, called osteoblasts and osteoclasts (Fig. 7-4), as well as an intercellular matrix. The intercellular matrix is composed of organic compounds, such as collagen and other proteins, and inorganic components responsible for bone rigidity. Minerals such as calcium phosphate, calcium carbonate, magnesium, fluoride, sulfate, and other trace elements form crystalline structures called "hydroxyapatites" (NAMS, 2010a).

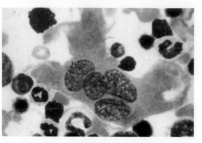

Figure 7-4 Osteoclast. (Venes, D. [2009]. *Taber's cycolpedic medical dictionary* [22nd ed., p. 1655]. Philadelphia, PA: F.A. Davis.)

A & P review **The Bone Remodeling Unit**

The bone-remodeling unit is the site on the surface of the bone where osteoblasts and osteoclasts act to form and resorb bone. Bone is constantly being remodeled to provide

optimal support and to repair damage occurring from daily activities. An osteoblast (from the Greek words for "bone" and "germ," or embryonic) is a mononucleate cell that is responsible for bone formation. Osteoblasts produce osteoid, which is composed mainly of collagen. Osteoblasts are also responsible for mineralization of the osteoid matrix. Bone is a dynamic tissue that is constantly being reshaped by osteoblasts, which build bone, and osteoclasts, which resorb bone. An osteoclast (from the Greek words for "bone" and "broken") is a type of bone cell that removes bone tissue by removing its mineralized matrix and breaking up the organic bone. This process is termed *bone resorption*. Osteoclasts and osteoblasts are instrumental in controlling the amount of bone tissue: osteoblasts form bone; osteoclasts resorb bone. Osteoblast cells tend to decrease as individuals age, thus decreasing the natural renovation of bone tissue (Fig. 7-5) (ACOG, 2012b; NAMS, 2010a).◆

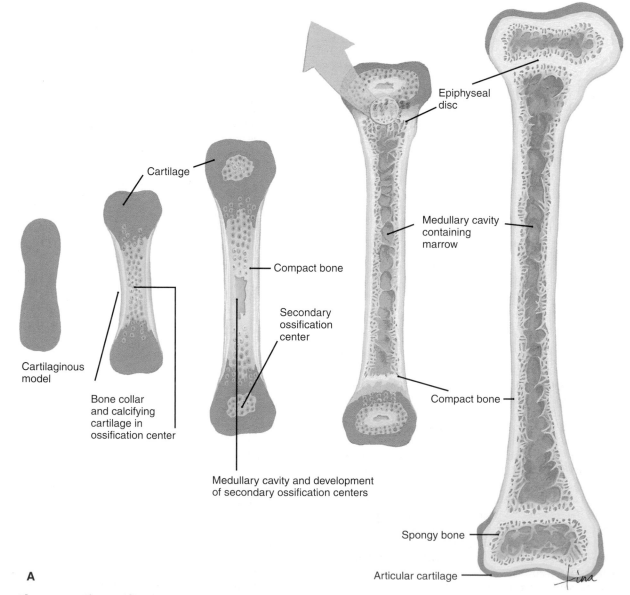

Figure 7-5 The ossification process in a long bone. *A,* Progression of ossification from the cartilage model of the embryo to the bone of a young adult.

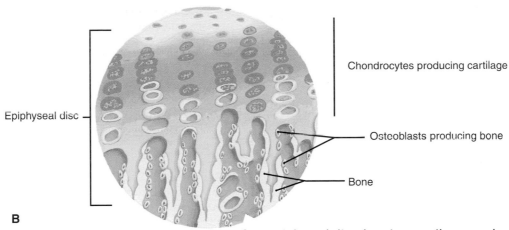

Epiphyseal disc

Chondrocytes producing cartilage

Osteoblasts producing bone

Bone

B

Figure 7-5—cont'd B, Microscopic view of an epiphyseal disc showing cartilage production and bone replacement. (Scanlon, V.C., & Sanders, T. [2007]. *Essentials of anatomy and physiology* [5th ed., p. 110]. Philadelphia, PA: F.A. Davis.)

Nursing Insight— *Gonadal hormones and bone metabolism*

Estrogen inhibits bone resorption by binding to estrogen receptors in bone tissue and also by blocking the production of cytokines, substances that increase the number of osteoclasts. Estrogen, however, is not the only hormone that has an important influence on the health of bone. Two other hormones produced by the ovaries, progesterone and dehydroepiandrosterone (DHEA), influence bone metabolism as well. Testosterone (one of the male hormones also produced by women) may also play a role in bone health (ACOG, 2012b; NOF, 2013a).

There are two major types of bone: cortical and trabecular. Cortical bone forms the outer shell of all bones and accounts for 75% of total bone mass. Trabecular bone is the spongy, interlacing network of struts that forms the internal support within the cortical bone. Trabecular bone is concentrated in the vertebral bodies and pelvis and at the ends of the long bones. Trabecular bone accounts for 25% of total bone mass, but because of its spongy, open architectural structure, it accounts for most of the volume in bone. Bone remodeling units are limited to the bone surface. Because trabecular bone has a larger surface area, it has a higher turnover rate than cortical bone. Trabecular bone is most likely to show early bone loss, but it also is the first bone type to show response to therapy (ACOG, 2012b).

Bone formation and resorption are ongoing processes that are usually "in balance" in young adults who have adequate nutrition and exercise and experience normal puberty. Bone mass peaks at approximately 19 years in Caucasian females and at 20.5 years in Caucasian males, a fact that underscores the importance of bone health promotion during adolescence. After reaching peak bone mass, approximately 0.4% of bone is lost per year in both genders. Bone strength is determined by the total bone mass and the integrity of its protein and crystal matrix. Bone strength is also related to the efficiency of bone repair in response to mild trauma, which produces microfractures. Remodeling tends to occur along lines of stress, increasing the strength in those weakened areas (ACOG, 2012b; NOF, 2013a).

Nursing Insight— *The menopause–bone loss link*

In addition to the bone loss with aging that naturally occurs in both genders, women lose approximately 2% of cortical bone and 5% of trabecular bone per year for the first 5 to 8 years after menopause. With menopause and aging, the coordinated "balance" between osteoclasts and osteoblasts may be disturbed, resulting in excessive bone resorption and loss of both bone density and structure. The time of most rapid bone loss coincides with the marked decline in estrogen levels during the periomenopausal period. Rapid bone loss begins 1 year before the final menses and lasts approximately 3 years, and during this time, there is a 6% bone loss at the femoral neck and a 7% bone loss in the lumbar spine. In women who are recently menopausal, excess bone loss commonly is caused by excessive osteoclast-mediated resorption. In later postmenopausal years, suppressed osteoblast activity and inadequate formation of bone may play a major role in the progression of osteoporosis, providing an opportunity for new therapeutic approaches, such as stimulating bone formation. Osteoporosis is more common in women than men in part because of the accelerated loss of bone that occurs after menopause (ACOG, 2012b).

Bone health promotion typically centers on methods to ensure adequate intake of calcium. However, bone health maintenance and the prevention of fractures should encompass other strategies, such as preventing the loss of calcium and other minerals from the bone, maintaining the soft tissue components around the bone, and promoting the efficiency of bone repair (NOF, 2013a; Speroff & Fritz, 2011).

Nursing Insight— *Fractures commonly associated with osteoporosis*

Three major types of fractures may occur as a result of osteoporosis:

Spontaneous vertebral crush fracture—the vertebrae become so weak that one vertebra collapses under the minimal stress of lifting or due to the weight of the woman's body. This action causes a loss of height and kyphosis, or dowager's hump, the curvature of the upper back often present in older people (Fig. 7-6).

Colle's fracture—a transverse fracture of the distal radial metaphysis with displacement of the hand posteriorly and outward. This fracture occurs when a person breaks a fall by landing on a hand, causing fracture of the radius (Venes, 2013).

Osteoporotic hip fracture—The hip fracture related to the osteoporotic process is the most severe form of these three types of fractures.

Tooth loss and periodontal disease represent other aspects of osteoporosis.

In the United States, it is estimated that more than 10 million individuals have osteoporosis and almost 18 million more are estimated to have osteopenia, or low bone mass, placing them at increased risk for osteoporosis. Of the 10 million Americans estimated to have osteoporosis, 8 million are women and 2 million are men. Although osteoporosis is often considered to be an older person's disease, it can strike at any age. Both osteopenia and osteoporosis increase the risk of fracture (ACOG, 2012b; NOF, 2013a).

Cultural Diversity: Osteoporosis

Osteoporosis varies among racial and ethnic groups. In the United States, much variation exists in hip fracture rates. Caucasian women have the highest rates of hip fractures, African American women have the lowest rates, and Mexican American women have rates in between the two other groups. Chinese American women typically have lower bone mineral density than Caucasian women but lower rates of hip and forearm fracture. It has been postulated that greater cortical density and thicker trabeculae compensate for less trabeculae in smaller bones. Hence, bone mineral density and microarchitecture appear to play distinct roles in fracture vulnerability. African American women have approximately a 6% higher bone mineral density than Caucasian women. Among non-Hispanic African American women who are older than age 50, 5% have osteoporosis and 35% have osteopenia. As African American women age, their risk for hip fracture doubles approximately every

7 years, and they are more likely than Caucasian women to die following a hip fracture. Among Hispanic women over age 50, 10% have osteoporosis and 49% have osteopenia. When compared with other ethnic/racial groups, the risk of osteoporosis is increasing most rapidly among Hispanic women. And among non-Hispanic white women and Asian American women who are 50 and older, approximately 20% have osteoporosis, while 52% have osteopenia (ACOG, 2012b; National Institutes of Health Osteoporosis and Related Bone Diseases, 2012; NOF, 2013a; Speroff & Fritz, 2011).

Osteoporosis constitutes a major health threat for women. In this country, the incidence of osteoporosis-related fractures has increased over the past 20 years. Most fractures occur at the femoral neck, the vertebrae, and the distal radius. Postmenopausal women who experience a hip or symptomatic vertebral fracture have a six- to eightfold increased risk of death in the year following their fracture. On an annual basis, the associated costs of osteoporosis-related fractures exceed $14 billion, and this figure is expected to increase as the life expectancy increases and the population ages. By 2025, annual direct costs from osteoporosis are expected to reach approximately $25.3 billion (Dempster, 2011; Nelson, 2011).

Nursing Insight— *Heredity and bone mass*

The single largest factor that influences a woman's peak bone mass (i.e., the maximal BMD gained during the skeletal development and maturation phase) is genetics. Up to 80% of the variability in peak bone mass is attributable to genetic factors alone. Female children of women with osteoporotic fractures have lower bone mass than would be expected for their age when compared with unrelated individuals. First-degree relatives of women with osteoporosis have lower bone mass than those with no family history of osteoporosis (ACOG, 2012b; NAMS, 2010a, 2010b).

CAUSES

Stated in simple terms, osteoporosis occurs when the normal balance of bone formation and bone resorption is disrupted. In women and young adults, bone growth and calcium deposition take place continuously throughout young adulthood. Bone mass generally reaches a peak around age 30. As women grow older, net bone loss gradually occurs due to an imbalance in bone tissue and metabolism. A deficiency of estrogen worsens the situation, as does the inefficiency in calcium and vitamin D assimilation that naturally occur as women age (NOF, 2013a; Nelson, 2011; Speroff & Fritz, 2011).

During the first 5 to 6 years following menopause, women lose bone density six times more rapidly than do men. By the age of 65, one-third of women have experienced a vertebral fracture; by the age of 80, women have lost approximately 47% of the trabecular bone, which is concentrated in the vertebrae, pelvis, and other flat bones, and the epiphyses. The most well-defined risk factor for the development of osteoporosis is the loss of the protective effects of estrogen, which occurs with declining ovarian function during perimenopause (NOF, 2013a).

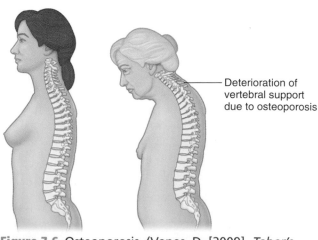

Deterioration of vertebral support due to osteoporosis

Figure 7-6 Osteoporosis. (Venes, D. [2009]. *Taber's cyclopedic medical dictionary* [22nd ed., p. 1695]. Philadelphia, PA: F.A. Davis.)

Osteoporosis may result from other causes, including rheumatoid arthritis, chronic lung disease, anorexia nervosa, and endocrine diseases such as diabetes, hypogonadism, overactive thyroid, and hyperparathyroidism. Also, certain prescription drugs, including glucocorticoids (e.g., prednisone), anticoagulants (e.g., heparin), chemotherapeutic agents, anticonvulsants (e.g., phenytoin), and some diuretics (e.g., furosemide), as well as some over-the-counter aluminum-containing antacids (e.g., Maalox), can contribute to bone loss. An excessive caffeine intake increases calcium excretion, and excessive alcohol use (i.e., three or more drinks per day) interferes with calcium absorption and depresses bone formation (Fontenot & Harris, 2014; NOF, 2013a).

Optimizing Outcomes— With routine postmenopausal osteoporosis risk assessment

All postmenopausal women should be assessed for risk factors associated with osteoporosis and fracture. This assessment requires a history, physical examination, and any necessary diagnostic tests. The goals of this evaluation are to evaluate fracture risk, to rule out secondary causes of osteoporosis, to identify modifiable risk factors, and to determine appropriate candidates for pharmacological therapy (NAMS, 2010a).

RISK FACTORS

There are a number of risk factors for osteoporosis. Nonmodifiable factors include genetic background and medical conditions; these are presented in Box 7-10. Modifiable risk factors related to lifestyle include smoking (active or passive), alcohol use, low dietary calcium, vitamin D insufficiency, high dietary intake of sodium, protein, caffeine, phosphates, sugar, colas, and refined flour products, lack of sun exposure or a deficiency of vitamin D, and lack of exercise (McEneaney, 2012; NOF, 2013a).

Nursing Insight— *Tobacco use and osteoporosis risk*

Compared with nonsmokers, women smokers tend to lose bone more rapidly, have lower bone mass, and reach menopause 2 years earlier, on average. The mechanisms by which smoking might adversely affect bone mass are not known, although some experts suggest that cigarette smokers may have impaired calcium absorption and lower estradiol levels (NAMS, 2010a).

DIAGNOSING OSTEOPOROSIS

A *clinical* diagnosis of osteoporosis is made when a postmenopausal woman suffers a nontraumatic, nonpathological fracture of the spine. A *radiological* diagnosis is based on the T-score, which is obtained from bone densitometry analysis. The first-line technique for assessing bone mineral density (BMD) (bone densitometry) is the central dual energy x-ray absorptiometry, or DXA. This test usually assesses BMD in the lumbar spine, total hip, and femoral neck. Osteoporosis objectives for the *Healthy People 2020* initiative track bone mineral density as a measure of the major risk factor for fractures (USDHHS, 2013a).

Diagnostic Tools Bone Density Scan (DXA)

Bone density scanning, also called "dual energy x-ray absorptiometry" or "bone densitometry," is an enhanced form of x-ray technology that is used to measure bone loss. Central DXA is today's established standard for measuring bone mineral density. DXA is most often performed on the lower spine and hips. Central DXA devices have a large, flat table and an "arm" suspended overhead; these machines are usually located in hospitals and medical offices. Peripheral devices (pDXA) that use x-ray or ultrasound are sometimes used to screen for low bone mass. Peripheral devices measure bone density in the wrist, heel, or finger, and are often available in drugstores and on mobile health vans in the community. The pDXA device, much smaller than the central DXA device, is a portable, boxlike structure with a space for the foot or forearm to be placed for imaging. Although bone tests at peripheral sites can identify women at risk of fracture, they are not useful for the diagnosis of osteoporosis and have limited or no value in the follow-up of patients. In some communities, a CT scan with special software can also be used to diagnose or monitor low bone mass. This is accurate but less commonly used than DXA scanning. DXA is effective in tracking the effects of treatment for osteoporosis and other conditions that cause bone loss; the DXA test can also assess an individual's risk for developing fractures (NAMS, 2010b).

DXA works by measuring a specific bone or bones (i.e., lumbar spine, total hip, femoral head). The density of these bones is then compared with an average index based on age, sex, and size. The resulting comparison is used to determine risk for fractures and the stage of osteoporosis in an individual. Results are generally scored by two measures, the T-score and the Z-score. The T-score refers to the extent of bone loss and is reflective of the number of standard deviations by which a patient's BMD falls below the expected BMD score for healthy young women. Every decrease of one standard deviation represents approximately a 12% reduction in BMD, which translates into a 1.5- to 3.0-fold increase in fracture risk (NOF, 2013a).

Box 7-10 Nonmodifiable Risk Factors for Osteoporosis

Gender—Eighty percent of the 10 million Americans who have osteoporosis are women

Race—Caucasian, Asian, and Latina women are at the highest risk; African American women have a lower risk

Advanced age

History of:

- Previous fractures that occurred without any major trauma, or fracture after the age of 50
- Poor absorption of calcium and other minerals or nutrients owing to celiac disease, chronic diarrhea, low stomach acid (common in older individuals), surgical removal of part of the stomach or intestines

Family history of female osteoporosis or fractures or both

Body build—women who are small boned and slim and have small muscle mass are at greater risk than women with other body builds

Current osteopenia

Early menopause (before age 40 years, or if surgically induced); amenorrhea; never having gone through a pregnancy

Diabetes; liver disease; kidney disease with dialysis; daily use of thyroid replacement medication (>2 grains); hyperthyroidism; hyperparathyroidism

Lactose intolerance—present in 60% of women with osteoporosis and in only 15% of the general population

Use of phenytoin sodium (Dilantin), a medication that interferes with the body's ability to absorb calcium; aluminum-containing antacids; steroid medications

Sources: ACOG (2012); NAMS (2010a, 2010b); NOF (2013a).

✿ *Nursing Insight*— *Understanding the BMD Z-score and T-score*

The Z-score is the number of standard deviations above or below the mean for the patient's age, sex, and ethnicity. The Z-score is used in premenopausal women, men under the age of 50, and in children. The T-score, which is also the number of standard deviations above or below the mean, is a comparison of a patient's BMD to that of a healthy 30-year-old of the same sex and ethnicity. This value is used in postmenopausal women and men over age 50 because it better predicts risk of future fracture. The World Health Organization's T-score criteria are as follows:

- Normal: a T-score of −1.0 or higher
- Low bone mass (osteopenia): a T-score less than −1.0 and greater than −2.5
- Osteoporosis: a T-score equal to or less than −2.5 (i.e., the bone density is two and a half standard deviations below the mean of a 30-year-old healthy woman)

Scores indicate the amount one's bone mineral density varies from the mean. Negative scores indicate lower bone density; positive scores indicate higher bone density.

❝**What to say**❞ — *Preparing patients for a DXA examination*

The nurse can do much to allay the patient's anxiety about a scheduled bone densitometry test. The nurse explains why the test is performed, how the test is performed, and what information will be gained from the test results. The nurse may also counsel the patient about how to prepare for the test. For example, the nurse may say:

- The bone density test is a quick, noninvasive, painless procedure.
- The amount of radiation used is extremely small—less than one-tenth the dose of a standard chest x-ray and less than a day's exposure to natural radiation.
- DXA bone density testing is the most accurate method available for the diagnosis of osteoporosis and is also considered an accurate estimator of fracture risk.
- No radiation remains in your body after an x-ray examination.
- On the day of the exam, you may eat normally. You should not take calcium supplements for at least 24 hours before your exam.
- You should wear loose, comfortable clothing, and avoid garments that have zippers, belts, or buttons made of metal. Objects such as keys or wallets that would be in the area being scanned should be removed.
- You may be asked to remove some or all of your clothes and to wear a gown during the exam. You may also be asked to remove jewelry, dentures, eyeglasses, and any metal objects or clothing that might interfere with the x-ray images.
- You will be positioned on a padded table and your legs will be supported on a padded box (to flatten the pelvis and lumbar spine). You must hold very still and you

may be asked to hold your breath for a few seconds while the x-ray picture is being taken.

- The DXA bone density test is usually completed within 10 to 30 minutes, depending on the equipment used and the parts of the body being examined.
- You should inform your health-care provider if you recently had a barium examination or have been injected with a contrast material for a computed tomography (CT) scan or radioisotope scan. In this event, you may have to wait 10 to 14 days before undergoing the DXA test.
- You should inform your health-care provider and the x-ray technologist if there is any possibility that you may be pregnant.

⟲ Optimizing Outcomes— **Routine height assessments to detect asymptomatic osteoporosis**

As women grow older, routine height assessments should become standard practice during annual examinations. Loss of height may indicate bone loss in asymptomatic women. Identifying height loss in women who are in their 40s or early 50s should signal a need for further testing to determine the cause. After achieving maximal height, women can lose up to 1.0 to 1.5 inches (2.0–3.8 cm) of height as part of the normal aging process, primarily as a result of degenerative arthritis and shrinkage of intervertebral disks. Height loss greater than 1.5 inches increases the likelihood that a vertebral fracture is present. The nurse should measure height using an accurate method such as a wall-mounted ruler or a stadiometer (an instrument used to measure both sitting and standing height) (NAMS, 2010b; NOF, 2013a).

According to recommendations established by the American College of Obstetricians and Gynecologists, the U.S. Preventive Services Task Force (USPSTF), The North American Menopause Society (NAMS), and the National Osteoporosis Foundation (NOF), health-care providers should routinely screen all women older than 65 for osteoporosis, regardless of risk factors. Women with risk factors should be screened beginning at age 60.

⟲ Optimizing Outcomes— **Teach women about osteoporosis early warning signs**

Teaching women about the early warning signs of osteoporosis constitutes an important nursing role in bone health promotion. Nurses should alert women to the following signs and symptoms that may signal bone loss, and advise them to promptly contact their health-care provider if they experience them:

- Sudden onset of insomnia and restlessness
- Leg and foot cramps that occur frequently during the night
- Persistent low back pain
- Gradual loss of height
- Development of gum disease or loose teeth

In this country, women typically reach menopause around age 51, and most bone loss occurs during the first

5 to 7 years after cessation of menses. Thus, it may be prudent to begin screening at an earlier age. It is generally recommended that the BMD be reassessed every 3 to 5 years. For certain women, including those who are undergoing treatment for osteoporosis and those who are immobilized, the BMD may need to be measured beginning at an earlier age, and more often, such as every 6 to 24 months (ACOG, 2012b; NAMS, 2010a; NOF, 2013a, USPSTF, 2011).

> ### ✿ *Nursing Insight*— *ACOG recommendations for bone mineral density (BMD) testing*
>
> The American College of Obstetricians and Gynecologists (2012) has published the following recommendations for BMD testing:
>
> - Bone mineral density testing should be recommended to all postmenopausal women aged 65 years or older regardless of risk factors.
> - Bone mineral density testing may be recommended for postmenopausal women younger than 65 years with any of the following risk factors: medical history of a fragility fracture; body weight less than 127 lb; medical causes of bone loss (medications or diseases); parental medical history of hip fracture; current smoker; alcoholism; rheumatoid arthritis.
> - Alternatively, FRAX can be used in women younger than 65 if they are postmenopausal and have other risk factors for fracture.
> - Routine screening of newly menopausal women is not recommended nor is a "baseline" screen recommended.

> ### ◯ Optimizing Outcomes— **With the FRAX assessment tool**
>
> The launch of the World Health Organization (WHO) technical report *Assessment of Osteoporosis at the Primary Health Care Level* and the related Fracture Risk Assessment Tool (FRAX) are major milestones toward helping health professionals worldwide to improve identification of patients at high risk of fracture. The practical Web-based tool FRAX assesses the 10-year risk of osteoporosis fracture in women older than 50 years who are postmenopausal, are not receiving osteoporosis treatment, have low bone mass, and have had no prior hip or vertebral fracture. An individual's risk factors such as age, sex, weight, height, and femoral neck BMD (if available) are entered into the Web site tool, followed by clinical risk factors, which include a prior fragility fracture, parental history of hip fracture, tobacco smoking, long-term use of glucocorticoids, rheumatoid arthritis, other causes of secondary osteoporosis, and daily alcohol consumption. The FRAX tool then provides a figure indicating a 10-year fracture probability as a percentage, which, together with a clinical assessment, provides guidance for determining access to treatment in health-care systems. Estimates are available for U.S. whites, blacks, Hispanics, and Asian Americans. The FRAX algorithm is intended for use with postmenopausal women and men aged 50 and older and applies only to previously untreated patients. The FRAX model is available on the National Osteoporosis Foundation (NOF) Web site (www.nof.org) or at the FRAX Web site (www.shef.ac.uk/FRAX/). It is also available on newer DXA machines or with software upgrades that provide the FRAX scores on the bone density report (Laster, 2014; Lewiecki, 2012; McKenzie, 2012; NOF, 2013a; Wright, 2011).

PROMOTING BONE HEALTH THROUGH OPTIMAL NUTRITION

Although it is impossible to determine the precise effect of diet on bone health, there is at least circumstantial evidence that the standard American diet, which frequently contains excessive sugar, refined grains, and caffeine, promotes the development of osteoporosis. Other dietary factors that adversely affect bone health include alcohol and protein, phosphorus, and sodium. The relationship between these substances and their impact on bone loss is presented in Box 7-11.

Nurses can empower women with information about the value of optimal nutrition in reducing osteoporosis risk. Consuming a diet that is composed primarily of plant-based, unprocessed whole foods is an important strategy in the promotion of bone health and the prevention of osteoporosis. Examples of plant-based nutritious substances include legumes, fresh fruits and vegetables, whole grains, nuts, and seeds. These foods provide a rich supply of nutrients in the right proportions to enhance their absorption and use. In addition to calcium, many vitamins, such as vitamins K, B_6, C, and D, and minerals, such as manganese, magnesium, boron, and zinc, play an important role in maintaining bone mass and in preventing bone loss (Box 7-12) (NAMS, 2010a; NOF, 2013a).

Calcium

Calcium deficiency is only one of the predisposing factors for the development of osteoporosis in women, and not everyone

---

> **Box 7-11** **Selected Dietary Substances and Their Association With Bone Loss**
>
> **Sugar:** The average American ingests 139 pounds of refined sugar each year. Sugar intake may be associated with large increases in urinary calcium excretion. Owing to the fact that 99% of the body's calcium is stored in bone, and the blood maintains a very narrow concentration range of calcium, when the body loses calcium, it is likely to be from bone.
>
> **Refined grains:** The nutrient-rich portions of grains have been removed through refinement, including vitamin B complex, calcium, magnesium, and zinc.
>
> **Caffeine:** Caffeine in coffee, tea, and soft drinks, as well as similar substances in chocolate and some drugs, causes calcium to be excreted in the urine. Increased calcium excretion causes a systemic acidosis that stimulates bone resorption.
>
> **Alcohol:** Excessive alcohol intake interferes with calcium absorption and depresses bone formation.
>
> **Protein, phosphorus, and sodium:** The typical American diet contains excessive amounts of protein, phosphorus, and sodium. Calcium is mobilized to neutralize the acidic by-products and is then excreted in the urine, causing a loss of calcium from the body. Phosphorus is an ingredient in many soft drinks, and excess protein results from the high consumption of meat and dairy products in the average American diet.
>
> **Oxalate and phytate sodium:** Foods with high amounts of oxalate and phytate reduce the absorption of calcium contained in those foods. Examples of foods high in oxalate include spinach, rhubarb, and beet greens. Legumes (e.g., pinto beans, navy beans, peas) are high in phytate. To reduce the phytate level, soak the legumes in water for several hours; discard the water; then cook them in fresh water. Wheat bran is also high in phytate; take calcium supplements 2 or more hours before eating any foods with 100% wheat bran.

Box 7-12 Selected Vitamins and Minerals and Their Role in Promoting Bone Health

Vitamin K: Along with calcium, vitamin K is involved in bone metabolism. This important vitamin attracts calcium into the matrix to form bone—the process of bone mineralization and fracture healing. The current adequate intake value for vitamin K is 90 units/day. Vitamin K is found in several forms: vitamin K_1 (phylloquinone), the form occurring naturally in plants; vitamin K_2 (menaquinone), the form produced by intestinal bacteria and also derived from putrefied fish meal; and synthetic vitamin K (menadione). Humans are unable to synthesize vitamin K. It must be acquired either from dietary sources or as metabolic by-products of intestinal bacteria. Sources of vitamin K include dark green, leafy vegetables (e.g., cabbage, broccoli, lettuce, spinach, cauliflower), soybeans, strawberries, liver, and certain dairy products such as egg yolks, butter, and cheese. Vitamin K supplements are contraindicated in women taking warfarin (Egan, 2010; NAMS, 2010b).

Vitamin B_6: Vitamin B_6 (pyridoxine) is believed to be involved in bone matrix formation. Sources of this vitamin include whole grains, fish, chicken, organ meats, nuts, watermelon, and tomatoes.

Vitamin C: It has been known from the days of widespread scurvy that vitamin C (ascorbic acid) is necessary for normal bone formation. This vitamin promotes the formation and cross-linking of some of the structural proteins found in bone. Vitamin C is present in citrus fruits, strawberries, melons, broccoli, tomatoes, potatoes, green peppers, and raw, deep-green leafy vegetables.

Vitamin D: Calcium metabolism and absorption depend on the presence of vitamin D. Vitamin D is made from either of two inert precursors: vitamin D_2 (ergocalciferol) or D_3 (cholecalciferol). D_2 is plant derived and obtained through diet; D_3 is produced in the skin with exposure to sunlight. Exposing the skin to ultraviolet rays from the sun causes the cholesterol beneath the skin's surface to be converted to vitamin D, which is then stored in the liver until needed. Vitamin D increases the absorption of calcium by the intestines and promotes calcium uptake into the bone. With aging, there is a decrease in the synthesis of vitamin D by the skin. This problem is exacerbated by the common tendency for older individuals to decrease their exposure to the sun. Sun exposure consisting of as little as 10 to 15 minutes each day can have a positive impact on bone health by improving calcium absorption and use. Vitamin D deficiency that stems from reduced sun exposure increases the risk of other conditions, including colorectal, breast, and pancreatic cancers. Wearing a sunscreen with a sun protection factor of 8 or more blocks the skin's ability to produce vitamin D by 95%. Risk factors for vitamin D deficiency or insufficiency include darkly pigmented skin or living at an increased distance from the equator. Women with pancreatic insufficiency, liver disease, and inflammatory bowel disease are at high risk for vitamin D deficiency, as are elderly institutionalized women with poor dietary intake of vitamin D and little sun exposure. Dietary sources of vitamin D include saltwater fish, egg yolks, butter, cod liver oil, fortified milk and orange juice, margarine, cereals and bread products, liver, and supplements. Fortified substances usually provide 100 IU per serving. Certain medications (e.g., anticonvulsants, thiazide diuretics, corticosteroids, cimetidine [Tagamet], heparin, and some cholesterol-lowering agents) can prevent vitamin D absorption, and in some individuals, malabsorption may be related to loss of GI acidity or malfunction of the proximal small bowel. The National Osteoporosis Foundation (NOF) (2013) recommends that adults under age 50 obtain 400 to 800 IU/day and that adults aged 50 and over obtain 800 to 1,000 IU/day. The Institute of Medicine (IOM) recommends 600 IU of vitamin D every day for most healthy adults under age 71; 800 IU for healthy people aged 71 and older, and set 4,000 IU/day as the upper tolerable limit for safety. According to the IOM, "More is not better," and emerging evidence suggests that excess intake of vitamin D is linked to all-cause mortality, cancer, cardiovascular risk, falls, and fractures. The NOF's recommendations for daily vitamin D intake remain higher than the IOM's, but fall well within the margin of safety. Vitamin D_3 (cholecalciferol) is the form of vitamin D that best supports bone health .

Sources: Athanasiadis & Simon (2011); Droste et al. (2010); Grasso & Rafferty (2012); IOM (2010); NAMS (2010a); NOF (2013a).

with osteoporosis is deficient in calcium. Calcium balance and metabolism in the body are complex and involve a number of factors, including ingestion, absorption, use, and excretion. In addition, calcium balance is modulated by various hormonal systems. Adequate calcium intake for osteoporosis prevention should begin early in life when bone mass is reaching its peak. This important period for bone health occurs during the late teens to the early 20s (Speroff & Fritz, 2011).

Optimizing Outcomes— **With skeletal health promotion in children and adolescents**

An important role for nurses who work with men, women, and families centers on promoting bone health and preventing osteoporosis. Ideally, protection against osteoporosis should begin in childhood and adolescence, with efforts focused on building bone mass. Children should be encouraged to eat calcium-rich foods, and nurses should teach parents to encourage regular exercise, including participation in school gym classes and sports programs, to build strong bones and establish healthy lifestyle habits. Parents also should be informed about the negative effects that eating disorders, excessive dieting, excessive exercise, alcohol consumption, and smoking have on bone density. From the mid-20s through age 35, focus should continue to be placed on building and maintaining bone mass through a calcium-rich diet. After age 35, bone resorption exceeds bone formation. At that time, emphasis should be placed on preventing bone loss through a healthy diet, use of calcium supplements, and engaging in weight-bearing exercises such as weight lifting, walking, jogging, dancing, and climbing stairs (Fontenot & Harris, 2014; Venes, 2013).

The National Institutes of Health, Office of Dietary Supplements (2013) recommend the following calcium dietary allowances for women, which represent the amounts of calcium required to maintain adequate rates of calcium retention and bone health in healthy individuals:

- 9–13 years: 1,300 mg/day
- 14–18 years: 1,300 mg/day (same amount for pregnant and lactating individuals)
- 19–50 years: 1,000 mg/day (same amount for pregnant and lactating individuals)
- 50+ years: 1,200 mg/day

When considering dietary sources of calcium, most people are aware that dairy products are rich in calcium, but many do not realize that the animal protein in these products can interfere with the body's ability to absorb the calcium. Other substances that can inhibit calcium absorption are found in wheat bran, raw spinach, salt, caffeine, alcohol and tobacco, and fructose (present in many soft drinks). An important nursing role in bone health promotion centers on teaching women about good nutritional sources of calcium.

"What to say" — *Educating women about dietary calcium*

Nurses can teach women about calcium-rich dietary sources. The nurse may offer the following information:

- Dietary sources are the preferred means of obtaining adequate calcium intake because there are other essential nutrients in high-calcium foods.

- Milk, yogurt, ice cream, and cheese are rich sources of calcium.
- Nondairy calcium sources include vegetables such as Chinese cabbage, kale, and broccoli.
- Most grains do not have high amounts of calcium unless they are fortified; however, they contribute calcium to the diet because they do have small amounts and people consume them frequently.
- Seafood, including sardines and salmon, are good sources of calcium.
- Puddings, instant breakfast drinks, cottage cheese, and sour cream are good sources of calcium.
- Many products, such as soymilk, rice, yogurt, cereals, and orange juice, are now available with extra calcium added.
- Reduced-fat or low-fat products contain at least as much calcium per serving as high-fat dairy products, and they offer an alternative for women concerned about body weight and lipid profiles.

(NOF, 2013a; NAMS, 2010b)

Some individuals are lactose intolerant and have difficulty digesting dairy products because they lack the enzyme lactase, which is needed to break down the milk sugar lactose. Lactose intolerance is fairly common in adults, particularly African Americans, Asians, Native Americans, and Inuits (Alaska Natives). Persons with lactose intolerance experience abdominal cramping, bloating, and diarrhea following milk consumption, although many can tolerate small amounts of milk without symptoms. Calcium sources such as yogurt, sweet acidophilus milk (fermented with certain bacteria), buttermilk, cheese, chocolate milk, and cocoa may be tolerated even when fresh milk is not. Lactase supplements such as Lactaid are available to consume with milk, and lactase-treated milk is also available in many markets. The lactase in these products digests the lactose in the milk so that lactose-intolerant persons can drink milk without experiencing unpleasant intestinal symptoms (NOF, 2013a).

Optimizing Outcomes— Teaching women about strategies to enhance calcium absorption

The absorption of calcium depends upon adequate acidity in the stomach. Low stomach acid is a common problem that becomes more prevalent with increasing age. When counseling women about strategies to optimize the absorption of calcium, the nurse can offer the following advice:

- Eat slowly and chew well.
- Limit fluid intake with meals.
- Consider the use of digestive enzymes.

Most women will need an additional 600 to 900 mg of calcium per day over their usual daily dietary intake to reach recommended levels. Many calcium supplements are available today. Various formulations are available, including oral tablets, chewable tablets, dissolvable oral tablets, and liquids. Patients should be advised that the "best" supplement for them is the one that best meets their needs, based on tolerance, convenience, cost, and availability.

Nurses can teach women that when choosing a calcium supplement, special consideration should be given to the product's purity, absorbability, tolerance, and possibility of interactions with other drugs. Although vitamin D is necessary for the absorption of calcium, it is not necessary that it be included in the calcium supplement. Calcium citrate tends to be better tolerated than calcium carbonate; however, it is a more expensive form of calcium supplement. Most individuals adequately absorb calcium carbonate, a less expensive calcium source, unless there is a problem with insufficient stomach acid. Antacids are not the best sources of calcium, as they can cause other problems, such as kidney stones, and they may aggravate other medical conditions as well. Furthermore, some antacids also contain aluminum, which can cause the body to lose calcium. Nurses can reassure women that total calcium intakes of up to 1,500 mg/day do not appear to increase the risk of developing renal calculi and may actually reduce it. Also, women should not exceed the recommended daily requirement for calcium, as there appears to be no benefit to consumption of amounts in excess of 1,500 mg/day (Institute of Medicine [IOM], 2010; NAMS, 2010a, 2010b; NOF, 2013a).

"What to say" — *Providing guidance to assist women in choosing calcium supplements*

When discussing calcium supplements, the nurse may offer the following advice:

- *Purity:* Choose only those supplements that are known brand names that have proven reliability. The product label should include the term *purified,* or have the USP (United States Pharmacopeia) symbol, although the USP label is voluntary and not all products display this symbol. Avoid calcium extracted from unrefined oyster shell, bone meal, or dolomite without the USP symbol— these products historically have contained higher lead levels or other toxic materials (NOF, 2013a).
- *Absorbability:* Most brand-name calcium products are readily absorbed by the body. If the product label does not state that it is absorbable, it is easy to determine absorbability by doing this: Place the tablet in a small amount of warm water for 30 minutes, and stir occasionally. If the tablet has not dissolved within this time period, it probably will not dissolve in the stomach. Calcium supplements in chewable and liquid form dissolve well because they are broken down before they enter the stomach. Calcium, whether in the diet or from supplements, is best absorbed when it is taken several times a day in amounts of 500 mg or less. Calcium carbonate is absorbed best when taken with food; calcium citrate can be taken any time (NOF, 2013a).
- *Tolerance:* Although calcium supplements are well tolerated by most people, certain preparations can cause side effects such as gas or constipation in some individuals. If simple strategies such as increased fluids and fiber intake do not resolve the symptoms, try another calcium source. A combined calcium-magnesium product may be helpful if constipation is a problem. It is best to increase the intake of any calcium supplement gradually, beginning with 500 mg a day for several days, and add additional calcium slowly (NOF, 2013a).

- *Interactions with other drugs:* Before taking any calcium supplement, it is important to talk with your health-care provider or pharmacist about possible interactions between prescription or over-the-counter medications and the calcium supplements. For example, calcium supplements may interfere with the absorption of the antibiotic tetracycline. Calcium also interferes with iron absorption and should not be taken at the same time as the iron supplement unless the iron supplement is taken with vitamin C or calcium citrate. Any medication that is to be taken on an empty stomach should not be taken with a calcium supplement (NOF, 2013a).

- *Dietary factors that limit calcium absorption:* Consumption of certain foods, including those that contain oxalic acid (found in spinach, rhubarb, and some other green vegetables), large amounts of grains that contain phytates (e.g., wheat bran, soy protein isolates), and possibly, tannins (found in tea), are known to limit calcium absorption from the intestines (NAMS, 2010b).

Optimizing Outcomes— With NOF resources for patients and health-care professionals

Boning Up on Osteoporosis is a 100+ patient care handbook that offers current information on the prevention, diagnosis, and treatment of osteoporosis. The handbook also includes detailed nutrition information and exercises for individuals with low bone density and osteoporosis. It may be purchased from the NOF online store at http://www.nofstore.org/.

The *Clinician's Guide to Prevention and Treatment of Osteoporosis* was first published in 2008, and an updated online version became available in 2013. This resource was developed to inform clinical decision making for the management of men and women at high fracture risk. It integrates the expression of a patient's fracture risk as a 10-year probability with current clinical recommendations for the management of osteoporosis. The *Clinician's Guide* document and *Clinician's Guide* app may be downloaded at http://nof.org/hcp/resources/913.

PROMOTING BONE HEALTH THROUGH PHYSICAL ACTIVITY

Immobilization and bedrest are associated with an increase in bone loss. During travel in space, astronauts have been shown to experience accelerated rates of bone loss. It is known that overall, bone mass is directly related to weight-bearing physical exercise. Women who regularly engage in exercise programs that include weight-bearing and muscle-strengthening elements can help prevent postmenopausal bone loss and reduce their risk of falling. Reducing the risk of falls with exercise training may occur through improvement of balance, gait, and muscular strength. The bone-building effect of exercise results mainly from the repetitive physical stress applied to the bones. With weight-bearing exercise, pressure is placed on the bones either by the weight of the body or by the force of muscular contractions. Effective exercises

for menopausal women that are generally safe and contribute to cardiovascular health and bone mass are walking, dancing, hiking, stair climbing, gardening, weight lifting, and low-impact aerobics. An effective program involves regular exercise for at least 30 minutes, every day of the week. Also, the 30 minutes do not need to be done all at once—physical activity may be divided into 10-minute segments, if desired. According to a recent (2011) Cochrane analysis, weight-bearing, resistance exercises, and aerobics have a beneficial effect on spine BMD, and walking is beneficial for hip BMD (Adams-Fryatt, 2010; Howe et al., 2011; Hurley & Armstrong, 2012; NOF, 2013a).

Optimizing Outcomes— With exercises to promote balance, posture, and function

Nonimpact exercises improve balance, posture, and movement and help to increase muscle strength and decrease the risk of falls and fractures. Balance exercises such as tai chi strengthen the legs and enhance the balance. Posture exercises that improve one's posture and help reduce rounded shoulders decrease the risk of fractures, especially in the spine. Functional exercises enhance the performance of daily activities and decrease the risk of falls and fractures. Yoga and Pilates can also improve strength, balance, and flexibility. Individuals with low bone mass (osteopenia) or osteoporosis should avoid certain positions such as forward-bending exercises to prevent fractures (Goldstein, 2013; NOF, 2013a).

When counseling older women, it is helpful to include information about safety and prevention of falls. Many factors, such as fragility, altered balance, poor vision, and use of certain medications can contribute to falls (Box 7-13). Strategies to minimize falls include lowering the bed, removing throw rugs, illuminating dark areas with night lights, using safety treads and safety rails in the bathroom, ensuring ready access to a telephone, eliminating exposed electrical cords, ensuring stair safety (handrails, good condition, nonslip surfaces), and removing all clutter from the floors. Also, older women should be advised to avoid wearing slippery-soled shoes or slippers, because they provide insufficient support, traction, and stability (Nelson, 2011; Zagaria, 2011).

Optimizing Outcomes— Potential nursing diagnoses for women with osteoporosis

Nursing diagnoses for women with osteoporosis may focus on potential or real problems such as trauma, pain, or impaired mobility:

Risk for Trauma (related to loss of bone density/integrity; increasing risk of fracture with minimal or no stress)

Acute/Chronic Pain (related to vertebral compression on spinal nerves/muscles/ligaments, spontaneous fractures, possibly evidenced by verbal reports, guarding/distraction behaviors, self-focus, and changes in sleep pattern)

Impaired Physical Mobility (related to pain and musculoskeletal impairment, possibly evidenced by limited range of motion, reluctance to attempt movement/expressed fear of reinjury, and imposed restrictions/limitations) (Venes, 2013)

Box 7-13 Medical Risk Factors for Falls

- Acute illness
- Age
- Anemia
- Anxiety and agitation
- Arthritis of the lower extremities
- Cardiac arrhythmias
- Dehydration
- Delirium
- Depression
- Female gender
- Hypoglycemia
- Impaired transfer and mobility
- Lower extremity pain or edema
- Kyphosis
- Malnutrition
- Medications that cause oversedation (e.g., narcotic analgesics, anticonvulsants, psychotropics)
- Muscle weakness
- Orthostatic hypotension
- Parkinson's disease
- Peripheral neuropathy
- Poor balance
- Poor vision and use of bifocals
- Previous fall
- Reduced problem-solving or mental acuity and diminished cognitive skills
- Reduced proprioception
- Stroke/transient ischemic attack
- Thyroid disorders
- Urgent urinary incontinence
- Vitamin D insufficiency

Sources: Kemle (2011); NOF (2013a); NAMS (2010a).

Collaboration in Caring— *An osteoporosis prevention and management model in a faith community*

Forster-Burke, Ritter, and Zimmer (2010) described a faith community–based osteoporosis prevention and management model provided by a parish nurse, family nurse practitioner, and registered dietitian. Incorporating education focused on lifestyle changes, nutrition, and pharmacological therapies, the model centered on the whole person perspective of osteoporosis prevention and management for females aged 11+ in the faith community. The collaborative team of health-care professionals provides education and support for community members who wish to make significant lifestyle changes. Ongoing evaluation of members' changing needs are assessed with continuous follow-up and evaluation, and choices in lifestyle change coupled with faith beliefs and religious readings provide important support and coping strategies for bone health promotion across the life span.

MEDICATIONS FOR THE PREVENTION AND/OR TREATMENT OF OSTEOPOROSIS

A number of medications are effective in preserving bone mineral density. FDA-approved osteoporosis treatments have been shown to decrease fracture risk in patients who have had fragility fractures and/or osteoporosis by DXA. The National Osteoporosis Foundation treatment guidelines state that treatment should be recommended to anyone who faces at least a 3% risk of suffering hip fracture in the next 10 years and to anyone who has at least a 20% risk of sustaining any major bone fractures in that time frame; this is based on a cost-effectiveness model. Pharmacotherapy may also reduce fractures in patients with low bone mass (osteopenia) without fractures. There is no consensus about when to initiate therapy to prevent fractures; the health-care provider should assess the potential benefits and risks of therapy in each patient on an individual basis (ACOG, 2012b; Goldstein, 2013; Nelson, 2011; NOF, 2013b).

Nursing Insight— *ACOG and NAMS recommendations for osteoporosis pharmacotherapy*

The American College of Obstetricians and Gynecologists (2012b) recommends osteoporosis pharmacotherapy for the following women:

- Women who have experienced a fragility or low-impact fracture, especially of the vertebra or hip, even in the absence of osteoporosis on the central dual energy x-ray absorptiometry (DXA) report
- Women who have a BMD T-score (determined by DXA) of less than or equal to –2.5
- For women in the low bone mass category (T-score between –1 and –2.5), the FRAX calculator can be used to make an informed treatment decision
- Women who are found to have a 10-year risk of major osteoporotic fracture greater than or equal to 3% using the FRAX calculator are candidates for medical pharmacological therapy

The North American Menopause Society (2010a) recommends osteoporosis pharmacotherapy for:

- All postmenopausal women who have had an osteoporotic vertebral or hip fracture
- All postmenopausal women who have BMD values consistent with osteoporosis (i.e., T-scores equal to or worse than –2.5 at the lumbar spine, femoral neck, or total hip region)
- All postmenopausal women who have T-scores from –1.0 to –2.5 and a 10-year risk, based on the FRAX calculator, of major osteoporotic fracture (spine, hip, shoulder, or wrist) of at least 20% or of hip fracture of at least 3%

The U.S. Food and Drug Administration has approved a number of medications for the prevention and/or treatment of postmenopausal osteoporosis. These include, in alphabetical order: bisphosphonates (alendronate, alendronate plus D, ibandronate, risedronate, risedronate with 500 mg of calcium carbonate and zoledronic acid), estrogens (estrogen and/or hormone therapy), estrogen agonist/antagonists (raloxifene), and parathyroid hormone (PTH). Certain medications are available in oral and IV forms; specific information about each medication is presented in Box 7-14.

Box 7-14 FDA-Approved Medications for the Prevention and/or Treatment of Postmenopausal Osteoporosis

BISPHOSPHONATES

Bisphosphonates are synthetic forms of a class of compounds found in the body. These compounds bind to the crystals in the bone matrix and inhibit bone resorption. Women who cannot or who choose not to take estrogen are good candidates for bisphosphonate therapy. Bisphosphonates inhibit normal physiological bone resorption as well as abnormal bone resorption, thereby halting bone loss, increasing bone mineral density, and reducing the risk of fractures (NOF, 2013b).

Alendronate (Fosamax, Fosamax Plus D, Binosto) is FDA approved for the prevention (5 mg PO daily or 35 mg PO weekly) and treatment (10 mg PO daily or 70 mg PO weekly) of postmenopausal osteoporosis. A liquid formulation and an effervescent tablet (Binosto) are available, as well as a formulation that contains 5,600 IU of vitamin D. Alendronate is also available as a generic preparation. Alendronate reduces the incidence of spine and hip fractures by about 50% over 3 years in patients with a prior vertebral fracture, and it reduces the incidence of vertebral fractures by about 48% over 3 years in patients without a prior vertebral fracture (NOF, 2013b).

Etidronate (Didrocal) is approved in Canada for osteoporosis prevention and treatment in postmenopausal women (400 mg/day for 14 days every 3 months, with calcium taken between cycles). In the United States, etidronate is approved only for treatment of Paget's disease, not for osteoporosis therapy (NAMS, 2010a).

Ibandronate (Boniva) is FDA approved for the treatment (2.5 mg daily tablet, 150 mg monthly tablet, and 3 mg every 3 months by IV injection) of postmenopausal osteoporosis. The oral preparations are also approved for the prevention of postmenopausal osteoporosis. Ibandronate reduces the incidence of vertebral fractures by about 50% over 3 years. It is available as a generic preparation in the United States (NOF, 2013b).

Risedronate (Actonel, Atelvia) is approved by the FDA for the prevention and treatment (5 mg daily tablet or 35 mg weekly tablet, packaged with five tablets of 500 mg calcium carbonate or 75 mg tablets taken on 2 consecutive days every month, or 150 mg monthly tablet) of postmenopausal osteoporosis. This medication reduces the incidence of vertebral fractures by about 41% to 49% and nonvertebral fractures by about 36% over 3 years, with significant risk reduction occurring after 1 year of treatment, in patients with a prior vertebral fracture (NOF, 2013b).

Zoledronic acid (Reclast, United States; Aclasta, Canada) is approved by the FDA for the treatment (5 mg by IV infusion over at least 15 minutes once yearly) and prevention (an infusion administered once every 2 years) of osteoporosis in postmenopausal women. Zoledronic acid reduces the incidence of vertebral fractures by about 70%, hip fractures by about 41%, and nonvertebral fractures by about 25% over 3 years. Zoledronic acid is also indicated for the prevention of new clinical fractures in patients who have recently had an osteoporosis-related hip fracture. Prior to administration, patients must have two blood tests: One is for creatinine to confirm that kidney function is normal; the other test is for calcium to confirm that the serum calcium level is within normal limits (NAMS, 2010a; NOF, 2013b).

CALCITONIN

Calcitonin salmon (Miacalcin, Fortical) received FDA approval for the treatment of osteoporosis in women who were at least 5 years postmenopausal in 1984. The medication is delivered as a single daily intranasal spray that provides 200 IU of the drug. Subcutaneous administration by injection also is available; side effects associated with this administration route include local inflammation and flushing of the face or hands. However, in 2013, FDA advisory panel experts opted to recommend that marketing of calcitonin-salmon for the treatment of osteoporosis in women greater than 5 years after menopause be stopped, owing to concerns over lack of benefit and the possibility of cancer (NAMS, 2010a; NOF, 2013b; U.S. FDA, 2013).

ESTROGEN/HORMONE THERAPY (ET/HT)

Estrogen therapy (Climara, Estrace, Estraderm, Estratab, Ogen, Ortho-Est, Premarin, Vivelle) and *hormone therapy* (Activella, Femhrt, Premphase, Prempro,

etc.) are approved by the FDA for the prevention of osteoporosis and relief of vasomotor symptoms and vulvovaginal atrophy associated with menopause. Women who have not had a hysterectomy require HT, which contains a progestin to protect the uterine lining. The Woman's Health Initiative (WHI) found that 5 years of HT (Prempro) reduced the risk of clinical vertebral fractures and hip fractures by 34% and other osteoporotic fractures by 23% (NOF, 2013b).

The WHI reported increased risks of myocardial infarction, stroke, invasive breast cancer, pulmonary emboli, and deep vein phlebitis during 5 years of treatment with conjugated equine estrogen and medroxyprogesterone (Prempro). Subsequent analysis of these data showed no increase in cardiovascular disease in women who started treatment within 10 years of menopause. In the estrogen-only arm of WHI, no increase in breast cancer incidence was noted over 7.1 years of treatment. Other doses and combinations of estrogen and progestins were not studied. Because of the risks, ET/HT should be used in the lowest effective doses for the shortest duration to meet treatment goals. When ET/HT use is considered solely for the prevention of osteoporosis, the FDA recommends that approved nonestrogen treatments should first be carefully considered (NOF, 2013b).

ESTROGEN AGONIST/ANTAGONIST (FORMERLY KNOWN AS SELECTIVE ESTROGEN-RECEPTOR MODULATORS [SERMS])

Raloxifene (Evista) is approved by the FDA for both prevention and treatment of osteoporosis in postmenopausal women. Raloxifene reduces the risk of vertebral fractures by about 30% in patients with a prior vertebral fracture and by about 55% in patients without a prior vertebral fracture over 3 years. Bone loss often resumes when raloxifene therapy is stopped. Raloxifene is indicated for the reduction in risk of invasive breast cancer in postmenopausal women with osteoporosis. This medication increases the risk of deep vein thrombosis to a degree similar to that observed with estrogen, and it also increases the frequency of night sweats and hot flashes (ACOG, 2012; NAMS, 2010a; NOF, 2013b).

PARATHYROID HORMONE (PTH)

Teriparatide (recombinant human PTH 1-34, marketed as Forteo) is approved by the FDA for the treatment of osteoporosis in postmenopausal women at high risk for fracture. It is a bone-building (anabolic) agent that directly stimulates osteoblastic bone formation, resulting in substantial increases in trabecular bone density and connectivity. This mechanism of action is very different from that of antiresorptive agents such as estrogen and bisphosphonates, which reduce bone resorption. It is administered by daily subcutaneous injection. Teriparatide in a dose of 20 mcg daily has been shown to decrease the risk of vertebral fractures by 65% and nonvertebral fractures by 53% in patients with osteoporosis, after an average of 18 months of therapy. This medication should only be used for a maximum of 2 years, and it is contraindicated in patients with an increased risk of osteosarcoma and those having prior radiation of the skeleton, bone metastases, hypercalcemia, or a history of skeletal malignancy. Teriparatide is also indicated for the treatment of glucocorticoid-induced osteoporosis and male osteoporosis.

RANK LIGAND INHIBITOR

Denosumab (Prolia) is approved for the treatment of postmenopausal osteoporosis in women who are at high risk for fracture and cannot use another osteoporosis medication. This medication has a different mechanism of action than the bisphosphonates. Denosumab inhibits RANK ligand (RANKL), which is a soluble protein needed for the formation of osteoclasts and is responsible for bone resorption. Administered in a 60 mg subcutaneous injection once every 6 months, the medication is contraindicated in patients with hypocalcemia and may be associated with serious adverse reactions including atypical femoral fractures; osteonecrosis of the jaw; and infections of the skin, urinary tract, ear, and abdomen. Patients using this medication should also be taking 1,000 mg of calcium and 400 IU of vitamin D (ACOG, 2012; NAMS, 2010a, 2010b; Wilton, 2011).

Combination therapy (usually a bisphosphonate with a nonbisphosphonate) can provide additional small increases in BMD when compared with monotherapy. However, the impact of combination therapy on fracture rates is unknown. At present, combination therapy is reserved for treatment failures when compliance has been assured (ACOG, 2012b; Fontenot & Harris, 2014; NAMS, 2010b).

> ### ✿ *Nursing Insight*— *Empowering women with information about osteoporosis medication options*
>
> An intravenous bisphosphonate may be an appropriate choice when a patient prefers less frequent dosing. Because an IV formulation must be administered by a health-care professional (in an infusion center or infusion-equipped office setting), use of an IV bisphosphonate ensures adherence for the indicated treatment period. Prior to the initiation of any therapy, it is important to inform the patient of various medication dosing and delivery options so that she may participate in the decision-making process, when possible (ACOG, 2012b).

The Nurse's Role in Fostering Safe Use of Osteoporosis Medications

An essential role for nurses who care for women who take prescribed osteoporosis medications centers on education and counseling about potential risks and side effects as well as the importance of adhering to specific dosing recommendations for the bisphosphonates. The oral bisphosphonates share a common risk profile in terms of their potential to cause gastrointestinal problems including difficulty swallowing, gastroesophageal reflux, inflammation of the esophagus, esophageal cancer, and gastric ulcer. Oral bisphosphonates are contraindicated in individuals with reflux, gastroesophageal reflux disease, and other esophageal abnormalities. Neither IV ibandronate nor IV zoledronic acid has been associated with upper GI adverse events. Side effects for all of the bisphosphonates may include abdominal, bone, joint, or muscle pain. The nurse should emphasize that deviating from the dosing instructions increases the likelihood of experiencing GI symptoms (ACOG, 2012b; Green et al., 2010; NAMS, 2010b; Wright, 2011).

It is essential that the oral bisphosphonates (with the exception of Atelvia) be taken on an empty stomach first thing in the morning with 8 ounces of plain water, with no additional food or drink consumption for at least 30 minutes (up to 2 hours, depending on the medication) and the patient remaining upright during this time. An enteric-coated bisphosphonate version of risedronate (Atelvia) is taken after breakfast. With this once-weekly medication, the patient does not need to have an empty stomach, but must still remain upright for 30 minutes after taking it with at least 4 ounces of water. Binosto, a new formulation of alendronate sodium, is supplied as an effervescent tablet that is to be dissolved in 4 ounces of plain (not flavored or mineral) water at room temperature. Not following the instruction to take the bisphosphonates with only plain water can substantially reduce medication absorption; substituting coffee or juice for water can reduce drug absorption by as much as 60%. Also, patients should exercise caution if taking the medications with well water, which can have a high mineral content that may decrease bisphosphonate absorption. Oral bisphosphonates are

contraindicated in women with uncorrected hypocalcemia, an inability to sit or stand for 30 to 60 minutes, esophageal stricture, or severe renal impairment. Side effects associated with the IV administration of bisphosphonates include flu-like symptoms: fever, pain in the muscles or joints, and headache. Eye inflammation (uveitis) is a rare side effect. There have been rare reports of osteonecrosis (death of the bone cells or tissue) of the jaw with bisphosphonate medications. Nearly all of these cases occurred in cancer patients receiving an intravenous bisphosphonate (ACOG, 2012b; Bechtle, 2013; NAMS, 2010b; Wilton, 2011; Wright, 2011).

Although unusual, patients being treated with the bisphosphonate tablets alendronate (Fosamax), ibandronate (Boniva), and risedronate (Actonel) for osteoporosis prevention or treatment have also been reported to have developed osteonecrosis of the jaw. Although the risk for this complication in healthy women is estimated as less than 1 in 100,000 treatment years, dental evaluation is recommended prior to the initiation of bisphosphonate therapy. Also, there have been rare reports of esophageal cancer in women taking oral bisphosphonates. Owing to this potential complication, patients with Barrett's esophagus (a premalignant condition caused by an abnormal change in the cells of the distal portion of the esophagus) should not use oral bisphosphonates. An essential component of health teaching for all women who take oral bisphosphonate tablets includes the warning that side effects such as chest pain, new or worsening heartburn, or difficulty or painful swallowing must be immediately reported to the health-care provider (ACOG, 2012b; Idzik & Krauss, 2013; NAMS, 2010b; Wright, 2011).

Other concerns center on the possibility of atypical femur fractures (AFFs) in patients taking alendronate, and possibly other bisphosphonates, for a prolonged period of time (i.e., 5–10 years). Atypical femur fractures linked to bisphosphonate use are termed "low energy fractures," meaning that minimal or no trauma has occurred. Owing to the possibility of AFFs, it is essential that nurses teach patients to be aware of the early signs of an impending fracture, such as prodromal groin, hip, or thigh pain. At present, the FDA requires labeling for all bisphosphonate preparations approved for osteoporosis that warn about the unusual femoral fractures (Hellier & Ross, 2012).

Because bisphosphonates are associated with esophageal irritation, it is important to provide detailed dosing information when counseling women about the use of these medications. Alendronate and risedronate tablets should be taken first thing in the morning with 8 ounces of plain water. Patients using the liquid formulation of alendronate should swallow one bottle (75 mL) and follow with at least 2 ounces of plain water. After taking these medications, patients must wait at least 30 minutes before eating, drinking, or taking any other medication. Patients should remain upright (sitting or standing) during this interval (NAMS, 2010b).

Oral ibandronate tablets should be taken on an empty stomach, the first thing in the morning, with 8 ounces of plain water (no other liquid). After taking this medication, patients should be instructed to wait at least 60 minutes before eating, drinking, or taking any other medication. Patients must remain upright for at least 1 hour after taking the medication. Ibandronate, 3 mg per 3 mL prefilled syringe, is given by IV injection over 15 to 30 seconds, once every 3 months. Patients should be advised that serum calcium and creatinine levels will be checked before each injection (ACOG, 2012b; NAMS, 2010b; Wright, 2011).

"What to say" — *Preparing patients for zoledronic acid infusion*

Nurses can help prepare patients who will be treated with an intravenous infusion of zoledronic acid (Reclast) by offering the following information:

- Eat normally and drink at least two glasses of fluids before the treatment
- Your treatment will take at least 15 minutes.
- You may resume your normal activities immediately after the treatment.
- After the first treatment, common side effects may include flu-like symptoms such as fever, muscle or joint pain, and headache.
- You may receive acetaminophen (Tylenol) prior to the infusion to reduce the risk of developing these symptoms; after the treatment, you may continue to use a mild pain reliever as needed for discomfort.
- Side effects are much less common after successive treatments.

(ACOG, 2012b; NAMS, 2010b)

The National Osteoporosis Foundation recommends BMD testing every 2 years. For women undergoing pharmacological therapy for osteoporosis, a repeat DXA scan should be performed 2 years after the initiation of treatment and at subsequent 2-year intervals (NAMS, 2010a).

Optimizing Outcomes— **Educating women about osteoporosis resources for consumers**

The U.S. Department of Health & Human Services (DHHS) Agency for Healthcare Research and Quality (AHRQ)'s Effective Health Care summary guides have produced *Osteoporosis Treatments That Help Prevent Broken Bones: A Guide for Women After Menopause*, a resource for consumers. The guide is based on a government-funded review of research reports about osteoporosis treatments to prevent broken bones and is available at http://www.effectivehealthcare.ahrq.gov /repFiles/LowBoneDensityConsumer.pdf.

Another publication, *The Surgeon General's Report on Bone Health and Osteoporosis: What It Means to You*, has been produced by the National Institutes of Health. This informative guide, which provides an in-depth discussion about strategies for promoting bone health, is available at http://www .niams.nih.gov/Health_Info/Bone/SGR/surgeon_generals _report.asp.

Optimizing Outcomes— **With professional resources to guide clinical care**

Several clinical and governmental organizations have published guidelines to assist clinicians in informing and

Where Research and Practice Meet: Strategies to Enhance Health After Hip Fracture

Singh and colleagues (2012) conducted a randomized controlled trial (n = 124) to compare individuals recovering from hip fracture who received usual surgery aftercare (the control group) with individuals who received targeted multidisciplinary interventions (the intervention group), which included the following: high-intensity progressive resistance and balance training twice a week; osteoporosis treatment with alendronate 10 mg/day or 70 mg/week; smoking cessation, moderation of alcohol consumption, calcium 1,200 mg/day, and vitamin D 1,000 IU/day supplementation; nutrition to include monthly weight checks, dietary counseling, and protein intake of 20 g/day; evaluation of depression monthly with the Geriatric Depression Scale; an evaluation of vision by an ophthalmologist; a home evaluation 2 to 7 days after discharge from an acute care facility to educate, evaluate, and modify fall hazards within the home; and social support to include information on community resources, social interactions during twice-weekly exercise sessions, and monthly visits or phone calls from investigators for 12 months.

The two groups did not differ at baseline, but at the end of the study, the intervention group's risk of death was reduced by 81%, nursing home admissions were reduced by 84%, activities of daily living declined less, and at 12 months, the intervention group had less assistive device use. Findings from this study underscore the importance of a multidisciplinary approach in developing interventions aimed to enhance recovery and quality of life and reduce morbidity and mortality following hip fracture.

guiding women toward appropriate treatments that will help to relieve their menopausal symptoms without placing their health in undue jeopardy. These organizations include the American College of Obstetricians and Gynecologists (ACOG), The North American Menopause Society (NAMS), the National Association of Nurse Practitioners in Women's Health (NPWH), the National Osteoporosis Foundation (NOF), the International Osteoporosis Foundation (IOF), the Association of Women's Health, Obstetric, and Neonatal Nurses (AWHONN), the U.S. Food and Drug Administration (FDA), and the U.S. Preventive Services Task Force (USPSTF). Nurses can use these recommendations to discuss options with their patients and provide current, evidence-based care.

Now Can You— **Discuss certain aspects of osteoporosis?**

1. Explain why menopausal women are at increased risk for osteoporosis and how to conduct a risk assessment for the condition?
2. Counsel a woman about preparing for a DXA examination?
3. Develop an osteoporosis educational program that includes strategies for reducing risk and tips for optimizing bone health?
4. Counsel a woman about the safe use of medications for the prevention and/or treatment of osteoporosis?

Summary Points

◆ Today, American women can expect to live to be 80 years old and spend close to one-third of their lives as menopausal women.

◆ Nurses can empower midlife women with factual, evidence-based information about menopause, the normal aging process, and strategies to optimize cardiovascular and skeletal health.

◆ Complementary and alternative medicine approaches such as stress management, guided imagery, biofeedback, yoga, and massage therapy may be useful in minimizing various menopausal symptoms.

◆ An important role for nurses centers on counseling women to become informed about any herbal preparations they are considering and to consult with their health-care providers before using any of them.

◆ Estrogen-containing drugs for menopausal use are divided into two categories: estrogen therapy (ET) and combined estrogen-progestogen therapy (EPT).

◆ The number one killer of older American women is cardiovascular disease, which includes coronary heart disease, stroke, congestive heart failure, hypertension, and other diseases of the heart and vascular system.

◆ Educating women about strategies to control the five cardiovascular risk factors (smoking, hyperlipidemia, diabetes mellitus, hypertension, obesity) can empower them to make changes that can greatly reduce their lifetime risk for CVD.

◆ Bone health promotion includes strategies such as optimizing calcium intake, preventing the loss of calcium and other minerals from the bone, maintaining the soft tissue components around the bone, and promoting the efficiency of bone repair.

◆ An essential role for nurses who care for women who take prescribed osteoporosis medications centers on education and counseling about potential risks and side effects as well as the importance of adhering to specific dosing recommendations for the bisphosphonates.

Review Questions

Multiple Choice

1. Normal physiological changes that accompany menopause include:
A. Vaginal lengthening with an increased production of cervical mucus
B. An increase in muscle mass
C. Less elastic skin with decreased melanin
D. Increased levels of estrogen and progesterone

2. Nurses can teach women about self-care strategies to help reduce menopausal symptoms, such as:
A. Dressing in layers
B. Consuming foods and beverages that contain caffeine
C. Reducing physical activity
D. Consuming foods that are highly seasoned

3. According to recommendations from The North American Menopause Society, recommendations for hormone therapy use include:
A. Prevention of diabetes mellitus
B. Short-term treatment for severe vasomotor symptoms
C. Prevention of coronary heart disease
D. Prevention of dementia

4. Risk factors for cardiovascular disease include:
A. Normal body weight
B. Parkinson's disease
C. Psychological stress
D. Regular dietary consumption of fiber, fruits, and vegetables

5. Risk factors for osteoporosis include:
A. Excessive sun exposure
B. Large body build
C. Late menopause
D. Caucasian ethnicity

REFERENCES

Adams-Fryatt, A. (2010). Facilitating successful aging: Encouraging older adults to be physically active. *The Journal for Nurse Practitioners, 6*(3), 187–192. doi:10.1016/j.nurpra.2009.11.007

Alexander, I.M. Overview of current HT recommendations using evidence-based decision making. *American Journal for Nurse Practitioners, 11*(10), 29-41

Allmen, T., & Moore, A. (2010). Attention and intervention: Responding to vaginal changes of menopause. *Women's Health Care: A Practical Journal for Nurse Practitioners, 9*(5), 38–51.

American College of Obstetricians and Gynecologists (ACOG). (2004). Hormone therapy: Cognition and dementia. *Obstetrics and Gynecology, 104*(Suppl.), 25S–40S.

American College of Obstetricians and Gynecologists (ACOG). (2005). Urinary incontinence in women. Practice Bulletin No. 63. (Reaffirmed 2013.) *Obstetrics & Gynecology, 105*(6), 1533–1545.

American College of Obstetricians and Gynecologists (ACOG). (2011). Tobacco use and women's health. Committee Opinion No. 503. *Obstetrics & Gynecology, 118*(3), 746–750.

American College of Obstetricians and Gynecologists (ACOG). (2012a). Compounded bioidentical hormones. Committee Opinion Number 532. *Obstetrics & Gynecology, 120*(2), 411–415.

American College of Obstetricians and Gynecologists (ACOG). (2012b). Osteoporosis. Practice Bulletin No. 129. *Obstetrics & Gynecology, 120*(9), 718–734.

American College of Obstetricians and Gynecologists (ACOG). (2013a). Hormone therapy and heart disease. Committee Opinion Number 565. *Obstetrics & Gynecology, 121*(6), 1407–1410.

American College of Obstetricians and Gynecologists (ACOG). (2013b). Postmenopausal estrogen therapy: Route of administration and risk of venous thromboembolism. Committee Opinion No. 556. *Obstetrics & Gynecology, 121*(4), 887–908.

American College of Obstetricians and Gynecologists (ACOG). (2014). Management of menopausal symptoms. Practice Bulletin No. 141. *Obstetrics & Gynecology, 123*(1), 202–216.

American Diabetes Association (ADA). (2013). *The cardiometabolic risk initiative: Moving beyond the metabolic syndrome.* Retrieved from http://professional.diabetes.org/ResourcesForProfessionals.aspx?cid=60379

American Heart Association (AHA). (2011). Effectiveness-based guidelines for the prevention of cardiovascular disease in women—2011 update: A guideline from the American Heart Association. *Circulation, 123*(2), 1243–1262. doi:10.1161/CIR.0b013e1820faaf8

American Heart Association (AHA). (2013a). *Heart disease & stroke statistics—2013 update.* Retrieved from http://circ.ahajournals.org/content/127/1/e6

American Heart Association (AHA). (2013b). *Medicines to help you quit smoking.* Retrieved from http://www.heart.org/HEARTORG/Getting Healthy/QuitSmoking/QuittingSmoking/Medicines-To-Help-You -Quit-Smoking_UCM_307921_Article.jsp

American Heart Association and American College of Cardiology Foundation. (2011). AHA/ACCF secondary prevention and risk reduction therapy for patients with coronary and other atherosclerotic vascular disease: 2011 update: A guideline from the American Heart Association and American College of Cardiology Foundation. *Circulation, 124*(11), 2458–2473. doi:10.1161/CIR.0b013e318235eb4d

Anastasi, J.K., Chang, M., & Capili, B. (2011). Herbal supplements: Talking with your patients. *The Journal for Nurse Practitioners—JNP, 7*(1), 29–35. doi:10.1016/j.nurpra.2010.06.004

Andelloux, M. (2011). Products for sexual lubrication. *Nursing for Women's Health, 15*(3), 253–257. doi:10.1111/j.1751-486X.2011.01642.x

Arslanian-Engoren, C. (2011). Women's risk factors and screening for coronary heart disease. *Journal of Obstetric, Gynecologic & Neonatal Nursing, 40*(3), 337–347. doi:10.1111/j.1552-6909.2011.01234.x

Artinin, N.T., Fletcher, G.F., Mozaffarian, D., Kris-Etherton, P., Van Horn, L., Lichtenstein, A.H., . . . Burke, L.E.; American Heart Association Prevention Committee of the Council on Cardiovascular Nursing. (2010). Interventions to promote physical activity and dietary lifestyle changes for cardiovascular risk factor reduction in adults: A scientific statement from the American Heart Association. *Circulation, 122*(8), 406–441. doi:10.1161/CIR.0b013e3181e8edf1

Association of Women's Health, Obstetric & Neonatal Nursing (AWHONN). (2011). Women's cardiovascular health. Position statement. *Journal of Obstetric, Gynecologic & Neonatal Nursing, 40*(6), 662–664. doi:10.1111/j.1552-6909.2011.01289.x

Athanasiadis, I., & Simon, J.A. (2011). Nonskeletal benefits of vitamin D beyond the media hype. *The Female Patient, 36*(6), 35–38.

Barbieri, R.L. (2013). When estrogen isn't an option, here is how I treat menopausal symptoms. *OBG Management, 25*(8), 13–14.

Bechtle, J. (2013). Osteoporosis risk reduction and bone health. *Nursing for Women's Health, 17*(3), 245–251. doi:10.1111/1751-486X.12039

Bradley, J., & Merz, C.N. (2011). Heart disease in women: What's new. *Consultant, 51*(5), 273–278.

Bulechek, G.M., Butcher, H.K., Dochterman, J.M., & Wagner, C. (2013). *Nursing interventions classification (NIC)* (6th ed.). St. Louis, MO: Elsevier Mosby.

Burns, D.S., & Carpenter, J.S. (2012). Paced respiration for hot flashes? *The Female Patient, 37*(8), 38–41.

Buster, J.E. (2010). Transdermal matters: Update on menopausal hormone replacement. *The Female Patient, 35*(9), 24–27.

Carey, S.A., & Gray, J.R. (2012). Women and heart disease: A diagnostic challenge. *The Journal for Nurse Practitioners—JNP, 8*(6), 458–463.

Centers for Disease Control and Prevention (2011). *Physical activity and health*. Retrieved from http://www.cdc.gov/physicalactivity/everyone /health/

Chichester, M., & Ciranni, P. (2011). Approaching menopause (But not there yet!). *Nursing for Women's Health, 15*(4), 320–324. doi:10.1111 /j.,1751-486X.2011.01652.x

Chlebowski, R.T., Anderson, G.L., Gass, M., Lane, D.S., Aragaki, A.K., Kuller, L.H., . . . Prentice, R.L. (2010). Estrogen plus progestin and breast cancer incidence and mortality in postmenopausal women. *Journal of the American Medical Association, 304*(15), 1684–1692. doi:10.1001/jama.2010.1500

Culligan, P.J. (2012). Nonsurgical management of pelvic organ prolapse. *Obstetrics and Gynecology, 119*(4), 852–860. doi:10.1097/AOG .0b013e31824c0806

Dempser, D.W. (2011). Osteoporosis and the burden of osteoporosis-related fractures. *American Journal of Managed Care, 17*(Suppl. 6), S164–S169.

DeVon, H.A., Saban, K.L., & Garrett, D.K. (2011). Recognizing and responding to symptoms of acute coronary syndromes and stroke in women. *Journal of Obstetric, Gynecologic & Neonatal Nursing, 40*(3), 372–382. doi:10.1111/j.1552-6909.2011.01241.x

Doering, L.V., & Eastwood, J. (2011). A literature review of depression, anxiety, and cardiovascular disease in women. *Journal of Obstetric, Gynecologic & Neonatal Nursing, 40*(3), 348–361. doi:10.1111/j.1552-6909 .2011.01236.x

Droste, L., Holmes, C., Hernandez, J.F., & Mahdjoubi, M. (2010). Diagnosis and management of vitamin D deficiency in adults. *The American Journal for Nurse Practitioners, 14*(7/8), 25–32.

Durham, E. (2012). Making the right choice in hormone therapy. *The Clinical Advisor, 15*(1), 34–45.

Edelman, J.S. (2012). Getting a good night's sleep in perimenopause and midlife. *The Female Patient, 37*(2), 27–31.

Egan, P. (2010). Nutrition interventions for healthy aging. *Advance for Nurse Practitioners, 18*(8), 14–23.

Elliott, C.S., & Sokol, E.R. (2011). New techniques for treating stress urinary incontinence. *Contemporary OB/GYN, 56*(1), 28–37.

Evans, J., & Karram, M. (2011). Evaluation and nonsurgical management of lower urinary tract symptoms. *The Female Patient, 36*(8), 14–20.

Fantasia, H.C., & Sutherland, M.A. (2014). Hormone therapy for the management of menopause symptoms. *Journal of Obstetric, Gynecologic & Neonatal Nursing, 43*(2), 226–234. doi:10.1111/1552-6909.12282

Fontenot, H.B., & Harris, A.L. (2014). Pharmacologic management of osteoporosis. *Journal of Obstetric, Gynecologic & Neonatal Nursing, 43*(2), 236–244. doi:10.1111/1552-6909.12295

Forster-Burke, D., Ritter, L., & Zimmer, S. (2010). Collaboration of a model osteoporosis prevention and management program in a faith community. *Journal of Obstetric, Gynecologic, & Neonatal Nursing, 39*(2), 212–219. doi:10.1111/j.1552-6909.2010.01111.x

Freeman, E.W., Sammel, M.D., Lin, H., Liu, Z., & Gracia, C.R. (2011). Duration of hot flushes and associated risk factors. *Obstetrics & Gynecology, 117*(5), 1095–1104. doi:10.1097/AOG.0b013e318214f0de

Freeman, S.B. (2010). Tissue changes associated with vaginal atrophy. *The Clinical Advisor, 13*(9), 32–38.

Freeman, S.B. (2012). Vaginal atrophy: Managing a chronic disorder. *Women's Health Care: A Practical Journal for Nurse Practitioners, 11*(5), 27–32.

Goldstein, S.R. (2013). Osteoporosis. *OBG Management, 25*(12), 35–39.

Grasso, D., & Rafferty, M.A. (2012). Vitamin D: Implications of the Institute of Medicine report for clinical practice. *The American Journal for Nurse Practitioners, 16*(1/2), 35–40.

Green, J., Czanner, G., Reeves, G., Watson, J., Wise, L., & Beral, V. (2010). Oral bisphosphonates and risk of cancer of oesophagus, stomach, and colorectum: Case control analysis within a UK primary care cohort. *British Medical Journal, 341*(9). doi:10/1136bmj.c4444

Grimes, D.A., Blankenship, O., Kremer, C., Reese, S., & Sonstein, F. (2011). Initial office evaluation of hair loss in adult women. *The Journal for Nurse Practitioners—JNP, 7*(6), 456–462. doi:10.1016/j.nurpra.2010.09.013

Guiltinan, J., & Reed, S.D. (2010). Herbal alternatives for menopausal symptoms. *Contemporary OB/GYN, 55*(11), 38–46.

Halloran, L. (2012). Sex and intimacy: Talking with your patients. *The Journal for Nurse Practitioners—JNP, 8*(6), 490–492.

Hamlin, A.S., & Robertson, T.M. (2013). Incontinence in women. *Advance for NPs & PAs, 4*(10), 21–24.

Hauser, L. (2012). Migraines and perimenopause. *Nursing for Women's Health, 16*(3), 247–250. doi:10.1111/j.1751-486X.2012.01737.x

Hellier, S., & Ross, C. (2012). Long-term bisphosphonate therapy: Possible link to rare femur fracture. *The American Journal for Nurse Practitioners, 16*(0/10), 12–18.

Henderson, V.W. (2011). Cognitive symptoms and disorders in the midlife woman. *The Female Patient, 36*(5), 49–54.

Higgs, D., & Kessenich, C. (2010). Complementary therapies in osteoporosis. *The Journal for Nurse Practitioners—JNP, 6*(3), 193–198.

Howe, T.E., Shea, B., Dawson, L.J., Downie, F., Murray, A., Ross, C., . . . Creed, G. (2011). Exercise for preventing and treating osteoporosis in postmenopausal women. *Cochrane Database of Systematic Reviews.* Issue 7. Art No.: CD000333. doi:10.1002/14651858.CD00033.pub2

Hsia, J., Langer, R.D., Manson, J.E., Kuller, J., Johnson, K.C., Hendrix, S.L., . . . Prentice, R.; Women's Health Initiative Investigators. (2006). Conjugated equine estrogens and coronary heart disease: The Women's Health Initiative. *Archives of Internal Medicine, 166*(3), 357–365.

Hurley, B., & Armstrong, T.J. (2012). Bisphosphonates vs exercise for the prevention and treatment of osteoporosis. *The Journal for Nurse Practitioners—JNP, 8*(3), 217–224. doi:10.1016/j.nurpra.2011.07.029

Idzik, S., & Krauss, E. (2013). Evaluating and managing dental complaints in primary and urgent care. *The Journal for Nurse Practitioners, 9*(6), 329–338. doi:10.16/j.nurpra.2013.04.015

Im, E., Lee, B., Chee, W., & Stuifbergen, A. (2012). Attitudes toward physical activity of white midlife women. *Journal of Obstetric, Gynecologic & Neonatal Nursing, 40*(3), 312–321. doi:10.1111/j.1552-6909 .2011.01249.x

Im, E., Young, K., Hwang, H., Chee, W., Stuifbergen, A., Lee, H., & Chee, E. (2012). Asian American midlife women's attitudes toward physical activity. *Journal of Obstetric, Gynecologic & Neonatal Nursing, 41*(5), 650–658. doi:10.1111/j.1552-6909.2012.01392.x

Institute of Medicine. (2010). *Dietary reference intakes for calcium and vitamin D.* Washington, DC: National Academies Press.

Johnson, H.L., & Seibert, D.C. (2011). Dispelling the myths of heart disease for women. *The Journal for Nurse Practitioners—JNP, 7*(5), 392–398.

Johnson, M., Moorhead, S., Bulechek, G., Butcher, H., Maas, M., & Swanson, E. (2012). *NIC and NOC linkages to NANDA-I and clinical conditions* (3rd ed.). St. Louis, MO: Elsevier Mosby.

Jones, K.A., Bryson, E., & Harmanli, O. (2010). Successful pelvic floor rehabilitation practice for the obstetrician/gynecologist. *The Female Patient, 35*(5), 41–43.

Jones, P.H. (2010). Dyslipidemia: Individualizing care of patients. *Consultant, 50*(Suppl. 20), S1–S10.

Jones, P.H., Ansell, B., & Bloch, M. (2014). Evaluating cardiovascular risk factors and treatment options. *Consultant, 26*(Suppl. 2), S12–S13.

Katz, A. (2011). Sex, health, and aging: What women need to know. *Nursing for Women's Health, 15*(6), 519–521. doi:10.1111/j.1751-486X.2011.01683.x

Kaunitz, A.M., Pinkerton, J.V., & Simon, J.A. (2014). When should a menopausal woman discontinue hormone therapy? *OBG Management, 26*(2), 59–65.

Keilman, L.J. (2011). Urinary incontinence in the older female population. *The Clinical Advisor, 14*(12), 67–77.

Kellogg-Spadt, S. (2012). Treatment for the genitourinary symptoms of vaginal atrophy: A perspective for nurse practitioners. *Women's Health Care: A Practical Journal for Nurse Practitioners, 11*(5), 33–39.

Kellogg-Spadt, S. (2011). Vaginal lubrication: Exploring options. *Women's Health Care: A Practical Journal for Nurse Practitioners, 10*(9), 49–50.

Kemle, K. (2011). Falls in older adults: Averting disaster. *The Clinical Advisor, 14*(2), 50–56.

Kenton, K. (2014). What is new in the evaluation and treatment of urinary incontinence? *Obstetrics & Gynecology, 123*(1), 179–182. doi:10.1097/AOG00000000067

Khouzam, H.R. (2012). Depression in the elderly: When to suspect. *Consultant, 52*(3), 225–240.

Kretzer, K. (2011). Integrating a CAM therapeutic strategy for hypertension. *The American Journal for Nurse Practitioners, 15*(11/12), 48–52.

Laster, A.J. (2014). Dual-energy x-ray absorptiometry: Overused, neglected, or just misunderstood? *North Carolina Medical Journal, 75*(2), 132–136.

Lewiecki, E.M. (2012). To treat or not to treat: Reducing fracture risk in postmenopausal women. *The Female Patient, 37*(1), 11–15.

Liu, J.H., & Minkin, M.J. (2013). Advances in transdermal estrogen-only therapy for vasomotor symptoms. *OBG Management, 33*(Suppl. 10), S1–S9.

McCracken, L.P., & Dunaway, A. (2012). Black cohosh. *Advance for NPs & PAs, 2*(5), 41–42.

McEneaney, M.J. (2012). Individualizing management for common concerns of postmenopausal women. *The Journal for Nurse Practitioners—JNP, 8*(6), 470–474. doi:10.1016/j.nurpra.2011.09.021

McKenzie, L.J. (2012). Osteoporosis: New recommendations and lingering questions. *Contemporary OB/GYN, 57*(12), 47–49.

McSweeney, J.C., Pettey, C.M., Souder, E., & Rhoads, S. (2011). Disparities in women's cardiovascular health. *Journal of Obstetric, Gynecologic & Neonatal Nursing, 40*(3), 348–361. doi:10.1111/j.1552-6909.2011.01239.x

Maes, C.A., & Louis, M. (2011). Nurse practitioners' sexual history-taking practices with adults 50 and older. *The Journal for Nurse Practitioners—JNP, 7*(3), 216–222. doi:10.1016/j.nurpra.2010.06.003

Main, C., Knight, B., Moxham, T., Sanchez, R., Sanchez Gomez, L., Roque i Figuls, M., & Cosp, X. (2013). Hormone therapy for preventing cardiovascular disease in post-menopausal women. *Cochrane Database of Systematic Reviews 2013.* Issue 4. Art. No.: CD002229. doi:10.1002/14651858.CD002229.pub3

Manson, J.E. (2013). What the KEEPS trial reveals about HT in younger menopausal women. *OBG Management, 25*(6), 38–39.

Manson, J.E., & Bassuk, S.S. (2011). Marine omega-3 fatty acids and cardiovascular disease. *The Female Patient, 36*(11), 12–16.

Mayhew, M.S. (2010). Aspirin for preventing cardiovascular damage. *The Journal for Nurse Practitioners—JNP, 6*(2), 147–148.

Mayo Clinic. (2013). *Nicotine dependence.* Retrieved from http://www.mayoclinic.com/health/nicotine-dependence/DS00307/DSECTION=treatments-and-drugs

Minkin, M.J. (2010). Transdermal estrogen therapy: Personalized treatment approaches. *The Female Patient, 35*(6), 16–18.

Minkin, M.J. (2013). Postmenopausal vulvovaginal atrophy: Communication and care. *The Clinical Advisor, 16*(10), 59–64.

Minkin, M.J., & Guess, M.K. (2012). Diagnosis and treatment of the non-sex-related symptoms of vulvovaginal atrophy. *The Female Patient, 37*(10), 33–41.

Monroe, J. (2012). Lichen sclerosus et atrophicus. *The Clinical Advisor, 15*(9), 71–72.

Moorhead, S., Johnson, M., Maas, M.L., & Swanson, E. (2013). *Nursing outcomes classification (NOC)* (5th ed.). St. Louis, MO: Elsevier Mosby.

Moran, B., & Walsh, T. (2013). Cardiovascular disease in women. *Nursing for Women's Health, 17*(3), 63–68. doi:10.1111/1751-486X.12008

Mosca, L., Benjamin, E.J., Berra, K., Bezanson, J.L., Dolor, R.J., Loyd-Jones, L., . . . Wenger, N.K. (2011). Effectiveness-based guidelines for the prevention of cardiovascular disease in women—2011 update: A guideline from the American Heart Association. *Circulation, 123*(2), 1243–1262. doi:10.1161/CIR.0b013e31820faaf8

Muffly, T.M., & Paraiso, M.F. (2012). Diagnosis and treatment of overactive bladder in midlife women. *The Female Patient, 37*(3), 17–22.

National Institutes of Health. (2005). National Institutes of Health State-of-the-Science conference statement: Management of menopause-related symptoms. *Annals of Internal Medicine, 142*(12, Part 1), 1003–1013.

National Institutes of Health. (2013). *Dietary supplement fact sheet: Calcium.* Retrieved from http://ods.od.nih.gov/factsheets/calcium.asp

National Institutes of Health Osteoporosis and Related Bone Diseases National Resource Center. (2012). *Osteoporosis and African American women.* Retrieved from http://www.niams.nih.gov/Health_Info/Bone/Osteoporosis/Background/

National Osteoporosis Foundation (NOF). (2013a). *Clinician's guide to prevention and treatment of osteoporosis.* Washington, DC: National Osteoporosis Foundation.

National Osteoporosis Foundation (NOF). (2013b). *Managing and treating osteoporosis.* Retrieved from http://nof.org/live/treating

National Women's Health Network. (2000). *Taking hormones and women's health: Choices, risks, and benefits* (5th ed.). Washington, DC: Author.

Nelson, A.L. (2011). Perimenopause, menopause, and postmenopause: Health promotion strategies. In R.A. Hatcher, J. Trussell, A.L. Nelson, W. Cates, D. Kowal, & M.S. Policar (Eds.), *Contraceptive technology* (20th ed., pp. 737–777). Decatur, GA: Bridging the Gap Communications.

O'Dell, K. (2014). Pharmacologic management of bladder dysfunction in adult women. *Journal of Obstetric, Gynecologic & Neonatal Nursing, 43*(2), 253–263. doi:10.1111/1552-6909.12287

Pearson, T. (2011). Atrophic vaginitis. *The Journal for Nurse Practitioners—JNP, 7*(6), 502–511. doi:10.1016/j.nurpra.2010.08.016

Pinkerton, J.V. (2012). The truth about bioidentical therapy. *The Female Patient, 37*(8), 16–20.

Pinkerton, J.V., Constantine, G., Hwang, E., & Cheng, J.R. (2013). Desvenlafaxine compared with placebo for treatment of menopausal vasomotor symptoms: A 12-week, multicenter, parallel-group, randomized, double-blind, placebo-controlled efficacy trial. *Menopause, 20*(1), 28–37.

Portman, D.J., Bachmann, G.A., & Simon, J.A. (2013). Ospemifene, a novel selective estrogen receptor modulator for treating dyspareunia associated with postmenopausal vulvar and vaginal atrophy. *Menopause, 20*(6), 623–630. doi:10.1097/gme.0b013e318279ba64

Rajki, M. (2011). Sleep problems in older adults. *Advance for NPs & PAs, 2*(12), 16–22.

Reed, S.D., & Guiltinan, J. (2010). Herbal alternatives for menopausal symptoms. *Contemporary OB/GYN, 55*(11), 38–42.

Ribowsky, J. (2011). Hormone therapy for menopause: A concise update of the benefits and risks. *Advance for NPs & PAs, 2*(8), 19–23.

Roberts, H. (2010). Long-term hormone therapy—a Cochrane summary. *The Female Patient, 36*(12), 50–54.

Roberts, M.E., & Davis, L.L. (2013). Cardiovascular disease in women: A nurse practitioner's guide to prevention. *The Journal for Nurse Practitioners, 9*(10), 679–687.

Rossow, J.E., Manson, J.E., Kaunitz, A.M., & Anderson, G.L. (2013). Lessons learned from the Women's Health Initiative trials of menopausal hormone therapy. *Obstetrics & Gynecology, 121*(1), 172–176. doi:10.1097/AOG.0b013e31827a08c8

Ruhl, C. (2010). Sleep is a vital sign: Why assessing sleep is an important part of women's health care. *Nursing for Women's Health, 14*(3), 243–247.

Salmoiago-Blotcher, E., Crawford, S., Jackson, E., Ockene, J., & Ockene, I. (2011). Constipation and risk of cardiovascular disease among postmenopausal women. *American Journal of Medicine, 124*(8), 714–723. doi:10.1016/j.amjmed.2011.03.026

Scheinfeld, N.S. (2011). Skin disorders in older adults: Cutaneous signs of normal aging. *Consultant, 51*(12), 933–936.

Sego, S. (2012). Wild yam. *The Clinical Advisor, 15*(2), 100–102.

Seidel, S.S. (2011). Urinary incontinence/overactive bladder in women: The role of sacral neuromodulation. *Women's Health Care: A Practical Journal for Nurse Practitioners, 10*(5), 38–41.

Sherman, C. (2011). Interventions to reduce CVD risk in adults. *The Clinical Advisor, 14*(6), 78–81.

Shifren, J.L., & Schiff, I. (2010). Role of hormone therapy in the management of menopause. *Obstetrics & Gynecology, 115*(4), 839–855.

Shoup, D. (2012). Individualizing hormone therapy: Weighing risks and benefits. *Contemporary OB-GYN, 57*(8), 16–24.

Singh, N.A., Quine, S., Clemson, L.M., Williams, E.J., Williamson, D.A., Stavrinos, T.M., . . . Singh, M.A. (2012). Effects of high-intensity progressive resistance training and targeted multidisciplinary treatment of frailty on mortality and nursing home admissions after hip fracture: A randomized controlled trial. *Journal of the American Medical Directors Association, 13*(1), 24–30. doi:10.1016/j.jamda.2011.08.005

Spencer, J. (2012). Continence promotion: How nurses can educate women. *Nursing for Women's Health, 16*(4), 337–340. doi:10.1111/j.1751-486X.2012.01753.x

Speroff, L., & Fritz, M.A. (2011). *Clinical gynecologic endocrinology and infertility* (8th ed.). Philadelphia, PA: Lippincott Williams & Wilkins.

Sprague, B.L., Terentham-Dietz, A., & Cronin, K.A. (2012). A sustained decline in postmenopausal hormone use. *Obstetrics & Gynecology, 120*(3), 595–603.

Sweitzer, V., Rondeau, D., Guido, V., & Rasmor, M. (2013). Interventions to improve outcomes in the elderly after hip fracture. *The Journal for Nurse Practitioners — JNP, 9*(4), 238–242. doi: http://dx.doi.org/10.1016/jnurpra2013.01.012

Tam, T., & Davies, M. (2013). Pessaries for vaginal prolapse: Critical factors to successful fit and continued use. *OBG Management, 25*(12), 42–59.

Teschke, R. (2010). Black cohosh and suspected hepatotoxicity: Inconsistencies, confounding variables, and prospective use of a diagnostic sausality algorithm. A critical review. *Menopause, 17*(2), 426–440.

The North American Menopause Society (NAMS). (2010a). Management of osteoporosis in postmenopausal women: 2010 position statement of The North American Menopause Society. *Menopause, 17*(1), 25–54.

The North American Menopause Society (NAMS). (2010b). *Menopause practice: A clinician's guide* (4th ed.). Mayfield Heights, OH: Author.

The North American Menopause Society (NAMS). (2012). The 2012 hormone therapy position statement of The North American Menopause Society. *Menopause: The Journal of The North American Menopause Society, 19*(3), 257–271. doi:10.1097/gme.0b013e31824b970a

The North American Menopause Society (NAMS). (2013). Management of symptomatic vulvovaginal atrophy: 2013 position statement of The North American Menopause Society. *Menopause, 20*(9), 886–887.

U.S. Department of Health and Human Services (USDHHS). (2013a). *Healthy People 2020: Topics & objectives; Arthritis, osteoporosis, and chronic back conditions.* Retrieved from http://healthypeople.gov/2020/topicsobjectives2020/overview.aspx?topicid=3

U.S. Department of Health and Human Services (USDHHS). (2013b). *Healthy People 2020: Topics & objectives; Heart disease and stroke.* Retrieved from http://www.healthypeople.gov/2020/topicsobjectives2020/objectiveslist.aspx?topicId=37

U.S. Food and Drug Administration. (2013). *Calcitonin salmon for the treatment of postmenopausal osteoporosis.* Retrieved from http://www.fda.gov/downloads/AdvisoryCommittees/CommitteesMeetingMaterials/Drugs/ReproductiveHealthDrugsAdvisoryCommittee/UCM343748.pdf

U.S. Preventive Services Task Force (USPSTF). (2009). Aspirin for the prevention of cardiovascular disease: Recommendation statement. *Annals of Internal Medicine, 150*(9), 396–404.

U.S. Preventive Services Task Force (USPSTF). (2011). *Screening for osteoporosis.* Recommendation statement. Retrieved from http://www.uspreventiveservicestaskforce.org/uspstf10/osteoporosis/osteors.htm

U.S. Preventive Services Task Force (USPSTF). (2012). *The guide to clinical preventive health services, 2012: Recommendations of the U.S. Preventive Services Task Force* (AHRQ Publication No. 10-05145). Washington, DC: AHRQ Publications Clearinghouse.

Venes, D. (2013). *Taber's cyclopedic medical dictionary* (22nd ed.). Philadelphia, PA: F.A. Davis.

Walker, E.M., Rodriguez, A.I., Kohn, B., Ball, R.M., Pegg, J., Pocock, J.R., . . . Levine, R.A. (2010). Acupuncture versus venlafaxine for the management of vasomotor symptoms in patients with hormone receptor-positive breast cancer: A randomized controlled trial. *Journal of Clinical Oncology, 28*(4), 634–640. doi:10.1200/JCO.2009.23.5150.

Weed, S. (2002). *New menopausal years, the wise woman way: Alternative approaches for women.* Woodstock, NY: Ash Tree.

Weinberg, N., Young, A., Hunter, C.J., Agrawal, N., Mao, S., & Budoff, M.J. (2012). Physical activity, hormone replacement therapy, and the presence of coronary calcium in midlife women. *Women & Health, 52*, 423–436.

Williams, J. K., & Brownlee, J. (2010). The dietary clinical trials of the Women's Health Initiative: Part 2. *The Female Patient, 35*(4), 39–41.

Wilton, J.M. (2011). Denosumab: New horizons in the treatment of osteoporosis. *Nursing for Women's Health, 15*(3), 249–252. doi:10.1111/j.1751-486X.2011.01641.x

Woods, N.F. (2013). An overview of chronic vaginal atrophy and options for symptom management. *Nursing for Women's Health, 16*(6), 483–494. doi:10.1111/j.1751-486X.2012.01776.x

Wright, W.L. (2011). Quantifying fracture risk. *Advance for NPs & PAs, 2*(3), 31–37.

Writing Group for the Women's Health Initiative Investigators. (2002). Risks and benefits of estrogen plus progestin in healthy postmenopausal women. *Journal of the American Medical Association, 288*(7), 321–333.

Zagaria, M.A. (2011). Proton pump inhibitors: Review of benefits and fracture risk. *The American Journal for Nurse Practitioners, 15*(7/8), 47–51.

DavisPlus | For more information, go to **http://www.davisplus.fadavis.com/.**

CONCEPT MAP

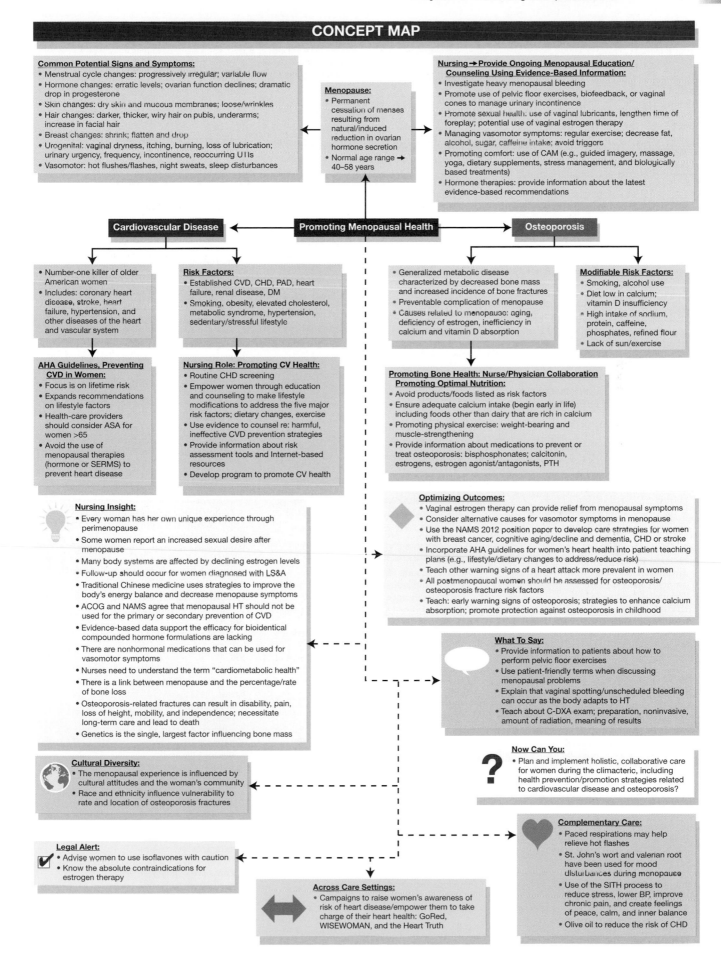

Common Potential Signs and Symptoms:
- Menstrual cycle changes: progressively irregular; variable flow
- Hormone changes: erratic levels; ovarian function declines; dramatic drop in progesterone
- Skin changes: dry skin and mucous membranes; loose/wrinkles
- Hair changes: darker, thicker, wiry hair on pubis, underarms; increase in facial hair
- Breast changes: shrink; flatten and drop
- Urogenital: vaginal dryness, itching, burning, loss of lubrication; urinary urgency, frequency, incontinence, reoccurring UTIs
- Vasomotor: hot flushes/flashes, night sweats, sleep disturbances

Menopause:
- Permanent cessation of menses resulting from natural/induced reduction in ovarian hormone secretion
- Normal age range → 40–58 years

Nursing → Provide Ongoing Menopausal Education/ Counseling Using Evidence-Based Information:
- Investigate heavy menopausal bleeding
- Promote use of pelvic floor exercises, biofeedback, or vaginal cones to manage urinary incontinence
- Promote sexual health: use of vaginal lubricants, lengthen time of foreplay; potential use of vaginal estrogen therapy
- Managing vasomotor symptoms: regular exercise; decrease fat, alcohol, sugar, caffeine intake; avoid triggers
- Promoting comfort: use of CAM (e.g., guided imagery, massage, yoga, dietary supplements, stress management, and biologically based treatments)
- Hormone therapies: provide information about the latest evidence-based recommendations

Promoting Menopausal Health

Cardiovascular Disease

- Number-one killer of older American women
- Includes: coronary heart disease, stroke, heart failure, hypertension, and other diseases of the heart and vascular system

Risk Factors:
- Established CVD, CHD, PAD, heart failure, renal disease, DM
- Smoking, obesity, elevated cholesterol, metabolic syndrome, hypertension, sedentary/stressful lifestyle

AHA Guidelines, Preventing CVD in Women:
- Focus is on lifetime risk
- Expands recommendations on lifestyle factors
- Health-care providers should consider ASA for women >65
- Avoid the use of menopausal therapies (hormone or SERMS) to prevent heart disease

Nursing Role: Promoting CV Health:
- Routine CHD screening
- Empower women through education and counseling to make lifestyle modifications to address the five major risk factors; dietary changes, exercise
- Use evidence to counsel re: harmful, ineffective CVD prevention strategies
- Provide information about risk assessment tools and Internet-based resources
- Develop program to promote CV health

Osteoporosis

- Generalized metabolic disease characterized by decreased bone mass and increased incidence of bone fractures
- Preventable complication of menopause
- Causes related to menopause: aging, deficiency of estrogen, inefficiency in calcium and vitamin D absorption

Modifiable Risk Factors:
- Smoking, alcohol use
- Diet low in calcium; vitamin D insufficiency
- High intake of sodium, protein, caffeine, phosphates, refined flour
- Lack of sun/exercise

Promoting Bone Health: Nurse/Physician Collaboration Promoting Optimal Nutrition:
- Avoid products/foods listed as risk factors
- Ensure adequate calcium intake (begin early in life) including foods other than dairy that are rich in calcium
- Promoting physical exercise: weight-bearing and muscle-strengthening
- Provide information about medications to prevent or treat osteoporosis: bisphosphonates; calcitonin, estrogens, estrogen agonist/antagonists, PTH

Nursing Insight:
- Every woman has her own unique experience through perimenopause
- Some women report an increased sexual desire after menopause
- Many body systems are affected by declining estrogen levels
- Follow-up should occur for women diagnosed with LS&A
- Traditional Chinese medicine uses strategies to improve the body's energy balance and decrease menopause symptoms
- ACOG and NAMS agree that menopausal HT should not be used for the primary or secondary prevention of CVD
- Evidence-based data support the efficacy for bioidentical compounded hormone formulations are lacking
- There are nonhormonal medications that can be used for vasomotor symptoms
- Nurses need to understand the term "cardiometabolic health"
- There is a link between menopause and the percentage/rate of bone loss
- Osteoporosis-related fractures can result in disability, pain, loss of height, mobility, and independence; necessitate long-term care and lead to death
- Genetics is the single, largest factor influencing bone mass

Optimizing Outcomes:
- Vaginal estrogen therapy can provide relief from menopausal symptoms
- Consider alternative causes for vasomotor symptoms in menopause
- Use the NAMS 2012 position paper to develop care strategies for women with breast cancer, cognitive aging/decline and dementia, CHD or stroke
- Incorporate AHA guidelines for women's heart health into patient teaching plans (e.g., lifestyle/dietary changes to address/reduce risk)
- Teach other warning signs of a heart attack more prevalent in women
- All postmenopausal women should be assessed for osteoporosis/ osteoporosis fracture risk factors
- Teach: early warning signs of osteoporosis; strategies to enhance calcium absorption; promote protection against osteoporosis in childhood

What To Say:
- Provide information to patients about how to perform pelvic floor exercises
- Use patient-friendly terms when discussing menopausal problems
- Explain that vaginal spotting/unscheduled bleeding can occur as the body adapts to HT
- Teach about C-DXA exam; preparation, noninvasive, amount of radiation, meaning of results

Now Can You:
- Plan and implement holistic, collaborative care for women during the climacteric, including health prevention/promotion strategies related to cardiovascular disease and osteoporosis?

Cultural Diversity:
- The menopausal experience is influenced by cultural attitudes and the woman's community
- Race and ethnicity influence vulnerability to rate and location of osteoporosis fractures

Legal Alert:
- Advise women to use isoflavones with caution
- Know the absolute contraindications for estrogen therapy

Across Care Settings:
- Campaigns to raise women's awareness of risk of heart disease/empower them to take charge of their heart health: GoRed, WISEWOMAN, and the Heart Truth

Complementary Care:
- Paced respirations may help relieve hot flashes
- St. John's wort and valerian root have been used for mood disturbances during menopause
- Use of the SITH process to reduce stress, lower BP, improve chronic pain, and create feelings of peace, calm, and inner balance
- Olive oil to reduce the risk of CHD

Index